Human Sleep
and Its Disorders

AN

INAUGURAL DISSERTATION

ON THE

CAUSES AND EFFECTS

OF

S L E E P.

SUBMITTED TO THE EXAMINATION OF THE

REV. JOHN EWING, S. T. P. PROVOST,

THE

TRUSTEES AND MEDICAL PROFESSORS

OF THE

UNIVERSITY OF PENNSYLVANIA,

ON THE SEVENTEENTH DAY OF MAY, 1796,

FOR THE DEGREE OF

DOCTOR OF MEDICINE.

By THOMAS BALL, OF VIRGINIA,

MEMBER OF THE PHILADELPHIA MEDICAL SOCIETY.

Tir'd Nature's fweet Reftorer—BALMY SLEEP!

YOUNG.

P H I L A D E L P H I A:

M.DCC.XCVI.

Title page of a dissertation on sleep written by Thomas Ball, an 18th century American physician. This fascinating work contains comments on such subjects as the effectiveness of hypnotics and causes of excessive sleepiness. (Courtesy of the Library of Congress)

Human Sleep
and Its Disorders

Wallace B. Mendelson, J. Christian Gillin,
and Richard Jed Wyatt

National Institute of Mental Health
Bethesda, Maryland

PLENUM PRESS · NEW YORK AND LONDON

Library of Congress Cataloging in Publication Data

Mendelson, Wallace B
  Human sleep and its disorders.

  Bibliography: p.
  Includes index.
  1. Sleep disorders. 2. Sleep. 3. Physiology, Pathological. I. Gillin, J. Christian, joint author. II. Wyatt, Richard Jed, joint author. III. Title. [DNLM: 1. Sleep. 2. Sleep disorders. 3. Pharmacology. WM188 M537h]
RC547.M46   616.8'49   76-48064
ISBN-13: 978-1-4684-2291-7

ISBN-13: 978-1-4684-2291-7   e-ISBN-13: 978-1-4684-2289-4
DOI: 10.1007/978-1-4684-2289-4

The authors have written this as private individuals.
Views expressed here do not necessarily reflect those
of the Public Health Service or the National Institute of Mental Health.

In Memoriam

Robert A. Woodruff

Preface

In this book we trace the development of several major themes in sleep research, from the first formal description of REM sleep in the early 1950s through the present. Chapter 1 provides those less familiar with this area with a perspective on the many possible ways to examine sleep. Chapter 2 describes in detail a major viewpoint of this book: that observations of pharmacological interventions affecting the neurotransmitters may aid in the understanding of sleep regulation. The remainder of the book is devoted to endocrine systems related to sleep (chap. 3) and to the contribution of sleep research to the understanding of various pathological states (chaps. 4–7). The areas of investigation open to those who wish to understand sleep are much broader than the traditional problems of insomnia and narcolepsy. Such disorders as depression, schizophrenia, and alcoholism have long been associated with disordered sleep. Our search for an understanding of the latter phenomena may clarify the nature of these conditions.

We have emphasized the study of *human* sleep. There are, of course, some scientific disadvantages to this approach. Because of ethical considerations, we obviously cannot, and do not wish to, employ the invasive procedures of the animal laboratory. Hence our inferences must often be indirect, and we may sometimes be observing epiphenomena, rather than the physiologic events themselves. On the other hand, there are several unique advantages to studying human sleep. First of all, sleep has a dual nature: It can be seen as both a physiological function and a subjective experience. In order to study the interworkings of these two phenomena, we must necessarily deal with humans. Second, it is our intention that our studies will ultimately be useful in solving human problems. In the absence of adequate animal models, we must study such conditions as the affective disorders and schizophrenia in persons suffering from them. Third, there is a technical advantage. The human REM-nonREM cycle lasts approximately 90 minutes, much longer than that of most laboratory animals. We are becoming more and more convinced that it is useful to study the effects of drugs that are infused briefly at different points in the sleep cycle. We also wish to examine substances in the blood that may appear in a specific stage of sleep. This can only be done when the cycle is long enough to be broken down into its constituent parts, as is the case in the human REM-nonREM cycle.

Finally, a few comments about our method of presentation are in order. We have tried to write in a manner that is understandable to the student as well as the professional researcher. For this reason, we have provided a section at the beginning of each chapter that outlines the basic concepts in the field. (In chapter 7, for example, we begin by briefly describing the symptoms and natural history of depressive disorders.) We have also tried to avoid giving the text a sedative quality of its own, which is often the result of narrating the results of one experiment after another. Since it is important that this information be available, however, we have made a series of tables describing the data from all the studies in a given area. In the text, we have emphasized the interplay of ideas derived from these studies. One approach that we found particularly useful was to determine the criteria needed to confirm or refute a hypothesis (e.g., that the secretion of a hormone is related to the occurrence of a sleep stage), and to determine how well these criteria have been met. Finally, we have tried to convey to the reader the sense of excitement we have experienced in studying the nature of sleep, a phenomenon both universal and exceedingly mysterious.

We wish to recognize the people who inspired and supported our work over the years: Drs. Frederick Snyder, William Bunney, Robert Cohen, Robert A. Woodruff, Donald W. Goodwin, Eli Robins, Irwin W. Feinberg, William Dement, and Alan Hobson.

In particular, we would like to thank Drs. Donald W. Goodwin, Lawrence S. Jacobs, and James F. Leckman for their valuable suggestions regarding various portions of this book. The responsibility for all statements in the text, however, lies with the authors.

Bethesda, Maryland   WALLACE B. MENDELSON
and   J. CHRISTIAN GILLIN
Washington, D.C.   RICHARD JED WYATT

Contents

An Introduction to Sleep Studies

Although spontaneous electrical discharges in the brains of animals were reported as early as 1875, the first recordings from humans were attributed to Hans Berger in 1929. Over the next decade he wrote a remarkable series of papers confirming previous animal studies and showing that the electrical activity was derived from neuronal tissue, that it responded to sensory stimulation, and that abnormal discharges occurred during epileptic seizures (Berger, 1929; Berger, 1938). He used the term *electroencephalogram* (EEG) to refer to his recordings of this electrical activity.

In 1937, Loomis, Harvey, and Hobart described the results of 30 all-night EEG recordings from humans. They discovered that, in terms of EEG observations, sleep is composed of a series of discontinuous stages. They pointed out that changes between these stages occurred spontaneously, apparently as a result of "internal stimuli." Although the classification of these stages has changed, the concept that sleep is made up of discrete, recurring stages, regulated by neural mechanisms, is basic to much of modern sleep research. These concepts led the way to the discovery some years later of rapid eye movement (REM) sleep.

The formal description of REM sleep, was anticipated by clinical observations of several of its characteristics prior to the advent of the electroencephalogram. Griesinger in 1868 (and others later) suggested that dreaming is associated with periods of eye movements. Freud (1895) mentioned that the major muscles of the body become very relaxed during dreaming. MacWilliam (1923) distinguished between

1

"undisturbed" and "disturbed" sleep. The latter was associated with increased blood pressure and pulse, and changes in respiratory rate.

In 1953, Aserinsky and Kleitman presented a polygraphic study demonstrating the occurrence of periods of sleep characterized by conjugate rapid eye movements. During these periods, the EEG showed an activated pattern consisting of low amplitude waves generally of 15–20 and 5–8 cycles per second frequencies. Associated with this sleep stage were increased rates of heartbeat and respiration. Aserinsky and Kleitman awakened patients during this REM sleep and found that about three-fourths of them reported that they were experiencing dreams involving visual imagery. Another small percentage reported "the feeling of having dreamed" but could not recall details. When subjects were awakened during sleep that did not contain REMs (referred to as nonREM sleep), only about 9% described dreams and another 9% reported the feeling of having been dreaming.

In the next few years after the description of REM sleep, two findings in particular led to a more complete understanding of its physiology. Jouvet and Michel (1959) reported that in animals there was a marked decrease in muscle tone during REM sleep; this was confirmed in humans by Ralph Berger in 1961. The second finding was a report by Dement and Kleitman in 1957 that REM sleep appeared to recur in a cyclic fashion throughout the night, interspersed by periods of nonREM sleep. Each REM-nonREM cycle was thought to last 90–100 minutes. Dement and Kleitman then proposed a classification system, in which REM was differentiated from nonREM sleep, which in turn was divided into four stages. This was the basis of an approach to classification that, with some revisions (Rechtschaffen and Kales, 1968) is still in use. Authors such as Oswald (1962) and Jouvet (1962) began to emphasize the concept that sleep is not a unitary process, but rather is composed of REM and nonREM sleep, which differ fundamentally in most physiological parameters when measured over time. Thus, REM sleep, nonREM sleep, and waking have come to be thought of as the three *states of consciousness.*

An improved understanding of the sleep stages has resulted from studies of a number of physiological systems that vary with them, differences between species, changes with age, and effects of depriving people of them. The results of some of these approaches will be described briefly in this chapter. For further information on the development of sleep research, the reader may wish to see historical reviews written by some of the men who helped create that history (Dement and Mitler, 1974; Bremer, 1974; Jouvet, 1969).

TECHNIQUES OF HUMAN SLEEP STUDIES

Sleep studies on humans are usually performed by using a polygraph to record three types of data: the electroencephalogram (EEG), electromyogram (EMG), and electrooculogram (EOG). Each of these procedures, which are described by Rechtschaffen and Kales (1968), may be summarized as follows:

EEG: Electrodes (generally concave metallic disks) are put next to the scalp and held in place by small cotton gauze patches that have been covered with collodion, a sticky proteinaceous substance. The surface of the electrode that touches the skin has been coated with an electrolytic jelly that facilitates transmission of the electric potentials. The electrode is usually attached to the scalp above the ear, two inches below the top of the skull (technically referred to as C_3 or C_4). Recordings may be made from either the left or right sides, as the signals from the two homologous areas are generally the same. The polygraph amplifies and traces on paper an electrical signal that represents the difference between voltage from this electrode and a relatively electrically neutral area (the *reference* lead). The latter is usually placed on the earlobe or on the mastoid bone behind the ear (A_1 or A_2). This arrangement is referred to as *unipolar recording*.

EOG: Electrodes are attached with plastic tape to the skin beside the outer corners (canthi) of the eyes. The signal that represents the difference between each eye lead and the reference electrode is amplified and displayed on paper. When the eyes move conjugately (as if following a moving object), the tracings of the two eye channels appear as mirror images of each other.

EMG: Two electrodes are attached beneath the chin. The difference between the potentials of these two electrically active electrodes is amplified and displayed on paper (bipolar recording). The amplitude (vertical height) of the signal is considered to be directly proportionate to the degree of muscle tone.

THE SLEEP STAGES

A determination of the sleep stage is based on the combined information from the EEG EOG, and EMG. The records are read in *epochs,* usually of 20 or 30 seconds; i.e., a determination is made of what the dominant sleep stage is for each sequential 20- or 30-second period. The most widely accepted criteria for defining the stages are those of Rechtschaffen and Kales (1968), and these should be studied in detail by any serious student of the subject. In summary, sleep stages may be defined as follows:

Waking (Fig. 1-1)

During relaxed wakefulness, with the eyes closed, the record is predominantly one of sinusoidal alpha waves (8–14 cycles per second) intermixed with lower amplitude irregular beta waves (15–35 cycles per second). Muscle tone is generally high, and eye movements may be present. As the subject becomes more drowsy, alpha activity decreases. The eyes may make slow rolling movements.

NonREM Sleep (Figs. 1-2 to 1-5)

Stage 1

Alpha activity is greatly decreased (less than 50% of the record). There is a low-amplitude mixed-frequency signal, primarily made up of beta and the slower theta (4–7 cycles per second) activity. As the subject progresses toward stage 2, the slower activity predominates.

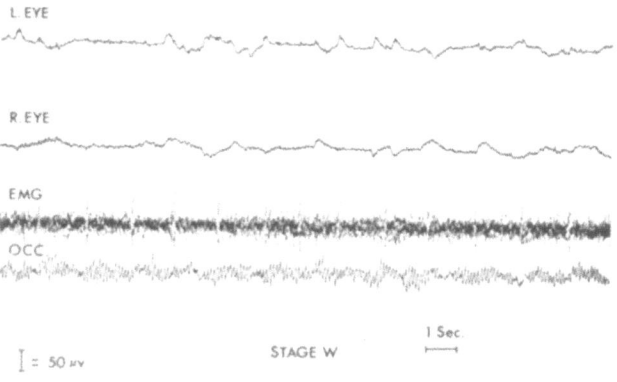

FIGURE 1-1. Polygraphic recording of relaxed wakefulness in a normal young adult male, whose eyes are closed. In Figures 1-1 through 1-5, the following abbreviations are used: L-EYE = electro-oculogram of left eye; R-EYE = electro-oculogram of right eye; EMG = submental electromyogram; OCC = unipolar electroencephalogram recorded from occipital area.

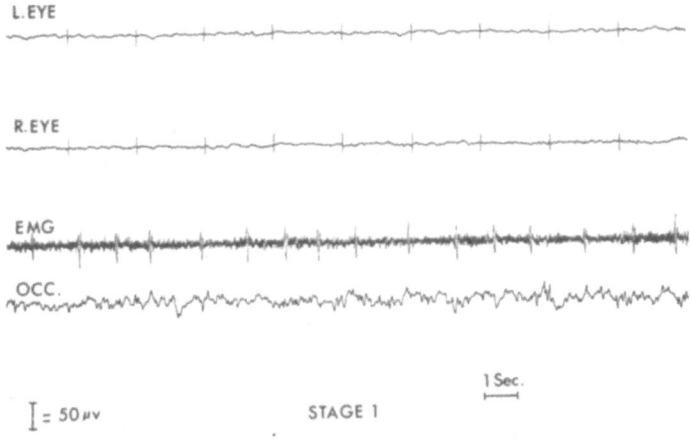

FIGURE 1-2. Polygraphic recording of stage 1 sleep.

Stage 2

This is composed of a largely theta background, and is character-ized by the appearance of two types of intermittent events, the spindles and K-complexes. Spindles are brief bursts of rhythmic 12–14 cycles per second waves, lasting at least 0.5 second. K-complexes are composed of a high-amplitude negative wave followed by a positive wave. Some-times brief bursts of low-amplitude 12–14 cycle per second activity may

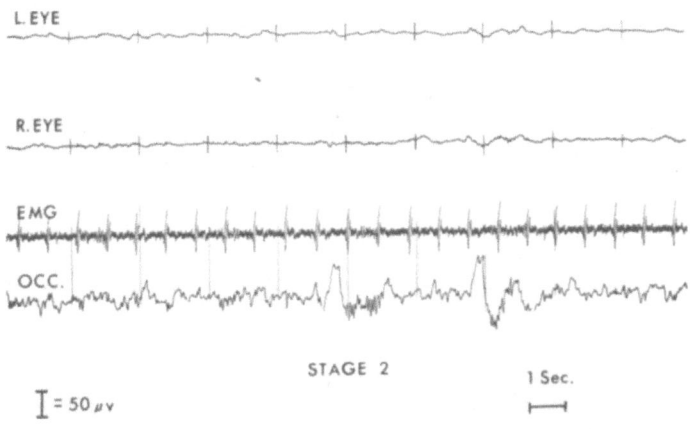

FIGURE 1-3. Polygraphic recording of stage 2 sleep.

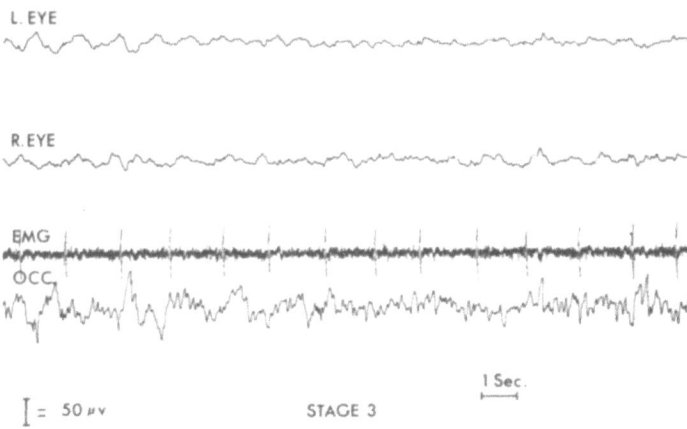

FIGURE 1-4.   Polygraphic recording of stage 3 sleep.

be superimposed on the K-complex. It should be noted that in addition to its spontaneous appearance during stage 2 sleep, the K-complex can occur at other times in a sleeping person in response to auditory stimuli.

Stages 3 and 4

These stages are characterized by the appearance of delta waves, which are high amplitude (at least 75 microvolts) and slow (0.5–3 cycles

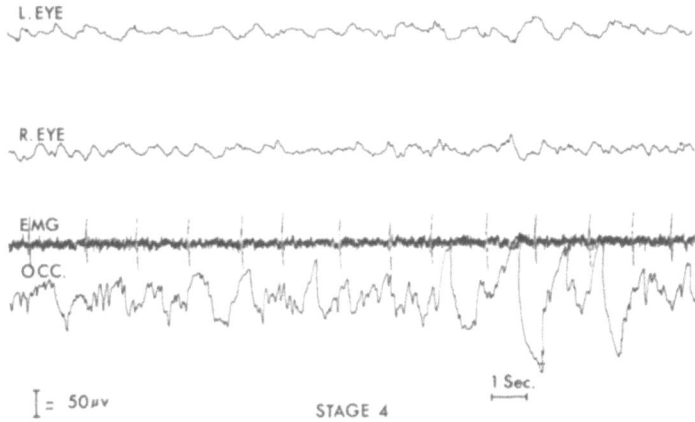

FIGURE 1-5.   Polygraphic recording of stage 4 sleep.

per second). Collectively, these stages are often referred to as *slow-wave sleep* or *delta sleep*. When delta activity is between 20–50% of the record, stage 3 is scored. In stage 4 delta activity makes up more than 50% of the epoch. Sleep spindles may or may not be present during stages 3 or 4.

REM Sleep (Fig. 1-6)

During REM sleep the EEG returns to a mixed frequency pattern similar to stage 1. In contrast to stage 2, there are no sleep spindles or K-complexes. The EMG drops to very low amplitude, indicating the decrease in tone of the submental muscles. Conjugate rapid eye movements appear. The frequency of eye movements in each epoch of REM sleep is often recorded, and is referred to as *REM density*.

THE REM-NONREM CYCLE

As was mentioned earlier, the sleep stages do not occur at random, but rather appear in cyclic fashion (Fig. 1-7). In general, a normal young adult goes from waking into a period of nonREM sleep lasting 70 to 90 minutes prior to the first REM period. (The duration of this portion of sleep is referred to as *REM latency*.) In an idealized situation, the sequence of stages during this period of REM latency is: waking, stage 1, stage 2, stage 3, stage 4, stage 3, stage 2. At the point the first REM period occurs, followed by a repetition of the nonREM stages (stage 2, stage 3, stage 4, stage 3, stage 2) and then another REM episode. This

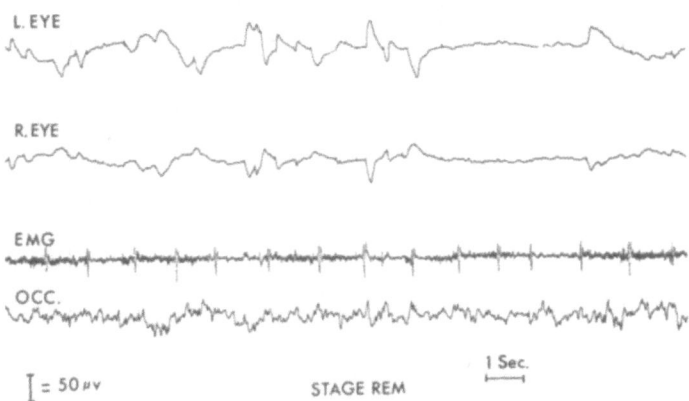

FIGURE 1-6. Polygraphic recording of REM sleep.

interval—from the beginning of one REM period to the beginning of the next—is the definition of a sleep cycle employed in this book. It should be noted, however, that it can also be defined in other ways, such as from the beginning of one nonREM sleep episode to the next (Feinberg, 1974). The latter method, though less widely used, has some benefit in that it includes evaluation of the first episode of slow-wave sleep in calculations involving cyclic phenomena.

The duration of the REM-to-REM cycle is generally thought to be about 90 minutes, but may vary from 70 to 120 minutes. Feinberg (1976) has emphasized that the mean duration of sleep cycles may change during the night in curvilinear fashion, with different patterns of change in different age groups.

The content of the sleep cycle changes as the night progresses (Feinberg, 1974). Excluding the first cycle of the night, subsequent cycles show progressively decreasing amounts of slow-wave sleep. The amount of slow-wave sleep in the first cycle is age dependent, decreasing with progressing age. With the exception of the elderly, the REM episode in the first cycle is shorter than those in subsequent cycles, in which it gets progressively longer. In general, then (and with the exception of the elderly), slow-wave sleep is greatest early at night and decreases as the night advances; REM sleep is in relatively small amounts early at night, but increases as the night advances.

SLEEP STAGES AND AGE

As can be seen in Figure 1-8, total sleep time and total nightly amounts of individual sleep stages, are age dependent (Feinberg and Carlson, 1968; Roffwarg, Muzio, and Dement, 1966). In general, total

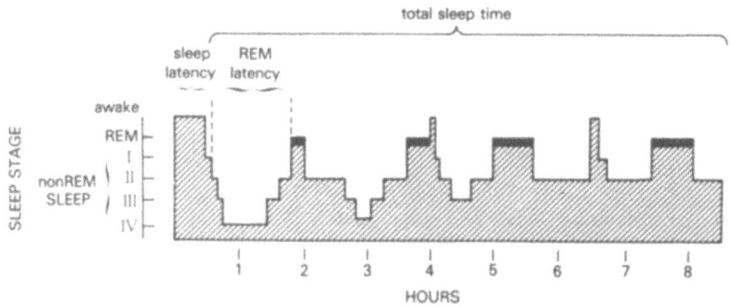

FIGURE 1-7. Graph of an idealized sequence of sleep stages in a normal young adult.

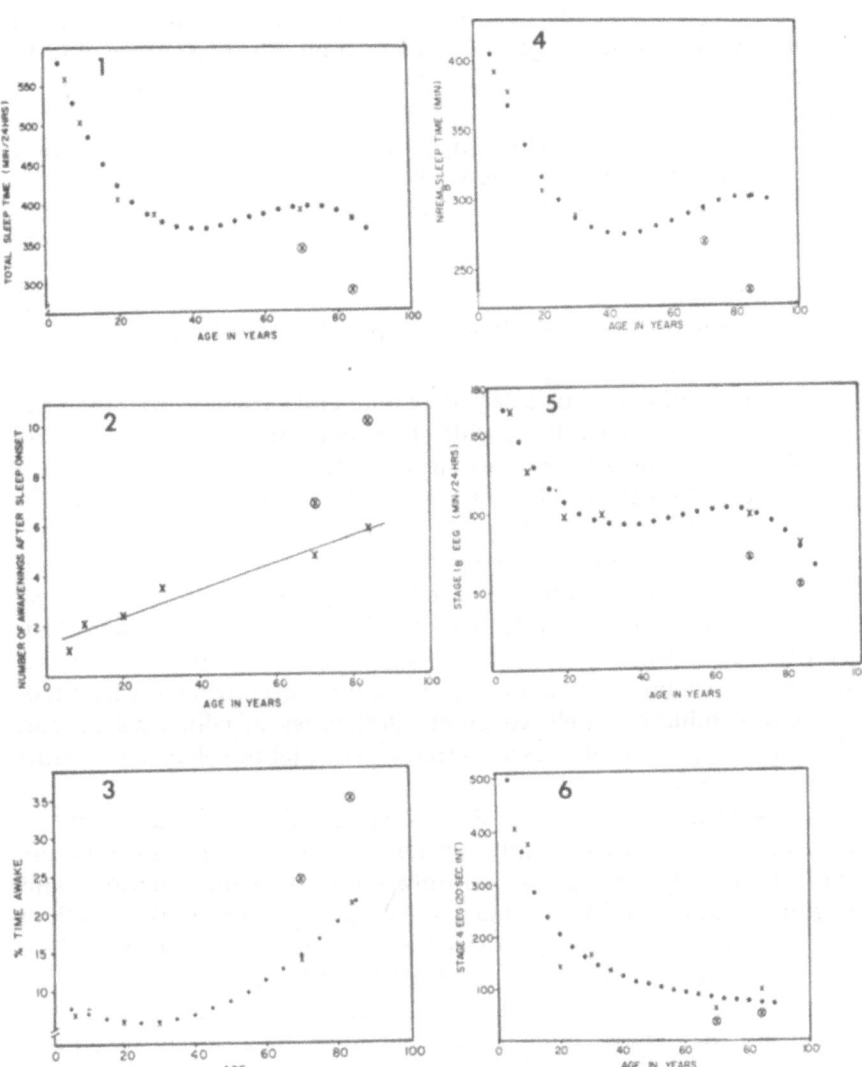

FIGURE 1-8. Changes in major sleep parameters with age. (From I. Feinberg. The ontogenesis of human sleep and the relationship of sleep variables to intellectual function in the aged, *Comprehensive Psychiatry* 9:138–147, 1968. Reprinted by permission.)

sleep time is greatest in infancy, and then decreases in childhood. It remains relatively stable starting in the young adult years until old age, where it declines. In contrast, the number of awakenings during the night may increase with age in a linear fashion. The percentage of REM sleep is highest in infancy and childhood, drops and then levels off in adulthood, and declines in old age. Stage 4 sleep is highest in infancy, and may be thought of as changing in a hyperbolic curve that decreases with age. Typical values for the whole night in a young adult might be as follows: 50% stage 2, 25% REM, 10% stage 3, 10% stage 4, and 5% stage 1.

EFFECTS OF TEMPORAL VARIABLES ON SLEEP

Sleep is influenced by a variety of temporal variables other than age and the length of time asleep, which have been mentioned already. The length of wakefulness prior to sleep is directly related to the total amount of delta sleep (Webb and Agnew, 1971) and inversely related to the time required to fall asleep (the *sleep latency*) (Agnew and Webb, 1971). While it is not surprising that the longer a person has been awake, the more quickly he falls asleep, it is perhaps surprising that the sleep latency is strongly influenced by the time of day at which sleep occurs, a so-called circadian effect (Webb and Agnew, 1975). It is easier to fall asleep at midnight than at, say, 4:00 P.M., even when the length of prior wakefulness is held constant. Difficulties in falling asleep and staying asleep are well known to transoceanic jet travelers and to shift workers.

In contrast to delta sleep, REM sleep is influenced much more by time of day than by the length of prior wakefulness. REM sleep occurs more frequently during the morning hours than the afternoon and evening hours, and this effect is relatively independent of the length of wakefulness prior to going to sleep and to the amount of prior sleep (Weitzman *et al.*, 1970, 1974; Carskadon and Dement, 1975; Taub and Berger, 1973; Hume and Mills, 1975). Thus, naps in the morning have been shown to have more REM sleep than naps in the afternoon (Karacan *et al.*, 1970). On the other hand, naps in the afternoon have more delta sleep than naps in the morning because of the increased period of wakefulness since arising in the morning. Furthermore, following an afternoon nap, delta sleep is reduced during nocturnal sleep for similar reasons.

In summary, temporal variables—age, length of time asleep, length of wakefulness prior to the sleep period, and time of day at which sleep

occurs—are important determinants of sleep characteristics. The underlying physiological and biochemical mechanisms for these temporal
effects are unknown.

PHYSIOLOGICAL VARIABLES RELATED TO THE SLEEP STAGES

In addition to the physiological changes that largely define REM
sleep, such as decreased muscle tone, a variety of metabolic and autonomic nervous system changes occur (Berger, 1969). During REM sleep
there is increased cerebral blood flow (Reivich et al., 1968) brain temperature (Kawamura and Sawyer, 1965) and oxygen consumption (Brebbia
and Altshuler, 1965). Erections may occur in the male during REM sleep.
It will be recalled from the historical review earlier in this chapter that
periodic increases in blood pressure, pulse, and respirations during
sleep were noted even before the use of the EEG (MacWilliam, 1923).
Subsequent polygraphic studies found increases in rate and variability
of these measures during REM sleep (Snyder et al., 1964). There has
been recent increased interest in respiratory changes in sleep following
reports that they may be related to some types of insomnia and hypersomnia (chap. 4).

SLEEP DEPRIVATION

A classic technique for determining the function of a physiological
process has been to remove it or prevent it from occurring, and see what
happens. Sleep deprivation studies, however, have not revealed the
hidden function of sleep. Investigators have performed three different
types of sleep deprivation studies: total sleep deprivation, selective
sleep stage deprivation, and partial sleep deprivation.

Total Sleep Deprivation

Total sleep deprivation of 150–200 hours has been associated with
the development of brief psychotic episodes in some subjects, but
apparently does not result in long-term psychological effects (Pasnau et
al., 1968; Gulevich, Dement, and Johnson, 1966). These findings have
led some authors to speculate that sleep deprivation psychoses might
be an aid in the understanding of schizophrenia (Luby and Gottlieb,
1966). It has become apparent, however, that florid psychotic states
following sleep deprivation occur in only a very small portion of cases.

Tyler (1955), for instance, found such changes in only seven of 350 subjects kept awake for 112 hours. They are very infrequent in persons who have been sleep deprived for less than 100 hours (Johnson, 1969).

Changes in mood and performance, in contrast to obvious psychotic states, do occur fairly consistently in persons undergoing prolonged sleep deprivation. Fatigue, irritability, feelings of persecution, and episodes of misinterpretation of stimuli have been reported (Johnson, 1969). Morris and Singer (1961), using projective tests on subjects kept awake for 72 to 98 hours, emphasized that the various disturbances in perception, orientation, and attentiveness were functions of the previous personality of the subject. Williams, Lubin, and Goodnow (1959) concluded that the unevenness of test results in sleep-deprived subjects was primarily due to a defect in attentiveness.

EEG studies of sleep-deprived subjects show decreases in amounts of alpha activity, which has been interpreted by various authors as demonstrating increased or decreased activation (Johnson, Slye, and Dement, 1965.) During periods of decreased alpha activity, there may be decreased tracking performance and deterioration of subjective ratings of feeling and effort, in combination with an EEG described as similar to stage 1 (Naitoh *et al.*, 1969). During recovery sleep after extremely long periods of sleep deprivation, there may be increases in percentage stage 4 and REM sleep above baseline values (Kales *et al.*, 1970b).

In contrast to the extremely long deprivation periods described above, most persons have experienced the uncomfortable feelings that occur after one or two nights of sleep loss. Although complaints of irritability, fatigue, poor concentration, and feelings of depersonalization are commonly described, objective psychological testing has been less consistent in showing changes in mood. Roth *et al.* (1974) deprived 11 normal males of one night's sleep, and found that tests showed higher scores on "sleepiness," "friendliness," and "aggression." After 24 hours of deprivation, there may be decreased "vigor" and increased "fatigue" and "confusion" (Hartmann, Orzack, and Branconnier, 1974b). Performance on a variety of psychological tests may be impaired; it has been suggested that this is due to periodic lapses, in which the encoding of data into short-term memory is decreased (Polzella, 1975). Whether a person remains inactive or exercises periodically during two nights of sleep deprivation seems to make little difference on performance scores (Webb and Agnew, 1973).

Sleep deprivation may result in the development of transient neurological symptoms. Sassin (1970) found that subjects deprived for 60 hours developed weakness of neck flexion, hand tremors, horizontal nystagmus, and other signs. Gunderson, Dunne, and Feyer (1973) described seizures in nonepileptic soldiers who had been continuously awake for at least 24 hours while traveling. In patients with a known seizure disorder, EEG recordings done during sleep may accentuate epileptic discharges that are otherwise poorly seen. Recent observations suggest that this effect may be enhanced even more by doing sleep recordings following a full day and night of wakefulness (Scollo-Lavizzari, Pralle, and de la Cruz, 1975).

Selective Sleep Stage Deprivation

If subjects are deprived of a sleep stage, an excessive amount of that stage will occur upon cessation of the deprivation. This is referred to as the *rebound phenomenon,* and may be seen following either REM (Clemes and Dement, 1967; Dement, Greenberg, and Klein, 1966a) or stage 4 (Agnew, Webb, and Williams, 1964) deprivation. Decreases in REM or stage 4 sleep can be produced by mechanically arousing a subject whenever the polygraph indicates that he is entering that stage. When a subject is deprived of REM sleep in this manner for several nights, it is found that he must be aroused progressively more and more often. This is considered to be a manifestation of an increase in a hypothetical *REM pressure.* Another method of producing decreased REM sleep is to administer a variety of medications, including alcohol, many hypnotics, stimulants, and the antidepressants. When such agents are discontinued, a REM sleep rebound usually occurs. During this period the subject may complain of disturbed sleep characterized by multiple awakenings and increased dreaming. REM sleep may also be decreased by causing a subject to sleep for a fewer number of hours, (partial sleep deprivation) since most REM sleep occurs in the later hours of sleep.

REM sleep deprivation studies have been reviewed by Vogel (1975). Animal studies suggest that REM deprivation leads to increased cortical excitability (Owen and Bliss, 1970; Cohen, Thomas, and Dement, 1970) and may increase stimulus-evoked aggressive (Morden et al., 1968) and sexual (Dement, 1965) behavior. REM sleep deprivation has been reported to impair memory of past events and acquisition of new data (Stern, 1970). As Vogel (1975) points out, there are a variety of methodological issues involved in studies in this area that have not yet been resolved.

In 1963, Dement and Fisher described a study in which 21 subjects were REM sleep deprived for two to seven nights. Both they and

Sampson (1965) described psychological difficulties that developed in these subjects. In a later study, Dement (1964) described even more dramatic psychological disturbances in two subjects who were REM sleep deprived for 15 and 16 nights by a combination of awakenings and amphetamine administration. A variety of studies have failed to confirm these findings (Kales *et al.*, 1964; Snyder, 1963; Foulkes *et al.*, 1968), and make it seem unlikely that REM sleep deprivation produces serious psychological problems. On the contrary, more recent studies suggest that REM deprivation may in fact be beneficial for depressed patients (Vogel, 1975). This hypothesis will be discussed in chapter 7.

NATURAL LONG, SHORT, AND VARIABLE SLEEPERS

The sleep deprivation studies demonstrate the great difficulty encountered by most people who are denied more than a few hours of sleep per day. There are some people, however, who normally sleep very little without difficulty. Napoleon, Thomas Edison, and Chou En-lai were all said to require little sleep. Meddis *et al.* (1973) studies a 70-year-old lady who claimed to have slept for only an hour per night for many years. She seemed puzzled why other people slept for long periods and "wasted so much time." During a 5-day study period in the laboratory, she averaged 67 minutes of sleep per 24 hours without any indication that she felt fatigued. Her sleep consisted of 16.5% REM sleep, 9.3% stage 4, 23.3% stage 3, and 50.9% stage 2. Likewise, Jones and Oswald (1968) studied two unusually short sleepers, men who had slept about 2¾ hours per day for many years. When studied in the laboratory, both men showed high proportions of delta sleep and REM sleep, as well as short REM latencies.

In contrast, there are also natural long sleepers. Albert Einstein was said to sleep a great deal. Little is known about why one person sleeps a long time, while another sleeps only a short time. Laboratory sleep studies indicate that natural long and short sleepers have equal amounts of delta sleep, but that the long sleepers have much more REM sleep than the short sleepers (Webb and Agnew, 1970; Webb and Friel, 1971; Hartmann, Chung, and Chien, 1971). Using a variety of scholastic, personality, and medical measures, Webb and his associates found no revealing differences between their natural long sleepers (greater than 9½ hours sleep per day) and the short sleepers (less than 5½ hours sleep per day). Hartmann and his associates (1972), however, described their short sleepers (defined by less than 6 hours sleep per day) to be more efficient, hardworking, conformist, and less creative than their long sleepers (defined by more than 9 hours). Hartmann's subjects were older and more set in their sleep habits than Webb's subjects and were obtained by newspaper advertisements rather than by population surveys. Hartmann (1973) has also described a group whom he calls variable sleepers, who need more sleep than normal at times of stress, worry, depression, and increased mental activity, and who require less sleep than normal at times when everything is going well.

In summary, people differ in their subjective sleep requirements, but it is not known why this should be. Questions such as "How much sleep should I get?" cannot be answered with reference to tables, like looking up ideal body weight for a given height. Each person seems to have his own individual requirement for sleep. In terms of factors known to determine human sleep characteristics, age, sex, and temporal variables are important in addition to individual differences. Theories about the function and regulation of sleep must ultimately account for these known variables.

REGULATION OF SLEEP

Passive versus Active Regulation

As early as the last quarter of the 19th century, there began to be interest in the possibility that areas of the brainstem are concerned with the regulation of sleep and wakefulness. After the worldwide epidemic of viral encephalitis in the 1920s, von Economo (1929) described two syndromes—one of excessive sleep and the other of sleeplessness—and attributed these to lesions of the mesencephalic tegmentum and posterior hypothalamus, and of the basal forebrain and striate structures, respectively. In 1935, Bremer reported that if the midbrain of a cat is severed at the intercollicular level below the nucleus of the third cranial nerve, the animal appears to be sleeping, has the high-amplitude slow EEG waves characteristic of sleep, and cannot be aroused by ordinary sensory stimulation (Bremer, 1974; Brazier, 1973). This type of preparation, which in effect separates the cerebrum from the rest of the brain, is referred to as *cerveau isolé*. In contrast, a lower transection at the first cervical segment of the spinal cord *(encephale isolé)* allows the animal to retain behavioral and EEG signs of wakefulness. Bremer and others writing in this period believed that the sleep of the *cerveau isolé* cat was due to lack of adequate sensory stimulation, which they felt was necessary for the maintenance of wakefulness. Sleep was thus considered to be a passive phenomenon. Although sleep might be regulated by specific neuronanatomical loci, it was thought to be primarily a resting state that the brain naturally went into when there was inadequate stimulation from a number of specific sensory modalities.

One of the major advances in the understanding of sleep came with the discovery by Moruzzi and Magoun in 1949 of the reticular activating system. This is an anatomically diffuse system running the entire length of the brainstem, which histologically shows cellular poly-morphism, dendrites lacking regional characteristics, and other fea-tures (Morgane and Stern, 1974). Electrical stimulation of the reticular activating system by a current with a frequency of 100–300 cycles per second was shown to arouse sleeping animals. It was thought that stimulation of this diffuse system (rather than of specific sensory tracts) led to arousal; when the reticular activating system was not actively stimulating the cerebrum, mechanisms in the thalamus and lower pons tended to produce synchronization of firing of cortical neurons, result-ing in the slow waves seen in sleep. This, too, is a basically passive concept of sleep.

Several types of studies, outlined by Jouvet (1969), brought the passive view of sleep into question. First, it was shown that electrical stimulation of various areas of the brain could produce sleep (Hess, 1929, 1944; see Parmegianni, 1964). These studies militated against sleep being a passive process, rather, it appeared that some types of stimulation resulted in sleep. There were many difficulties, however; only certain low frequencies were effective, and formal analyses dem-onstrating that the occurrence of sleep was statistically significant (rather than having occurred randomly) were often lacking. A second support for an "active" view of sleep came from studies demonstrating that lesions of the mid-pontine region resulted in insomnia (Batini *et al.*, 1958, 1959). Although this region was poorly localized, it seemed likely that there were brain loci that could actively inhibit the reticular activating system. Perhaps the final, strongest support for an "active" view of sleep was the discovery of REM sleep, discussed earlier in this chapter (Aserinsky and Kleitman, 1953). It became clear that sleep was not a unitary phenomenon, but that rather it was composed of at least two distinct types: REM and nonREM sleep. Thus, there appeared to be mechanisms not only for changing from sleep to wakefulness, but between different types of sleep.

As Jouvet (1969) points out, while sleep was conceived of as a passive phenomenon, its regulation could be thought of in terms of "dry" neurophysiology. This is a concept of F. O. Schmidt (1962) refer-ring to those aspects of neurophysiology that are essentially electrical in nature. Hence, in the passive concept of sleep, decreased activity of the

reticular activating system was considered to be due to such phenomena as decreased afferent input and neuronal fatigue. With the active
concept of sleep, many phenomena were observed that were difficult to
explain in terms of "dry" neurophysiology. First of all, the circadian
and ultradian rhythms of the sleep stages, and the REM rebound
phenomenon that may occur over many days time, ran very different
time courses than electrical potentials of the brain, which are measured
in milliseconds. It seemed more likely that issues of regulation of these
phenomena could be resolved in the realm of "wet" neurophysiology
(the study of neurohumors). As it turned out, this approach was very
fruitful.

The Neurotransmitters

Pharmacologic and Anatomic Approaches

Two types of studies yielded valuable information on the possible
role of neurotransmitters in the regulation of sleep. The first involved
infusions into animals of acetylcholine, the catecholamines norepinephrine and dopamine, and the indoleamine serotonin. These were
often done in young birds, whose blood brain barrier is permeable to
these substances (e.g., Spooner and Winters, 1965). Alternatively, precursors of these substances, which can enter the brain, have been given
to a variety of animals and to humans. Such studies showed that these
compounds, which presumably transmit impulses between neurons,
are profoundly involved in the regulation of sleep. It is this pharmacologic approach that is the basis of much of the work described in this
book.

The second type of study employing a biochemical approach to
neurochemical control mechanisms resulted from the discovery that
certain monoamines, when exposed to formaldehyde vapor, produced
compounds that fluoresce (Falck *et al.*, 1962). Thus, the histological
localization of these compounds in sections of brain tissue became
possible. Prior to the development of this technique, the diffuse, poly-
morphous nature of the reticular formation had made the discovery of
neuroanatomical pathways very difficult. By using histofluorescence it
became possible to identify cellular pathways on the basis of their
neurotransmitters. Using these techniques, it was found that serotonin-
containing neurons are located largely in a group of nuclei in the lower
midbrain and upper pons, referred to as the *raphe* nuclei. Noradrenergic neurons are found throughout the brainstem reticular formation,

but achieve their highest concentration in the locus coeruleus in the pons (Ungerstedt, 1971).

Studies of the cholinergic system have not had the benefit of a histological technique comparable to histofluorescence staining (Morgane and Stern, 1974). At present cholinergic tracts are identified indirectly, by testing for the presence of the enzyme acetylcholinesterase. These tracts are relatively diffuse. Shute and Lewis (1967) suggest that they fall into two general pathways. The *dorsal tegmental pathway* is centered in the nucleus cuneiformis of the midbrain tegmentum but also includes nuclear areas extending into the pons. Fibers from these tracts go to many areas, but ascending fibers are known to travel to the nonspecific nuclei and nucleus reticularis of the thalamus. The *ventral tegmental pathway* is centered in parts of the substantia nigra and ventral tegmental area of Tsai in the anterior midbrain. Ascending fibers go to the lateral nuclei of the hypothalamus, the striatum, septal nuclei, and hippocampus.

Neurotransmitters and the REM-NonREM Cycle

Once some sense of localization of neurons using these transmitters was obtained, it became possible to test the effects of lesions made in some of these areas. It was found that damage to 80–90% of the raphe area, for instance, produces total insomnia. With somewhat smaller lesions, slow-wave sleep appears; in lesions that allow a certain amount of slow-wave sleep to occur, some REM sleep will appear (Jouvet and Renault, 1966). Analysis of the tissue after such a lesion has revealed decreases in cerebral serotonin with no change in norepinephrine. Conversely, lesions of the locus coeruleus produce a decrease in REM sleep, with depletion of norepinephrine in the rostral part of the brain (Jouvet and Delorme, 1965). Studies such as these bring morphological, chemical, and electrophysiological data together and aid in formulating hypotheses on the control of sleep. Jouvet (1972) has combined these lines of evidence to suggest a control mechanism as follows: The caudal two-thirds of the locus coeruleus are responsible for the inhibition of muscle tone during REM sleep. The medial third of the locus coeruleus deals with such "tonic" aspects of REM as the cortical activation and such "phasic" events as eye movements and pontine-geniculate-occipital (PGO) spiking. Serotonergic neurons of the anterior part of the raphe system are related to behavioral and EEG aspects of slow-wave sleep. Fibers from the caudal raphe travel to the area of the locus coeruleus. Activity of such fibers both "primes" the initiation of REM sleep and inhibits the appearance of PGO spikes. An inibitory pathway from the locus coeruleus, however, decreases firing in the raphe, and allows PGO spikes to occur during REM sleep. In summary, Jouvet suggests that serotonergic activity may be related to the maintenance of slow-wave sleep and the priming of REM sleep. Adrenergic activity may be related to both tonic and phasic aspects of REM sleep.

Neurotransmitters and Arousal

The initiation and maintenace of arousal may involve somewhat different systems than those that govern the REM-nonREM cycle. As we have described, cortical activation of the EEG is related to the noradrenergic fibers of the pontine tegmentum and mesencephalic reticular formation. Jones (1969) distinguishes between such EEG indications of arousal and the maintenance of behavioral arousal, which may be mediated by dopaminergic fibers in the ventral tegmentum of the mesencephalon. Lesions of this area may produce animals with ataxia, akinesia, and lack of behavioral arousal, which may be in contrast to the level of arousal indicated by the EEG. Cholinergic mechanisms are also involved (Jouvet, 1972). Administration of physostigmine (which results in increases in acetylcholine by blocking its degradation) produces decreases in sleeping time in mice (Barnes and Meyers, 1964). Intravenous injection of acetylcholine itself stimulates arousal in EEG animal studies (Yamamoto and Domino, 1967). Similarly, cortical arousal induced by stimulation of the midbrain reticular formation is associated with increased release of acetylcholine at the cortical level (Kanai and Szerb, 1965). Serotonergic systems seem less related to regulation of the waking state in a direct sense, though as mentioned earlier, lesion studies suggest that disruption of serotonergic neurons involved in sleep regulation results in insomnia (Jouvet and Renault, 1966).

It should be noted that although study of adrenergic, serotonergic, and cholinergic systems has provided some basic understanding of the states of consciousness, these systems account for only a very small fraction of the pathways in the brain. It seems likely that a more complete understanding will have to include knowledge of pathways using other neurotransmitters. These might include glycine, gamma aminobutyric acid, histamine, and others.

Circulating Humors and Sleep

One intriguing hypothesis that has been in the sleep studies literature for some years is that a circulating substance (the *hypnotoxin*) is responsible for regulation of sleep. The first report of this finding in modern times comes from Legendre and Pieron (1910), who reported that a circulating material from sleep-deprived dogs could induce sleep when injected into recipients. Subsequent studies have suggested that such a material may be a protein of molecular weight between 355 and 1500 (Schoenenberger *et al.*, 1972; Monnier *et al.*, 1975). One of the difficulties with this hypothesis is that studies confirming the existence of a hypnotoxin have generally not used EEG criteria acceptable to most researchers (see review by Mendelson, 1974). The hypothesis is also weakened by the observations of Lenard and Schulte (1972) on the sleep of "Siamese" twins joined at the skull. Although their circulations were interconnected, their patterns of sleep onset and REM sleep were independent.

Some hormones may influence the occurrence of the sleep stages. This may be manifested either in subjects with diseases of oversecretion (e.g., hyperthyroidism) or in studies that involve administration of exogenous hormones. The possibility exists that some hormones such as growth hormone may in fact be involved in the physiologic regulation of sleep. These issues are discussed at length in chapter 3.

SUMMARY

Human sleep is not a passive state that occurs in the absence of stimulation; rather, it is an active process reflecting the interaction of complex structures in the diencephalon and brainstem. Electroencephalographically it is composed of four nonREM stages and of REM sleep. These stages occur in a series of cycles, lasting approximately 90 minutes in young adults. The content of the cycles varies somewhat as the night progresses. In a general sense, slow-wave sleep is most heavily concentrated early in sleep. In contrast, REM sleep occurs in greater amounts after some hours of sleep. The total amount of each stage for the whole night varies with the age of the subject. One approach to understanding the physiology of sleep is to examine the role of neurotransmitters involved in the neural pathways that regulate the sleep stages.

CHAPTER 2

A Pharmacologic Approach to Sleep Studies

In chapter 1 we outlined the development of the concept of "wet" neurophysiology, which emphasizes understanding neural systems by the examination of synaptic transmitters. As we discussed, initial animal experiments seemed to indicate that serotonergic, noradrenergic, and cholinergic systems are involved in the regulation of sleep. In this chapter we will describe human studies in which the activity of these systems has been pharmacologically altered. Several types of manipulations are usually employed. Chemical precursors of a transmitter are given to raise its concentration. Drugs that block its metabolism may also raise the concentration, and in addition will prevent formation of metabolites that themselves may be biologically active. The amount of available transmitter can be decreased by administering compounds that inhibit its synthesis. Receptor blockers are used to decrease the activity of a particular transmitter.

The function of a neurotransmitter may be studied by observing the sleep of normal volunteers who have received the sorts of drugs that we have just outlined. In some cases, however, the drug can have undesirable side effects, and ethical considerations militate against its use in normal subjects. Fortunately, some of the drugs in question are clinically used as medications that are of benefit in certain disease states. In these cases, sleep recordings are often done on patients receiving therapy with these agents. The problem, of course, is that patients with a particular disease may respond to a drug in a different manner than a normal person. In this chapter, emphasis will be placed on pharmacologic studies of normal volunteers, and medical patients will be discussed in those cases where data on normals is not available. The emphasis, then, is on the changes in normal sleep induced by administration of drugs that modify neurotransmitters in a relatively specific manner. Drugs that may be less specific in their actions, but that are important because of their clinical usefulness, will be discussed in subsequent chapters dealing with specific disease states.

SEROTONERGIC SYSTEM

L-Tryptophan and Sleep

Effects of Administration on Sleep

L-Tryptophan is an amino acid that may be metabolized to become serotonin (Fig. 2-1). Although synthesis of serotonin accounts for only a small amount of the total tryptophan used by the body, it is the major metabolic route found in the brain. L-Tryptophan cannot be synthesized in humans, but is found in the normal diet in amounts of 0.5–2 gm per day.

Even before EEG studies were performed it had been observed that L-tryptophan possesses sedative qualities (Oates and Sjoerdsma, 1960). Authors such as Greenwood *et al.* (1974) have documented slowing of

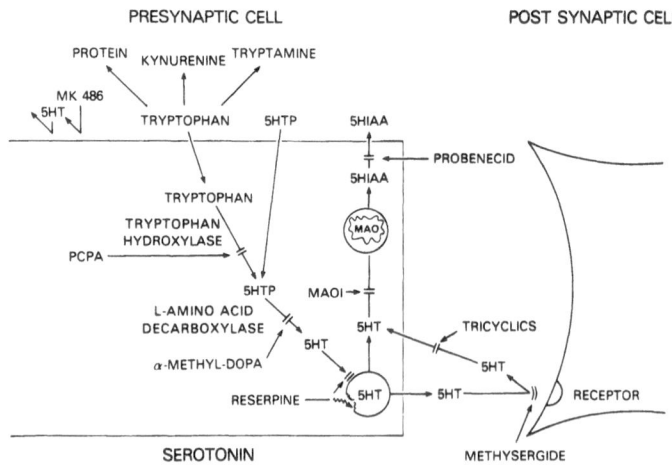

FIGURE 2-1. Synthesis and degradation of serotonin. Hypothesized actions of drugs discussed in text are shown.

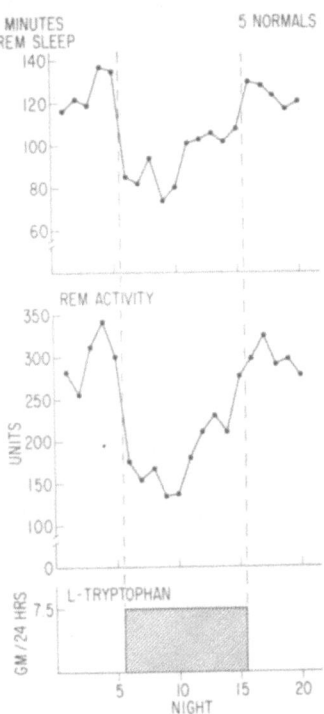

FIGURE 2-2.   Effects of 7.5 gm/24 hr of L-tryptophan on the REM sleep of five normal volunteers. (From Wyatt, 1972. Reprinted by permission.)

the clinical EEG and drowsiness (but not euphoria) following parenteral administration. Ten EEG studies have examined its effects on sleep (Table 2-1). Four studies reported increases in total sleep time, while three reported no effect on this parameter. Reports on REM latency have been variable, describing decreases (Oswald et al., 1964), no change (Hartmann et al., 1971) or increases (Wyatt et al., 1970a). Griffiths et al. (1972) reported variable changes at relatively low doses, but a consistent decrease in REM latency at higher doses (12 mg).

As in the case of REM latency, there are conflicting accounts of the effects on total REM sleep time. Four studies report no change and two report decreases following moderate doses of less than 10 gm (Fig. 2-2). One study each reports decreases (Hartmann et al., 1974a) or increases (Griffiths et al., 1972) at higher doses (10 and 12 gm, respectively). Thus, there seems to be no real agreement on the effects of L-tryptophan on REM sleep, and the differences do not seem to be resolved by examination of possible dose-dependent effects.

TABLE 2-1. The Effects of L-Tryptophan on Human EEG Sleep

Study	Dosage (mg/kg)*	Subjects	Total sleep	NREM sleep	Delta sleep	REM sleep	REM %	REM latency	No. of eye movements	REM density
Oswald et al., 1964, 1966	70–140	16 normal males	0	N.S.	N.S.	N.S.	N.S.	+ in 5 of 16	N.S.	N.S.
Evans and Oswald, 1966	70	7 narcoleptics	N.S.	N.S.	N.S.	Length of 1st REM period	N.S.	N.S.	N.S.	?
Cazzullo et al., 1969	N.S.	6 severe depressives	↑	↑	↑ ↓	↓	→	N.S.	N.S.	N.S.
Williams et al., 1969	109	15 normals	N.S.	N.S.	↑	0	0	0	N.S.	N.S.
Wyatt et al., 1970a	109	5 normal females	↑	↑	↑	→	→	↑	→	
	109	7 insomniacs (3 had affective disorders)	↑	↑	0	0	0	0	0	
Hartmann et al., 1971	120	10 normals	0	0	N.S.	0	0	0	N.S.	N.S.
Murri et al., 1971	100	7 chronic schizophrenics	0	0	0	0	0	0	N.S.	0
Griffiths et al., 1972	171	8 normals	N.S.	N.S.	↑ in 6 of 8 subjects	↑	↑	↑	N.S.	0
Mendels and Chernick, 1972	107	4 psychiatric pts. 4 normal controls	↑	N.S.	N.S.	N.S.	N.S.	N.S.	N.S.	N.S.
Hartmann et al., 1974a	14–214	10 normal men	0	N.S.	↑ at 140 mg/kg	↓ >140 mg/kg	N.S.	N.S.	N.S.	→

N.S. = not stated.
* When dosage was not reported as mg/kg, it was recalculated assuming a 70-kg subject.

Most studies suggest that L-tryptophan increases slow-wave sleep (Fig. 2-3). This feature and its ability to increase total sleep time seem to be the most consistent findings. It is possible that L-tryptophan may in fact be a natural sedative (Wyatt *et al.*, 1970a; Hartmann *et al.*, 1971). This position would seem to be strengthened by the report by Hartmann, Cravens, and List (1974a) that 1 gm—an amount comparable to that which is found in 0.5 kg of meat—can markedly reduce sleep latency. Subjects in this study were men with prolonged sleep latencies, but no subjective complaints about their sleep. The examination of effects of L-tryptophan in entirely normal subjects presents a methodological problem; since the normal sleep latency is so short (perhaps five or ten minutes), it is difficult to tell if a medication can reduce it further. For this reason, and because of interest in L-tryptophan as a "natural" sedative, it has been given to insomniacs in several studies. In general, it has produced decreased sleep latencies (see chap. 5).

In view of the possibility that dietary L-tryptophan intake may influence the sleep–waking cycle, it should be noted that different amino acids may compete for the same metabolic and transport mechanisms. Thus, when compared to fasting values, a balanced diet may produce decreases, and a carbohydrate diet may produce increases, in brain tryptophan levels (Perez-Cruit, Chase, and Murphy, 1974). It would also have to be determined if tolerance develops to the sedative effects of L-tryptophan. In one study that has examined this point (Wyatt *et al.*, 1970a), the effects on delta sleep decreased over a 10-day period of administration.

Metabolic Considerations

Other approaches to understanding the relation of L-tryptophan to sleep include measurement of plasma levels and determination of rates of metabolism during sleep. Chen *et al.* (1974), using the former approach, measured plasma tryptophan levels during the sleep of six normal women. Data was reported in terms of total plasma tryptophan, the fraction that is bound to albumin (90% of the total plasma tryptophan) and the free tryptophan fraction. The latter portion is thought to be particularly related to changes in turnover and total amount of brain serotonin (Knott and Curzon, 1972; Moir and Eccleston, 1968). Neither free nor bound tryptophan showed a direct temporal relationship to the sleep stages. On the other hand, the mean free tryptophan levels for the whole night were positively correlated with total percentage of REM sleep, and were correlated inversely with percentage nonREM sleep. The reverse was true for bound plasma tryptophan: Levels were related

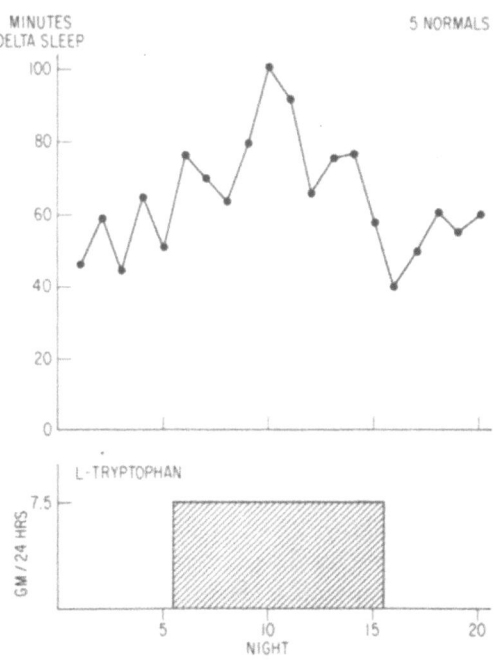

FIGURE 2-3. Slow-wave sleep in same subjects as in Figure 2-2. (From Wyatt, 1972. Reprinted by permission.)

positively to nonREM sleep and negatively to REM sleep. Overall free plasma tryptophan levels decreased as the night progressed, particularly after 4:00 A.M. The authors suggested that this latter finding is related to the increased levels of adrenocorticosteroids toward the next morning. Adrenocorticosteroids have been shown to induce liver tryptophan pyrrolase, an enzyme that catalyzes the first step of the pathway leading to formation of kynurenine. Thus, it may be that the increased levels of corticosteroids indirectly result in more tryptophan entering this alternate pathway rather than being available for serotonin synthesis. Tryptophan levels may also be influenced by dietary intake of tryptophan and other dietary substances such as nonesterified fatty acids and carbohydrates. The correlation of levels of free tryptophan and REM sleep once again may suggest some role of serotonergic systems in the control of REM sleep. It seems clear, however, that this study will have to be reevaluated in the light of recent work that suggests that it is not the free plasma tryptophan, but rather the ratio of free tryptophan to neutral amino acids that is related to levels of tryptophan and 5-hydroxyindoleacetic acid in the cerebrospinal fluid. (Perez-Cruet, Chase, and Murphy, 1974).

Rodden et al., (1973) administered tryptophan and tyrosine that had been labeled with radioactive carbon (^{14}C) to normal volunteers. By measuring the amount of $^{14}CO_2$ in the subjects' breath, an estimate of rate of metabolism was obtained. It was found that there was no difference between waking and sleeping rates of metabolism of tyrosine. In the case of tryptophan, however, it was found that in waking subjects the maximum excretion was at about 42 minutes, whereas in sleeping subjects maximum excretion occurred in 125 minutes. Although there are several possible explanations for these observations, it seems likely that tryptophan is metabolized more slowly during sleep.

The question arises as to which (if any) metabolic pathway of L-tryptophan may be related to its effects on sleep. In addition to conversion to serotonin, it may follow a pathway leading to kynurenine and its derivatives (including nicotinamide), or it may be converted to tryptamine and ultimately indoleacetic acid. There are difficulties in relating the effects of tryptophan on sleep to each of the three major metabolic routes. In order to determine if its effects are produced by increased levels of serotonin, Wyatt et al. (1970a) and Wyatt (1972) administered tryptophan to patients in whom synthesis of serotonin was partially blocked by parachlorophenylalanine (PCPA). As a result of the PCPA pretreatment, REM sleep was decreased. During each of four trials in three patients, administration of L-tryptophan resulted in increases in nonREM and decreases in REM sleep (Fig. 2-4). Thus, although PCPA partially blocked serotinin synthesis, L-tryptophan still had major effects on sleep. It seemed less likely, then, that its effects on sleep are mediated by changes in serotonin levels.

As with the case of serotonin synthesis, there is also some evidence that the effects of L-tryptophan on sleep are not mediated by tryptamine. Hodge, Oates, and Sjoerdsma (1964) gave L-tryptophan to subjects who had been pretreated with a monoamine oxidase inhibitor (MAOI), resulting in an increase in tryptamine levels. The subjects were observed to become sedated and intoxicated. Subjects were then pretreated with a MAOI plus RO4-4602. (The latter is a centrally active L-aromatic decarboxylase inhibitor, which partially blocks the conversion of tryptophan to tryptamine.) When tryptophan was given to these subjects, it still produced sedation, although intoxication did not occur.

The question as to whether L-tryptophan's effects on sleep are mediated by the kynurenine pathway is still unresolved. In an unpublished study, Gillin and Wyatt gave 2 gm/24 hr of L-kynurenine to three

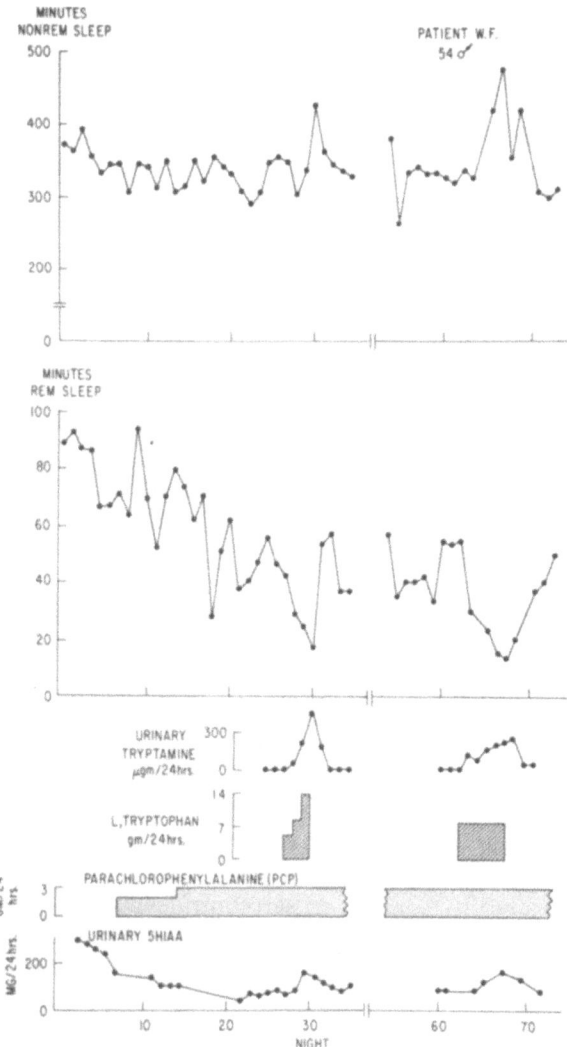

FIGURE 2-4.   The nonREM and REM sleep response to administration of L-tryptophan in one patient taking PCPA. (From Wyatt, 1972. Reprinted by permission.)

normal subjects for two days. There were no consistent effects on sleep. On the other hand, preliminary data by Pegram *et al.* (1975) suggests that nicotinamide, which may be derived from this pathway, increases REM sleep.

In summary, studies of the major metabolic routes of L-tryptophan have not entirely clarified the mechanism by which its sedative effects occur. Other possibilities are that its effects on sleep are due to some direct effect on the brain, or an action secondary to conversion to an unknown protein, or release of a hormone.

5-Hydroxytryptophan

Five-hydroxytryptophan (5-HTP), the immediate precursor of serotonin (Fig. 2-1), has been administered orally and intravenously to human subjects in both the racemate (D,L) and L forms (Table 2-2). In general, low doses in normal subjects have produced either no change (Hartmann, 1970) or increases (Mandell et al., 1964; Wyatt et al., 1971d) in REM sleep. Studies on schizophrenics include observations that low doses increase amounts of REM sleep in child (Zarcone et al., 1973) and adult (Murri et al., 1972) patients and that high doses may decrease both REM and delta sleep (Dawson et al., 1974). Gillin et al. (1972b) administered 5-HTP plus a peripheral decarboxylase inhibitor (which reduces metabolism of 5-HTP outside of the brain) to depressed patients. Intravenous infusion during REM and nonREM sleep produced no changes in sleep. High doses given inadvertently to a patient with Down's syndrome produced no effects on amounts of REM or delta sleep (Bazelon et al., 1968); low doses given to children with Down's syndrome have been reported to cause no change in total amounts of REM, but increases in REM density were noted (Petre-Quadrens and DeGreef, 1971). Zarcone and Hoddes (1975) administered 5-HTP to abstinent alcoholics. They found that although it did not change the total amount of REM sleep, it decreased the fragmentation of REM periods (a REM period was defined as two consecutive REM episodes separated by less than 25 minutes of nonREM sleep). This was taken to imply that 5-HTP may have helped correct sleep disturbances in alcoholics due to abnormal serotonergic regulation.

Wyatt (1972) administered a related drug, alpha-methyl-5-HTP to three hypertensive patients. This compound may be converted to alpha-methyl-serotonin, a poor substrate for monoamine oxidase. REM sleep was increased by 4–50% in doses over 0.75 gm (Fig. 2-5), although insomnia was produced in one patient.

Five-hydroxytryptophan has been given to patients with unusual sleep disorders due to various lesions of the central nervous system. Fischer-Perroudon, Mouret, and Jouvet (1974) gave 5-HTP to a patient who had had virtually no sleep since having a presumably viral illness four months previously. Doses of 2–12 gm/24 hr markedly increased total sleep time, restored slow-wave sleep, and resulted in some REM sleep.

TABLE 2-2. Effect of 5-HTP on Human EEG Sleep

Study	Dosage (mg/kg)	Subjects	Total sleep	NREM sleep	Delta sleep	REM sleep	REM %	REM latency	No. of eye movements	REM density
Mandell et al., 1964	0.7–2.1 (D, L) combined oral and I.V.	2 males	N.S.	N.S.	N.S.	N.S.	↑	N.S.	N.S.	N.S.
Oswald et al., 1966	0.6 mg I.V.	N.S.	N.S.	N.S.	N.S.	N.S.	N.S.	↓ in 1 of 6 observations	N.S.	N.S.
Bazelon et al., 1968	2.4–85.5	1 female with Down's syndrome	N.S.	0	0	0	0	N.S.	N.S.	N.S.
Hartmann, 1970	0.7 (D, L)	4 subjects	0	0	0	0	0	N.S.	N.S.	N.S
Petre-Quadrens et al., 1971	0.3–0.75	4 children with Down's syndrome	N.S.	N.S.	N.S.	N.S.	N.S.	N.S.	N.S.	↑
Wyatt et al., 1971d	8.6 (D, L)	8 normals	0	0	0	↑	↑	0	N.S.	↑
Gillin et al., 1972b	0.35–0.7 (D, L) and L) I.V. MK-486	3 depressed subjects	0	0	0	↑	↑	0	N.S.	↑
		I.V. infusion during NREM at REM onset	0	0	0	0	0	0	N.S.	N.S.
Murri et al., 1972	7.1 (D, L)	6 chronic schizophrenics	0	0	0 →	0 ↑	0	0	N.S.	N.S.
Guilleminault et al., 1973a	21 (D, L)	1 man with brainstem lesion	↑	↑	0	0	→	0	N.S.	N.S.
Zarcone et al., 1973b	3.0 (D, L)	2 childhood schizophrenics	0	→	0	↑	↑	0	↑	↑
Zarcone et al., 1973a	21/24 hr over 14 days	2 narcoleptics	0	—	0	—	→	0	—	—
Dawson et al., 1974	51.5–80.7/24 hr + MK 486	18 chronic schizophrenics	↓ (at high doses)	—	→	→	0	↑	—	0
Zarcone and Hoddes, 1975	4.3	12 alcoholics	—	—	0	0	0	—	—	—

N.S. = not stated.

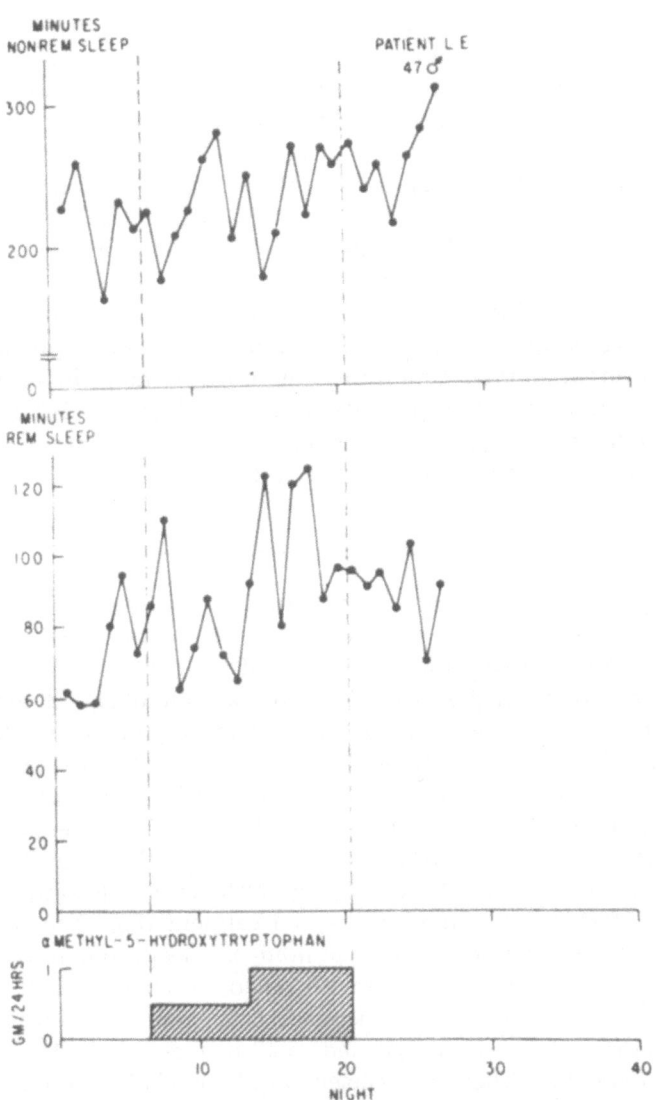

FIGURE 2-5.   Sleep response in patient taking AM-5-HTP. REM response seen primarily when drug dosage is above 0.75 gm/24 hr. (From Wyatt, 1972. Reprinted by permission.)

Guilleminault, Cathala, and Castaigne (1973a) administered 5-HTP to a patient with a posttraumatic brainstem lesion that had produced a state of hyposomnia (four hours sleep per night). Administration of the drug resulted in increases in total sleep time, essentially by increasing nonREM sleep. Higher doses (1500 mg) resulted in decreased sleep latencies, and also caused decreases in REM sleep. The decrease in REM sleep at higher doses seems consistent with the experience of other studies. Comparable high doses in other hands have not generally caused changes in total sleep time in narcoleptics (Zarcone, Hoddes, and Smythe, 1973a), nor have there been changes in total sleep time at lower doses in a variety of patients. The explanation for these findings may lie in the unusual nature of the patient, or in possible actions of 5-HTP other than producing increases in serotonin. Some animal data, for instance, suggests that exogenous 5-HTP may not act as a precursor of serotonin under normal conditions, although it may do so in cats pretreated with parachlorophenylalanine (Pujol *et al.*, 1971). Other possible actions might include functioning as a false neurotransmitter or interfering with metabolism of catecholamines.

Parachlorophenylalanine

Parachlorophenylalanine (PCPA) interferes with the synthesis of serotonin by inhibiting the enzyme tryptophan hydroxylase (Fig. 2-1). Because of the relatively high incidence of toxic effects, studies with PCPA have not been performed on normal volunteers. It has been studied, however, in medical patients undergoing therapeutic trials of PCPA. Wyatt (1972) administered PCPA to 17 patients, including those with carcinoid tumors, migraine headaches, Huntington's chorea, and dystonia musculorum deformans. Doses of 2–4 gm/24 hr were given for periods ranging from 14 days to three years. PCPA was found to decrease amounts of REM sleep by 20–70% with a maximum effect occurring after two to three weeks of treatment (Fig. 2-6). In some patients there was a small increase in nonREM sleep, so that total sleep time was not disturbed. These patients had only small amounts of delta sleep, and usually there was no change in this parameter with administration of drug. Some, however, had small increases in delta sleep, an effect also noted by Chernik, Ramsey, and Mendels (1973) in a patient receiving both methadone and PCPA.

In contrast to experience with many REM sleep suppressing drugs, there was no "rebound" increase in REM sleep above normal amounts upon withdrawal of PCPA. In fact, amounts of REM sleep did not return to normal levels for about three weeks. This might suggest that PCPA

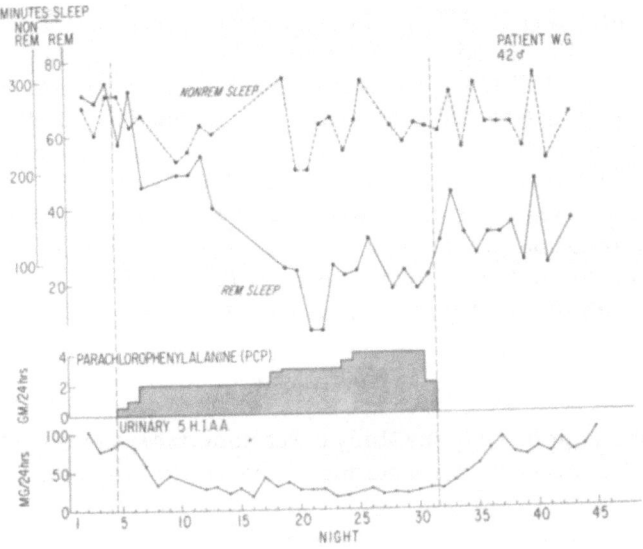

FIGURE 2-6.   Comparison of the effect of REM and nonREM sleep of PCPA. (From Wyatt, 1972. Reprinted by permission.)

interferes with a fundamental aspect of REM sleep production, rather than suppressing its occurrence.

PCPA was found to have effects on the phasic aspects of REM sleep. The number of eye movements per minute of REM sleep (*REM density*) and the total number of eye movements over the whole night (*REM activity*) were decreased. On the other hand, there was an increase in the number of isolated rapid eye movements occurring in stage 2 sleep. Similarly, PCPA administration was related to an increase in phasic integrated potentials (PIPs) occurring in nonREM sleep in two patients. [PIPs are a measure of the integrated potential of eye movement activity, and are thought to be analogous to the pontine-geniculate-occipital (PGO) spikes in cats.] These observations with rapid eye movements and PIPs have been taken to imply that one of the functions of the serotonergic system is to confine such phasic events to REM sleep.

Since PCPA has been found to have effects on several biochemical systems, the question arises as to whether its effects on REM sleep are in fact due to inhibition of serotonin synthesis. Wyatt (1972) approached this problem by adminstering 5-HTP to four patients with carcinoid tumors who were being treated with PCPA. (The principle involved was that 5-HTP is the immediate precursor of serotonin; hence, when it is added, it may be possible to synthesize serotonin in the presence of PCPA.) It was found that in three of the four patients, administration of 400–800 mg of D, L-5-HTP resulted in a partial or total recovery of REM sleep (Fig. 2-7). Total rapid eye movement activity also returned toward normal. Upon withdrawal of 5-HTP, the amount of REM sleep decreased to the lower level associated with PCPA treatment. NonREM sleep was unaffected by this procedure. This experiment seems to imply that the effects of PCPA on REM sleep are in fact due to its inhibition of serotonin synthesis.

Methysergide

Another approach to the study of serotonergic systems in sleep is to examine the effects of administering methysergide, a serotonin receptor

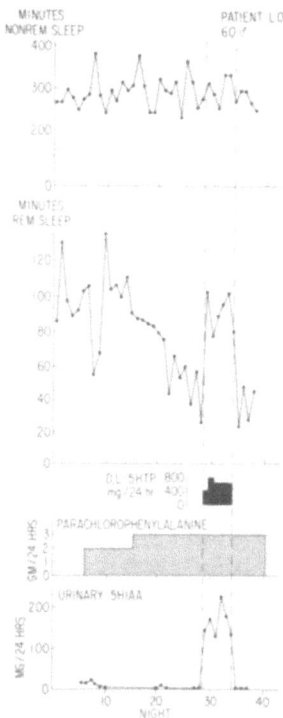

FIGURE 2-7.   REM sleep response to 5-HTP in patient taking PCPA. (From Wyatt, 1972. Reprinted by permission.)

blocker. Methysergide is a drug structurally similar to serotonin, used clinically for the prevention of migraine headaches. One preliminary study has suggested that it may be beneficial in the treatment of narcolepsy (Wyler, Wilkus, and Troupin, 1975).

Methysergide has been shown to reverse the effects of serotonin in a variety of systems (Douglas, 1970), to block the central toxic effect of 5-HTP in mice (Karfa, Karki, and Tala, 1961), and to compete with serotonin in binding to a subcellular fraction of hypothalamic tissue thought to contain "nerve-ending membranes" (Fiszer and DeRobertis, 1969). It should, of course, be noted that it may have other actions besides serotonin inhibition. These may include feeble vasoconstrictor and oxytocic effects (Douglas, 1970) and the ability to block the inhibitory action of dopamine on insulin release (Feldman and Lebovitz, 1972).

In 1966, Oswald *et al.* observed that pretreatment with methysergide (3 mg/24 hr for 72 hr) could prevent the reduction in REM latency that is usually produced by a single dose of 5–10 gm of L-tryptophan. Mendelson, Reichman, and Othmer (1975a) administered methysergide to normal volunteers for 48 hours, at a dose of 8 mg per 24 hr. There was no change in total sleep time, sleep latency, or REM latency. Stage 4 decreased and stage 3 increased, with no change in total slow-wave sleep. Total REM sleep time, however, was reduced by 36%. There was a small but significant increase in total nonREM sleep. This pattern—a decrease in REM, with a small "compensatory" increase in nonREM sleep, and no change in total sleep time—is similar to that observed by Wyatt (1972) with PCPA in humans. These studies are in contrast to a report that administration of PCPA or methysergide to rabbits resulted in a marked decrease in REM sleep and a smaller decrease in nonRem sleep (Tabushi and Himwich, 1971). Thus, in rabbits and humans these drugs have been reported to have different effects; within each species, however, their effects are similar. In humans, the implication would seem to be that both an inhibitor of serotonin synthesis and a blocker of its receptors result in decreased amounts of REM sleep.

Lysergic Acid Diethylamide

Lysergic acid diethylamide (LSD) is a hallucinogen that has profound effects on the serotonergic system. Neurons in the raphe nuclei may have either an increased or decreased firing rate in response to LSD, depending on dose and method of administration. Although earlier theories suggested that it acts by blocking serotonin receptors, more recent work suggests that in doses that produce psychological effects it may mimic serotonin at central synapses (Byck, 1975). Muzio, Roffwarg, and Kaufman (1966) administered 0.08–0.73 gm/kg of LSD orally to normal volunteers either just before going to bed or one hour after falling asleep, and found increases in the length of the first or second REM period. Similarly, Torda (1968) observed that intravenous infusions of LSD 30–50 minutes after the onset of the third REM period of the night reduced the latency prior to the next REM period.

Ventricular Fluid 5-HIAA

Another approach to understanding the relation of serotonergic activity to sleep is to examine levels of the serotonin metabolite 5-hydroxyindoleacetic acid (5-HIAA) in the cerebral ventricles during sleep. This is possible in patients with presenile dementias in whom ventricular cannulas have been surgically installed for therapeutic purposes. As it is thought that production of 5-HIAA is proportional to serotonergic neuronal activity (Aghajanian, Rosecrans, and Sheard, 1967), it seems possible that 5-HIAA levels might give an indication of the relative activity of serotonergic neurons in different stages of sleep. Wyatt et al. (1974) found that 5-HIAA concentrations were higher during nonREM sleep than in waking or REM sleep. Levels during REM sleep were lowest, and were significantly less than waking levels. This finding seems compatible with the hypothesis that serotonergic activity is related to restricting phasic events (rapid eye movements) to REM sleep. It is also compatible with the concept, largely derived from animal studies, that serotonergic neurons initiate or sustain nonREM sleep (Jouvet, 1972).

NORADRENERGIC SYSTEM

L-Dihydroxyphenylalanine (L-DOPA)

Effects on REM Sleep

L-DOPA, which may be converted into dopamine and norepinephrine (Fig. 2-8), has been administered in 17 sleep studies (Table 2-3). Its effects seemed most marked on REM sleep, although studies differed on the direction of these effects. There were no consistent changes in REM sleep in four studies, an increase in seven studies, and decreases in four studies. One showed differing effects on REM sleep at different doses (Bergonzi et al., 1974) and another reported differences between acute and chronic administration (Schneider et al., 1974a).

Wyatt et al. (1970b) administered L-DOPA to seven medical and

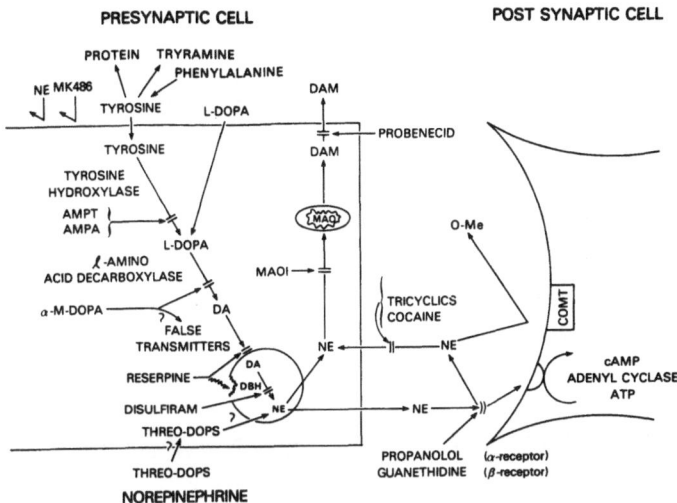

FIGURE 2-8. Synthesis and degradation of norepinephrine. Hypothesized actions of drugs discussed in text are shown.

neurologic patients. Three patients also received MK-485, a peripheral decarboxylase inhibitor that decreases the amount of L-DOPA converted to dopamine outside the nervous system. REM sleep was decreased, and REM latency increased (Fig. 2-9). When L-DOPA was discontinued, a REM rebound occurred. In some patients receiving submaximal doses, it was noted that REM sleep was decreased during the first half of the night and increased during the second half. The net effect was that the total REM sleep for the whole night was unchanged. This phenomenon of a "partial withdrawal," which has also been observed with alcohol (see chap. 6), may help to explain why some studies report decreases in REM sleep while others reported no systematic change. In an effort to evaluate the phenomenon of the "partial drug withdrawal" effect, two patients were given L-DOPA on a schedule that omitted the drug during the two hours prior to bedtime (Wyatt, 1972). Under these conditions, REM sleep time did not differ from placebo. When the same total dosage was given so that a 500-mg dose was given 30 minutes prior to bedtime, REM sleep was markedly reduced. A similar phenomenon was reported by Yules et al. (1967) using ethanol; decreases in REM sleep were much more striking when administration occurred shortly before bedtime, rather than four hours earlier. Thus, it seems important that time of administration should be considered in evaluating agents that have relatively short-lived effects on REM sleep.

TABLE 2-3. The Effect of L-DOPA on Human Sleep

Study	Dosage (mg/kg)	Subjects	Total sleep	NREM sleep	Delta sleep	REM sleep	REM %	REM latency	No. of eye movements	REM density
Bonasegla and Menegati, 1968	1.4 I.V. prior to bed	3	N.S.	N.S.	↑	↑	↑	↑	N.S.	N.S.
Bricolo et al., 1970	28–80	14 Parkinson patients	0	0	↓	↑	↑	↓	0	0
Fram et al., 1970	Up to 180	8 depressed patients	↑	N.S.	N.S.	↓	↓	N.S.	N.S.	N.S.
Greenberg and Perlman, 1970	Up to 86	6 Parkinson patients	0	0	0	0	0	N.S.	N.S.	N.S.
Wyatt et al., 1970b	7–126 with and without a peripheral decarboxylase inhibitor	7 patients with medical and neurological disorders	↓	↓	0	↓	↓	↑	↓	↓
Zarcone et al., 1970	57	2 depressed patients	↑	0	0	↑	↑	N.S.	N.S.	N.S.
Gunne et al., 1971	10–34	6 narcoleptics (1 hr afternoon recording)	0	0	0	0	0	N.S.	N.S.	N.S.
Kales et al., 1971a	43–71	4 Parkinson patients	0	0	0	0	0	0	N.S.	N.S.
		4 normals	0	0	0	0	0	0	N.S.	N.S.
Schmidt and Knopp, 1972	N.S.	2 Parkinson patients	0 / N.S.	0 / N.S.	0 / N.S	0 / ↑		N.S.	N.S. / N.S.	N.S. / N.S.
Azumi et al., 1972	29–36	15 normal males	0					N.S.	N.S.	N.S.
Kales et al., 1972	N.S.	3 autistic children	N.S.	N.S.	N.S.	0	0	N.S.	N.S.	N.S.
Kendel et al., 1972	28–71	24 Parkinson patients	0	↓	↑	↑	↑	↑	N.S.	N.S.

Reference	Dose (mg/kg)	Subjects				↑ length of 1st REM period			
Castaldo et al., 1973	2.8	4 normals	N.S.	N.S.	N.S.	↑ length of 1st REM period	0	N.S.	N.S.
	7.1	10 normals	N.S.	N.S.	N.S.	0	0	N.S.	N.S.
	1.8	2 mental retardates	N.S.	N.S.	N.S.	0	↑	N.S.	N.S.
Gillin et al., 1973	0.33–0.66 I.V. with a peripheral decarboxylase inhibitor, MK-486, given during 1st NREM sleep period At REM onset	10 patients with affective disorders in partial remission	0	0	0	0	0	↑	0	0
Nakazawa et al., 1973	14.3	5 normal males	0	N.S.	0	0	0	0	N.S.	0
Bergonzi et al., 1974*	21.4–64.3 for 15–66 days	24 Parkinson patients	N.S.	↑(21.4–42.8 mg/kg) ↓(64.3 mg/kg)	N.S.	N.S.	↑(21.4–42.8 mg/kg) ↓(64.3 mg/kg)	N.S.	N.S.
Schneider et al., 1974a	28.6–57.2 or 2.1 plus decarboxylase inhibitor	26 Parkinson patients	N.S.	↑ (pts. who improved)	↑ (pts. who improved)	N.S.	↑	↑	N.S.

N.S. = not stated.
* Formal tests for significance not reported.

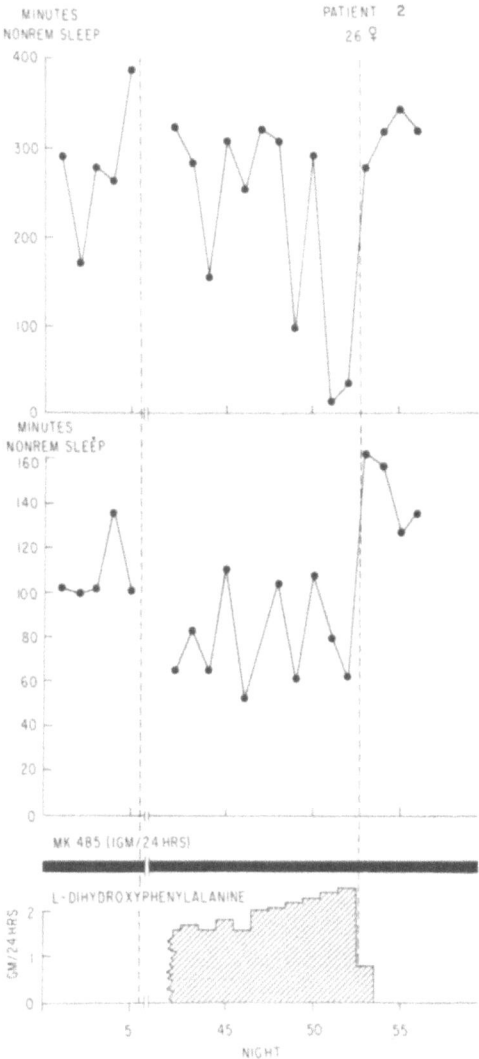

FIGURE 2-9. Sleep response during administration of L-DOPA in combination with the peripheral decarboxylase inhibitor MK485. (From Wyatt, 1972. Reprinted by permission.)

Bergonzi *et al.* (1974), treating parkinsonian patients, observed that L-DOPA exerted dose-dependent effects. Without medication, the patients appeared to have less stage 4 and REM sleep than might have been expected. When given 1.5–3.0 gm of L-DOPA, these stages increased; with 4.5 gm, however, the disturbances seen in the drug-free recording began to reappear. Although differing responses at various doses may help explain the conflicting reports regarding REM sleep, an evaluation of Table 2-3 does not reveal a simple dose-related pattern.

Differing effects of L-DOPA on sleep in parkinsonian patients may be related to degree of clinical improvement. Kendel *et al.* (1972) observed that patients who improved clinically developed an increased amount of REM sleep; those patients who showed no improvement had no consistent change in this parameter. REM latency was increased in all patients. Schneider *et al.* (1974a), like Kendel *et al.* (1972), found increases in REM latency, but found increases in percentage REM in all patients regardless of prognosis. On the other hand, those that improved showed decreases in sleep latency and wakefulness and increases in slow-wave sleep; there was little change in these parameters in patients who did not improve. They considered the small increases in REM sleep to be an "indirect" effect related to increased mobility, as opposed to the "direct" effect of increasing REM latency.

One approach to differentiate "indirect" effects due to clinical improvement from "direct" effects is, of course, to study the effects of L-DOPA on normal subjects. There are three studies available on acute oral doses of L-DOPA (2.8–71 mg/kg) in normals (Nakazawa *et al.*, 1973; Castaldo *et al.*, 1973; Kales *et al.*, 1971a). All three showed no statistically significant change in percentage of REM sleep following administration of L-DOPA. Nakazawa *et al.* (1973), however, did note decreased total minutes of REM sleep. Chronic administration of L-DOPA to normal subjects has been reported in two studies. Azumi *et al.* (1972) found increases in percentage REM sleep at doses of 29–36 mg/kg; Kales *et al.* (1971a) found no change at doses of 43–71 mg/kg. Aside from the difference in dosage, there seems no obvious explanation for the differing results in these two chronic studies. It should be noted that neither, however, provided formal statistical analysis of REM sleep data on the normal subjects before and after treatment. In summary, the data on oral administration of L-DOPA to normal subjects does not suggest a well-defined influence on REM sleep.

Intravenous L-DOPA, in contrast to oral administration, seems clearly to affect REM sleep. Gillin *et al.* (1973) administered L-DOPA intravenously to recovered depressed patients while they were sleeping. When infused 25 minutes after sleep onset, L-DOPA significantly delayed the onset of REM sleep from 44 to 71 minutes. When L-DOPA was given immediately after the onset of the first REM period, the length of the REM period was reduced by about half. The second REM episode was increased to about the same extent that the first one had been reduced.

Nakazawa *et al.* (1973) studied the effects of an oral dose of 1 gm of

L-DOPA on normal subjects recovering from "partially differential REM sleep deprivation." These subjects had been awakened at 5:30 A.M. every morning for three days, and consequently had reduced their REM sleep by about half, as well as decreasing stages 1 and 2. During a recovery night in which they received a placebo, there was a rebound increase in the total duration of REM sleep. This effect was blocked by L-DOPA. Thus, when given intravenously or when given orally to subjects who previously had been partially REM-deprived, L-DOPA shows REM-inhibiting effects.

Effects on NonREM Sleep

L-DOPA at low or moderate doses produces no consistent effects on total nonREM sleep (Table 2-3). Insomnia often develops in parkinsonian patients who receive L-DOPA, but may decrease along with clinical improvement (Kendel *et al.*, 1972). Bergonzi *et al.* (1974) found decreases in intermittent wakefulness when moderate doses were given to parkinsonian patients, but a resumption of high levels occurred with higher doses.

Threo-dihydroxyphenylserine (DOPS)

It is not clear which metabolite of L-DOPA may be having the effects on sleep that we have just described. One approach to clarifying this problem is to administer DOPS, a synthetic amino acid that is converted directly to norepinephrine without first being converted to dopamine. Gillin *et al.* (1972b) gave 50–150 mg of DOPS intravenously to depressed patients who had been pretreated with the decarboxylase inhibitor MK-486 (150 mg/24 hr). Infusions prior to and during the first REM period did not affect sleep. In an experiment performed in conjunction with Dr. T. N. Chase, up to 5000 mg/24 hr of DOPS was given orally to a patient with a hereditary cerebellar degenerative disease. There was no effect on sleep or on spinal fluid levels of the main metabolite of norepinephrine, 3-methoxy-4-hydroxyphenylglycol (MHPG). Since there is no direct evidence that DOPS is converted into norepinephrine in the human brain, this study leaves unsettled the question of whether dopamine or norepinephrine may exert effects on sleep.

Alpha-Methyl-Paratyrosine (AMPT) and Alpha-Methyl-Phenylalanine (AMPA)

Catecholamine synthesis may be decreased by AMPT and AMPA, which inhibit the rate-limiting conversion catalyzed by tyrosine hydroxylase (Figs. 2-8 and 2-10). The effects of AMPT on sleep have been examined in five medical or neurologic patients (Wyatt *et al.*, 1971a) and five patients with nonpsychotic depressions (Vaughn, Wyatt, and Green, 1972). During the first five nights of administration, total REM sleep was increased by 3–52% (Fig. 2-11). The return to baseline was variable when the drug was discontinued, but in general there was a drop in REM sleep below baseline. There were no striking changes in nonREM sleep; since the patients were allowed to sleep for a limited period (eight hours), however, large changes in total sleep could not occur. In these studies, as well as a report on sleep time estimated by nursing observations (Brodie *et al.*, 1971) there was a decrease in total sleep during the first few nights after AMPT was discontinued.

A study of the effects of AMPA on three medical and neurologic patients (Wyatt, 1972) showed increases in REM sleep of 8–48%. In the one patient examined after the drug was discontinued, REM sleep decreased 25% below baseline levels, with a "compensatory" increase in nonREM sleep. There were no major changes in nonREM sleep during AMPA administration.

The studies with AMPT and AMPA would seem to suggest that decreases in catecholamine synthesis are related to increases in total amount of REM sleep. It should be noted, of course, that the different monoamine systems are interrelated, and that a decrease in synthesis in one system could have its effects directly, or indirectly by influencing

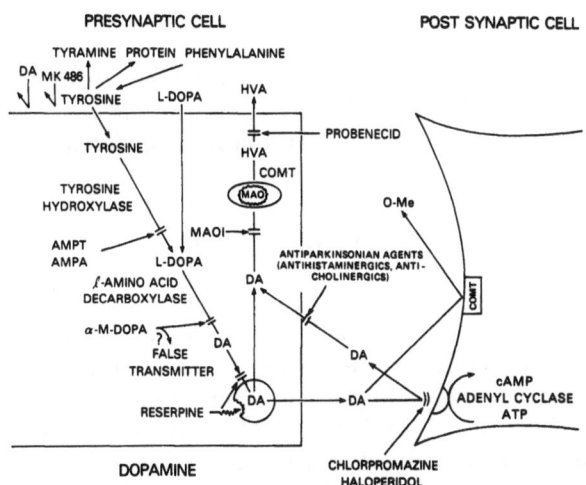

FIGURE 2-10.   Synthesis and degradation of dopamine. Hypothesized actions of drugs discussed in text are shown.

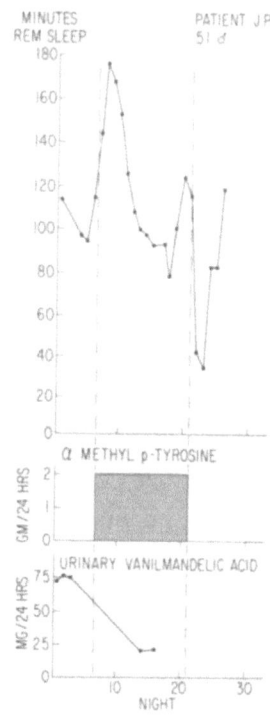

FIGURE 2-11. Sleep response during administration of AMPT. (From Wyatt, 1972. Reprinted by permission.)

other biochemical systems. Stein, Jouvet, and Pujol (1974), for instance, have shown that injections of AMPT in cats result in both decreases in catecholamines and increases in serotonin in different areas of the brain.

Alpha-Methyl-DOPA

Alpha-methyl-DOPA, clinically used for the treatment of hypertension, inhibits aromatic-L-amino acid decarboxylase, which is involved in the synthesis of both norepinephrine and serotonin. When 1.25 gm/24 hr was administered to 10 normal adults, total REM sleep for the night remained unaltered (Baekeland and Lundwall, 1971). During the first three hours of sleep, however, REM sleep was increased and stage 4 was decreased. Oswald *et al.* (1966) found that alpha-methyl-DOPA did not block the ability of L-tryptophan to shorten REM latency.

Pimozide

Another way to examine the role of catecholamines in sleep is to study the effects of receptor blockers. Pimozide, a neuroleptic agent chemically related to haloperidol, has been used for this purpose. As it is a central dopamine blocker that does not seem to affect noradrenergic transmission (Anden *et al.*, 1970), it is also of interest in that it might help distinguish between the roles played by dopamine and norepinephrine. Sagales and Erill (1975) administered 1–4 mg of pimozide to six normal subjects. During the first night, there was a small decrease in stage 1; there was no change in percentages of stages 2, 3, 4 or REM sleep. Although there was no change in REM latency, there was some increase in the mean duration of the first REM episode. In general, then, possible dopaminergic blockade with pimozide seemed to have little effect on sleep.

Adrenergic Receptor Blockers

Propanolol, which is used to treat certain cardiac arrhythmias, acts by blocking beta-adrenergic receptors. It is known to readily enter the brain. MacLean and Oswald administered 120 mg of propanolol before bedtime to three men for 13 days. There was no effect on total sleep time, percentage REM sleep, or other measures. Unpublished data from this laboratory also found no effect from 100 mg/24 hr of propanolol.

An alpha-adrenergic blocking agent, thymoxamine, has been reported to increase REM sleep (Oswald *et al.*, 1974). This seems consistent with the studies of AMPT previously described, in which this inhibitor of norepinephrine synthesis produced increases in REM sleep.

Other Drugs Influencing Amines

Monoamine Oxidase Inhibitors

Monoamine oxidase inhibitors (MAOI) block the breakdown of serotonin and norepinephrine (Figs. 2-1 and 2-8). Although both substances have alternate routes of metabolism (methylation), very little serotonin is in fact metabolized by this pathway (Snyder, 1972). Hence, it has been suggested that MAOIs have a greater influence on levels of serotonin than norepinephrine (Sourkes, 1972; Pscheidt, 1964). As can be seen in Figure 2-12, high doses of the hydrazine MAOI phenelzine (60–105 mg) as well as isocarboxazid (60 mg), mebamazine (15 mg), and

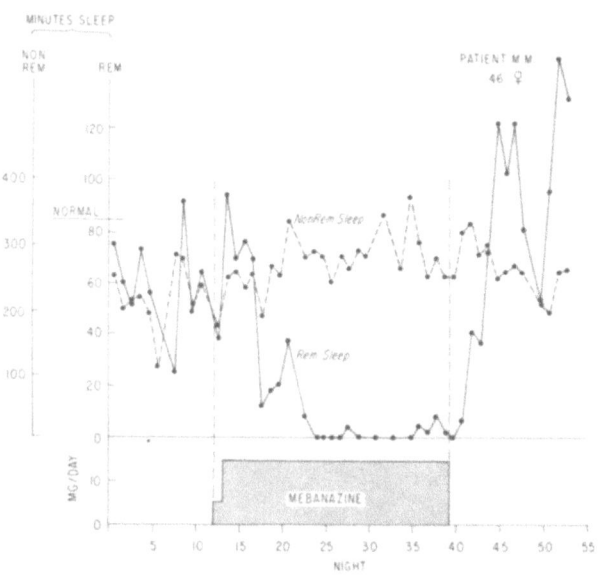

FIGURE 2-12. Typical nonREM and REM sleep response in a patient receiving the MAOI mebamazine. (From Wyatt, 1972. Reprinted by permission.)

the nonhydrazine MAOI pargyline (60–100 mg) markedly decreased REM sleep when given for 10 days to depressed or narcoleptic patients (Wyatt *et al.*, 1971b; Wyatt *et al.*, 1971c; Wyatt *et al.*, 1969). NonREM sleep was either unchanged or showed a small "compensatory" increase. The observation that the nonMAOI isoniazid (400 mg) did not suppress REM sleep suggests that the sleep-related effects of these drugs are in fact due to their inhibition of monoamine oxidase, rather than to some other property (Wyatt, 1972). Akindale, Evans, and Oswald (1970) also noted decreases in REM sleep following administration of 60–90 mg of phenelzine, but not after administration of nialamide.

The effects of MAOIs on REM sleep may be dose related. Wyatt (1972), noting that administration of large doses of MAOIs often resulted in a small increase in REM sleep that preceded the decreases (Fig. 2-13) administered low doses of phenelzine (5–15 mg/day) to four depressed patients. Consistent increases in REM sleep were observed (Fig. 2-14).

Kupfer and Bowers (1972) measured monoamine metabolite levels in the cerebrospinal fluid of nine psychotic patients, and found that phenelzine in relatively high doses (45–60 mg/day) decreased homovanilic acid (a metabolite of dopamine) more than 5-hydroxyindoleacetic acid (a metabolite of serotonin). During a REM rebound following discontinuation of phenelzine, spinal fluid HVA increased in four patients; in one patient who showed no rebound, HVA levels remained unchanged. Levels of 5-HIAA were not significantly changed during REM suppression or later REM rebound. These results seem to suggest a role for dopamine in the control of REM sleep.

Recent work has suggested that monoamine oxidase exists in two forms, depending on the preferred substrate (Neff and Yang, 1974). The type A enzyme generally metabolizes serotonin, norepinephrine, and normetanephrine. Type B preferentially metabolizes benzylamine and β-phenylethylamine. Some of the MAO inhibitors preferentially inhibit type A or B enzymes, and so it seems possible that they may have different effects on sleep-related phenomena. Examination of the

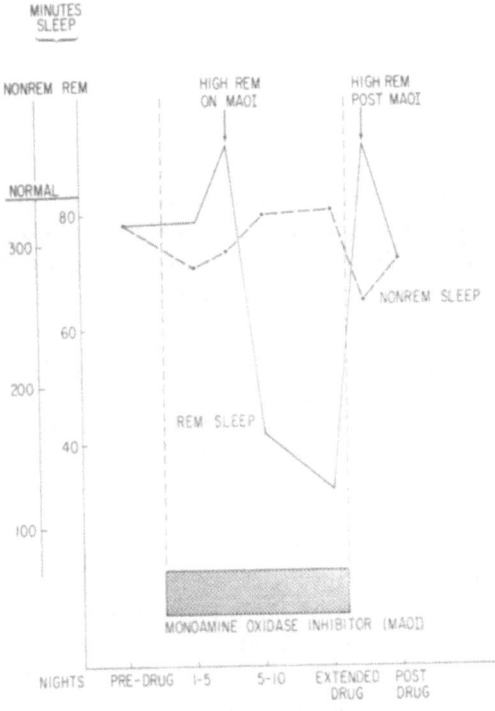

FIGURE 2-13. Composite of all subjects taking MAOI. High REM levels are significant (p < 0.001, two tailed t-test). (From Wyatt, 1972. Reprinted by permission.)

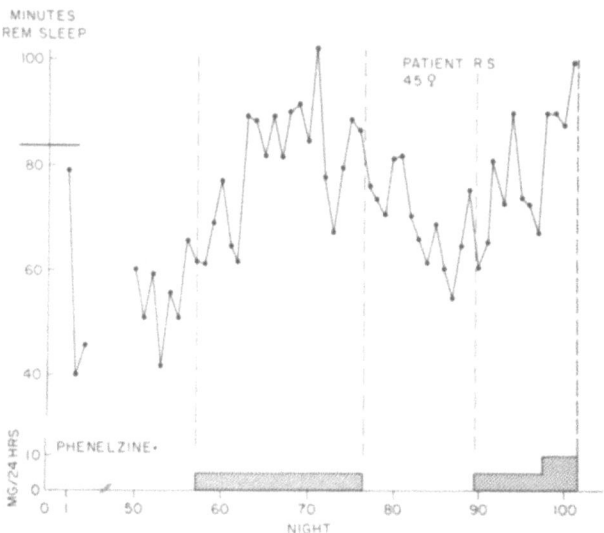

FIGURE 2-14.   REM sleep response in depressed patient given low dosage of the MAOI phenelzine. There was no therapeutic response at this dosage of the drug. (From Wyatt, 1972. Reprinted by permission.)

MAOIs that have been used in sleep studies shows that they are mostly of the "mixed" type, which inhibit both type A and B enzymes. The only exception is pargyline, which may preferentially inhibit the type B. Limited experience with pargyline, however, suggests that its effects on sleep are no different from those of the other MAOIs tested.

Tricyclic Antidepressants and Blockers of Amine Re-uptake

The tricyclic antidepressants and cocaine are thought to increase noradrenergic and serotonergic activity by blocking their re-uptake by the presynaptic neuron. In general, they have been found to suppress REM sleep. Post *et al.* (1972) described decreases in both total REM time and total sleep time when cocaine (65–200 mg/24 hr) was administered to depressed patients. The tricyclics have been studied by a number of investigators (Dunleavy *et al.*, 1972; Hartmann, 1969; Zung, 1969a; Ritvo *et al.*, 1967; Toyoda, 1964). Dunleavy *et al.* (1972) administered six tricyclics to normal volunteers over four weeks time. All of the drugs produced decreases in total REM sleep to varying degrees, with some increase in stage 2. With time, recovery toward normal occurred. Following discontinuation, a REM rebound occurred, which lasted up to a month. Slow-wave sleep was not systematically affected, although increases have been reported with desmethylimipramine (Zung, 1969a). Dunleavy et al. (1972) found that intrasleep restlessness (as determined by frequency of spontaneous shifts into stage 1 or wakefulness) was increased with imipramine, desipramine, and chlorimipramine, and did not go down during chronic administration. Some authors have suggested that the REM sleep inhibition of the tricyclics may be related to their antidepressant effect, a concept that is discussed in detail in chapter 7.

Of particular interest is chlorimipramine, a halogenated form of imipramine that is five times more potent than the parent compound in its ability to block serotonin re-uptake (Carlsson et al., 1969a). In comparison to other tricyclics such as protriptyline and desipramine, it is a relatively weak blocker of norepinephrine re-uptake (Carlsson et al., 1969b). It, too, is a powerful inhibitor of REM sleep, which, however, partially returns toward normal during chronic use (Dunleavy et al., 1972). Chlorimipramine has also been found useful in the treatment of cataplexy, sleep paralysis, and hypnogogic hallucinations in narcoleptic patients (Shapiro, 1975; Guilleminault et al., 1974) as discussed in chapter 4.

Reserpine

Reserpine administration results in decreased concentrations of norepinephrine and serotonin, and may also increase their rate of turnover (Brodie et al., 1966). In humans it is one of the few agents known to cause increases in REM sleep (Tissot, 1965; Hartmann, 1966; Hoffman and Domino, 1969; Coulter, Lester, and Williams, 1971). Reserpine administration has been associated with the development of depressive symptoms in some patients. In this regard it is interesting to note that reserpine administration results in decreased REM latency, an observation found in many depressed patients (see chapter 7).

Debrisoquine

The effects of debrisoquine on peripheral biogenic amines are dose related. At low concentrations it is an MAO inhibitor. At somewhat higher levels it is a noradrenergic blocker; and at even greater levels it causes depletion of norepinephrine (Medina, Grachetti, and Shore, 1969; Tomlinson and Mayor, 1973). Dunleavy, MacLean, and Oswald (1971) have reported that debrisoquine (20–80 mg/day) produced decreased REM sleep in three normal males. As this drug has been reported to be unable to cross the blood brain barrier (Medina, Grachetti, and Shore, 1969) and to have no influence on brain norepinephrine or serotonin levels (Karoum, Wyatt, and Costa, 1974), the mechanism of its possible action on sleep is unclear.

Amphetamines

Amphetamines are thought to enhance catecholaminergic activity. Administration of amphetamines has been reported to cause decreased percentage REM sleep (Gillin *et al.*, 1975b; Baekeland, 1967; Rechtschaffen and Maron, 1964). The d- and l-isomers may have somewhat different effects. Gillin *et al.* (1975b) gave single 30-mg doses of each isomer to seven depressed patients during the morning hours. Although both decreased percentage REM sleep, only the d-isomer delayed sleep onset, and reduced total sleep time and nonREM sleep.

Both Gillin *et al.* (1975b) and Feinberg *et al.* (1974a) found that d-amphetamine produced no change in REM density. The latter authors suggested that this quality may differentiate its effects from those of the sedative-hypnotics.

Withdrawal after chronic administration has been associated with large "rebound" increases in REM sleep that may last for some weeks (Watson, Hartmann, and Schildkraut, 1972; Oswald and Thacore, 1963). Feinberg *et al.* (1974a), studying the effects of chronic amphetamines on hyperactive children, suggested that the REM rebound is not necessarily a constant finding, and may be related (among other things) to changes in dosage before the drug is discontinued. Gillin *et al.* (1975b) noted no rebound during the first night following a single amphetamine night.

Amphetamine treatment is important in the management of narcolepsy, and will be discussed in chapter 4.

Chlorpromazine

Chlorpromazine, a phenothiazine used for the treatment of schizophrenia, has central dopaminergic-blocking activity as well as other actions including anticholinergic effects and changes in membrane permeability. Three studies describe the effects of single doses of chlorpromazine (100–150 mg orally and 0.4 mg/kg IM) on normal subjects (Lester and Guerrero-Figueroa, 1966; Lester *et al.*, 1971; Sagales, Erill, and Domino, 1969). There were no changes in total sleep time or amounts of REM sleep. Several studies report on multiple doses of chlorpromazine (25–100 mg) in normals (Okuma, Hata, and Fujii, 1975;

Hartmann and Cravens, 1973b; Naiman, Poitras, and Engelsmann, 1972; Lewis and Evans, 1969). They suggest an increase in total sleep time. Okuma et al. (1975) and Lewis and Evans (1969) reported some increase in REM sleep at 25 mg, whereas Hartmann and Cravens (1973b) reported no change at 50 mg. The study of Naiman et al. (1972) was oriented to the effects of chlorpromazine on REM rebound after REM deprivation. Predeprivation nights with no medication, however, were indistinguishable from predeprivation nights in which the subjects received 1 mg/kg of chlorpromazine. Thus, multiple low doses of chlorpromazine in normal subjects may have some effects on duration of sleep, but little effect on other parameters.

The results of these studies in normal subjects differ somewhat from reported effects in schizophrenics, which will be discussed in chapter 7. The changes in the latter studies may reflect higher dosages as well as the more disturbed sleep of the patients. The relative lack of actions of low doses of chlorpromazine on normal sleep is similar to observations with the more specific dopamine-blocker pimozide (Sagales and Erill, 1975). The lack of effect on total REM sleep with both of these agents is in contrast to the increased REM sleep seen after administration of AMPT, which may decrease catecholamine synthesis. It is possible that this difference, also, may be accounted for by the low doses of chlorpromazine used in these normal volunteer studies.

Hartmann and Cravens (1973b) have suggested that the increased sleep time with chlorpromazine is consistent with the view that a certain amount of dopaminergic activity is necessary for wakefulness (see Jones, 1969, and discussion in chapter 1).

Effect of Diets Deficient in Catecholamine Precursors

As part of a medical investigation, Lester, Chanes, and Condit (1969) placed three patients suffering from malignancies on a diet that was deficient in the catecholamine precursors tysosine and phenylalanine. REM sleep decreased in these patients, and returned to normal when these essential amino acids were once again added to the diet. Interpretation of this finding is difficult because the changes in REM sleep may also have been related to protein deficiency.

Metabolites of Norepinephrine and Dopamine in the CSF

Wyatt et al. (1976) examined metabolites in the CSF of patients who had ventriculo-atrial shunts, which are used for the treatment of normal-pressure hydrocephalus and presenile dementias. MHPG (3-meth-

oxy-4-hydroxyphenylglycol), a metabolite of norepinephrine, was measured during waking, nonREM, and REM sleep in five patients. It was
found that levels were highest in REM sleep, followed by waking and
nonREM sleep. HVA (homovanillic acid), a metabolite of dopamine
(Fig. 2-10), showed a similar pattern in six patients. In evaluating these
data, it should be recalled that these were patients with serious illnesses, in whom sleep patterns were disturbed. The increased levels of
MHPG during REM sleep may add further support to the view that
amounts of adrenergic activity are related to changes in the three states
of consciousness. These data are consistent with observations of Chu
and Bloom (1974) on unit cell firing in adrenergic neurons.

CHOLINERGIC SYSTEM

There is surprisingly little information available on the role of
acetylcholine in human sleep, although most over-the-counter sleeping
medications contain the anticholinergic agent, scopolamine. Scopolamine has been reported to decrease REM sleep in normal subjects,
although total sleep time remained unchanged (Sagales et al., 1969).
Methscopolamine, which is thought not to cross the blood brain barrier, has no effect on sleep (Sagales et al., 1969). Toyoda, Saraki, and
Kurihara (1966) observed that atropine administration resulted in
decreased REM sleep in the first two hours of sleep and increased REM
latency.

In contrast to the anticholinergic agents, anticholinesterases (which
increase acetylcholine) may cause increases in REM sleep. They have
been associated with nightmares and increased dreaming (Holmes and
Gaon, 1956; Grob and Harvey, 1958). Industrial workers exposed to
organophosphates, which have anticholinesterase properties, have
been reported to produce unusually long REM periods of particularly
rapid onset (Stoyva and Metcalf, 1968).

Recent work (Sitaram et al., 1976) suggests that the centrally acting
anticholinesterase agent physostigmine may influence the occurrence
of REM sleep. Seven normal volunteers were given physostigmine (0.5
mg) in nonREM sleep 35 minutes after sleep onset or during REM sleep.
Following nonREM infusions of physostigmine, REM sleep episodes
appeared within about 10 minutes, significantly more often than after
saline infusions (Fig. 2-15). The length and the number of eye movements during the induced REM period were not different from those of
the first REM period after saline infusions. When physostigmine was
infused during REM sleep, awakenings occurred more often than after

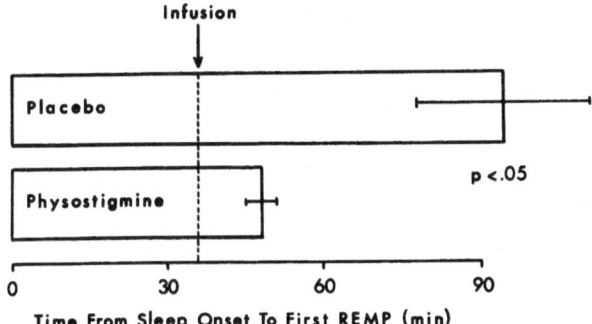

FIGURE 2-15. Effect of physostigmine infusion during nonREM sleep on REM latency. Physostigmine (0.5mg) or placebo was administered about 35 to 40 minutes after the onset of stage 2 sleep. (From Sitaram *et al.*, 1976. Copyright 1976 by the American Association for the Advancement of Science. Reprinted by permission.)

saline infusions. Total REM, nonREM, and delta sleep for the night were not altered. These data imply that cholinergic mechanisms may be related to the initiation of REM sleep episodes. They are consistent with the hypothesis that the nonREM, REM, and awake states form a continuum of progressively higher levels of arousal (Moruzzi, 1972) and that the shift between these levels may be mediated by cholinergic mechanisms.

HISTAMINERGIC SYSTEM

Administration of L-histadine, the precursor of histamine, seems to have little effect on human sleep. Gillin *et al.* (1975a) gave 20 gm/24 hr for three weeks to three narcoleptic patients and found no change in their clinical condition or the major sleep parameters. Similarly, 32.4 gm/24 hr had no effect on the sleep of four normal volunteers when given for five days.

DISCUSSION

The human studies described here are necessarily indirect, and open to varying interpretations. There are, however, some common themes that may be found throughout the data. We will now examine these, and suggest some hypotheses that may explain a number of the observations that have been described.

Serotonin

We have presented a variety of studies in which drugs that modify serotonergic activity were found to influence the amounts of the sleep stages. Questions that come to mind are:

1. Are these effects being exerted by serotonin or one of its metabolites?
2. What is the precise nature of the relation to the sleep stages?

Serotonin or a Metabolite?

Citing evidence that MAO inhibitors can completely suppress REM sleep, Jouvet (1972) has suggested that a serotonin metabolite is necessary for its occurrence. We have tried to test this hypothesis in two ways. In the first studies, low doses of phenelzine (5–15 mg) were found to *increase* REM sleep in depressed patients. Since it seems likely that phenelzine partially blocked monoamine oxidase, resulting in increased serotonin and decreases in its metabolites, it seems doubtful that the increase in REM was related to an oxidized-deaminated product. In a second study alpha-methyl-5-HTP (AM-5-HTP) was given to three patients with medical illnesses, and was found to increase REM sleep. It will be recalled that AM-5-HTP is converted in man to alpha-methyl serotonin, which cannot be metabolized by MAO. These studies would seem to suggest that it is serotonin, and not a metabolite, that produces the observed changes in REM sleep. Alternative considerations are that phenelzine may cause changes in other systems than that of serotonin, and that AM-5-HTP is also a tyrosine hydroxylase inhibitor, and thus may act similarly to AMPT.

It is not clear whether the effects of L-tryptophan on sleep are due to its conversion to serotonin, or are related to another metabolic route. Our studies in which L-tryptophan was administered to patients pretreated with PCPA suggest that an alternate metabolic route is related to its effects on nonREM and REM sleep. It seems likely, however, that PCPA only partially inhibits tryptophan hydroxylase, at least in certain areas of the brain (Aghajanian, Kuhar, and Roth, 1973; Deguchi, Sinha, and Barchas, 1973; Knapp and Mandell, 1972).

Relation to REM Sleep

PCPA, which decreases synthesis of serotonin, causes decreases in the amount of REM sleep, with little change in nonREM sleep. As this effect can be reversed by giving the serotonin precursor 5-HTP, it seems likely that decreases in serotonin were in fact related to the decrease in REM sleep. The effects of PCPA are all the more striking in that (1) REM sleep remains decreased as long as PCPA is given (in contrast to the experience with many REM-suppressing drugs such as the sedative-hypnotics); and (2) when PCPA is discontinued, REM sleep gradually returns to normal, with no evidence of a "rebound" increase. These findings seem to imply that PCPA interferes with the genesis of REM sleep in some very fundamental way. Conversely, raising serotonergic activity with low doses of 5-HTP or alpha-methyl-5-HTP (? or with high doses of L-tryptophan) results in increases in REM sleep. Within limits, then, there seems to be a linear correlation between serotonin concentrations and the total amount of REM sleep in humans.

Relation to NonREM Sleep

In contrast to the experience with humans, a variety of animal studies have suggested that the role of serotonin is more related to the triggering or maintenance of nonREM sleep. This hypothesis is based on studies of acute administration of PCPA and of short-term effects of lesions in the raphe nuclei. As can be seen in Table 2-4, most species

TABLE 2-4. Effects of Parachlorophenylalanine on Sleep

Study	Animal	NREM	REM	Dosage (mg/kg)
Delorme, 1966	Cat	↓	↓	100–300
Torda, 1967	Rat	↓	?	510
Crowley et al., 1969	Monkey	↓	?	1000
Florio et al., 1968	Cat, rat, rabbit	↓	↓	300
Koella et al., 1968; 1969	Cat	↓	↓	50–200
Mouret et al., 1968	Rat	↓	↓	500
Weitzman et al., 1968b	Monkey	↓	0	600–1000
Dement et al., 1969	Cat	↓	↓	75–300
Rechtschaffen et al., 1969	Rat	↓	↓ ∿	500
Wyatt et al., 1969	Man	0	↓	50
Pujol et al., 1971	Cat	↓	↓	500
Bert, 1972	Baboon	↓	↓	150–300
Ursin, 1972	Cat	↓	0 ↓	200
Chernik et al., 1973	Man	0	0*	30
Cohen et al., 1973	Cat	↓	↓	150

* Patient on methadone as well as PCPA; while REM sleep did not change, other measures of REM diminished.

(except man and possibly the rat) show large decreases in nonREM sleep and less striking decreases in REM sleep after acute administration of PCPA. In the cat, for instance, insomnia develops within 24–48 hours of receiving a large acute dose of PCPA, and persists for about a week. Lesions of the midbrain raphe nuclei, which result in decreases of cerebral serotonin concentrations, produce insomnia. On the other hand, several lines of evidence militate against the concept that serotonin is important in the maintenance of nonREM sleep. Chronic administration of PCPA suggests that sleep returns to normal after about a week, although serotonin levels remain suppressed (Dement *et al.*, 1969). Similarly, the insomnia produced by lesions of the dorsal raphe nucleus in cats is only temporary, later returning to normal (Morgane and Stern, 1972). Studies of children with phenylketonuria, in whom blood and CNS serotonin is low, show that their sleep is similar to that of controls (Schulte *et al.*, 1973). Thus, several lines of evidence suggest that normal concentrations of serotonin are not necessary for sleep. What mechanisms, then, might explain the insomnia produced by acute doses of PCPA in animals? Among many possible answers, two seem particularly likely: (1) that sudden *changes* in serotonin levels (rather than absolute amounts) are related to insomnia; or (2) that when serotonin levels are low, there is a disregulation of sleep, in which certain phasic events of REM sleep begin to occur in nonREM sleep and result in awakenings.

Rate of Change of Serotonin. In recent studies from this laboratory, 5-HTP and a decarboxylase inhibitor were given to 18 chronic schizophrenics (Wyatt and Gillin, 1975; Wyatt, Kaplan, and Vaughan, 1973; Wyatt, Gillin, and Vaughan, 1972a). Although two-thirds of the patients improved compared to placebo treatment, a number of side effects were noted, including automatic, gastrointestinal, psychic, and hypermotoric symptoms. It was found that these could be avoided by starting with very low doses, and increasing slowly as tolerance developed. When 5-HTP was discontinued, a withdrawal syndrome appeared, which included insomnia, tremulousness, delusions, hallucinations, and seizures in two cases. In our studies with phenelzine, which (like 5-HTP) raises serotonin concentrations, we also noted a withdrawal syndrome that included insomnia.

It can be seen, then, that in patients who are being withdrawn from 5-HTP or phenelzine, and cats who are treated with PCPA, there is a sudden decrease in brain serotonin concentration, accompanied by a syndrome of insomnia and hyperactivity. One implication might be that the rate of fall of serotonin, rather than absolute level, is related to insomnia. This approach may be relevant to the understanding of insomnia during withdrawal from alcohol and other addicting drugs (see chapter 6).

The Phasic Event Suppression Hypothesis. Dement *et al.* (1969) noted that PGO spikes, which are normally confined to REM sleep, occurred in nonREM sleep and waking in cats treated with PCPA. Based on this observation, they suggested that the function of serotonergic neurons is to confine phasic events such as PGO spikes to REM sleep. A corollary of this hypothesis is that when serotonin levels are decreased, PGO spikes enter nonREM sleep, where they serve as a disruptive influence resulting in decreased nonREM sleep.

As we discussed earlier, studies with PCPA seem to suggest a phenomenon similar to that described by Dement *et al.* (1969). These involve observations of phasic integrated potentials (PIPs) of extraocular muscle activity, which are thought to be a measure of phasic events analogous to PGO spikes in the cat. Wyatt (1972) observed that in two patients taking 2 gm of PCPA/24 hr, the amount of PIPs increased during nonREM sleep.

McGinty, Harper, and Fairbanks (1973) provided a test of the phasic event suppression hypothesis. They observed that the serotonergic neurons in the dorsal raphe nucleus in unanaesthetized cats ceased to fire when PGO spikes appeared. These neurons were found to have the highest firing rate during waking, an intermediate rate during nonREM sleep, and the lowest rate during REM sleep. This would seem to provide further support for the phasic event suppression hypothesis. (It should be noted that Bloom *et al.* (1973), examining other parts of the raphe system, the raphe magnus and median nuclei, have reported units firing at most rapid rates during REM sleep.)

If the insomnia seen in cats following PCPA treatment is in fact due to the release of PGO spikes into nonREM sleep and waking, then the lower dose of PCPA given to humans may permit a slower release of such phasic events into these stages. This may in turn allow for habituation to the apparently disturbing effects of the phasic events. Consistent with this notion is the slow rate of decline of REM sleep seen in the human studies. A test of this principle would be to study sleep of cats who have been given low, chronic doses of PCPA. Such studies are not available at this time.

As in the case of the PCPA data, the phasic event suppression hypothesis may also provide an explanation for several differences between animal and human data. In humans, low (600 mg) doses of 5-HTP (like low doses of phenelzine and alpha-methyl-5-HTP) increase percentage REM sleep and the amount of eye movement activity during REM (Wyatt *et al.*, 1971d). High doses of 5-HTP (3600–6000 mg) may decrease REM sleep, at least in neurologic patients and schizophrenics (Dawson *et al.*, 1974). One way to view these data is that increased serotonin, resulting from 5-HTP administration, prevents the occurrence of phasic events in nonREM sleep, forcing them to occur in REM sleep. As the amount of phasic events in a 24-hour period may be constant (Dusan-Peyrethon and Jouvet, 1967; Dement *et al.*, 1970), there is a limit to how many phasic events can be forced into REM sleep and potentially cause further increases in it.

Animal studies, which generally use high doses, suggest that 5-HTP suppresses REM sleep. This seems comparable to the REM sleep suppression seen with high doses in man. Animal studies employing low doses comparable to most human studies have not been performed.

Difficulties with the Phasic Event Suppression Hypothesis. Although the approach we have outlined does explain a variety of studies, there are also several observations that appear inconsistent with it. Weitzman *et al.* (1968b) and Crowley, Pegram, and Smith (1969) have reported that PCPA administration to rhesus monkeys causes decreases in nonREM sleep, but no change in REM sleep. Aside from the species difference, no obvious explanation can be made in terms of the phasic event suppression hypothesis.

It has been reported that serotonin applied to the area postrema produces slow waves (Koella, 1969). These studies are difficult to evaluate, as the cats that were studied had previously been chemically or surgically immobilized. As sleep is defined in behavioral as well as physiological terms, the interpretation of these studies must await more careful analysis of the behavioral aspects of "sleep" in these cats. Certainly, many agents such as some anticholinergic drugs may produce slow waves that do not seem to correspond to behavioral sleep.

Noradrenergic System

Norepinephrine or a Precursor?

The most striking feature of studies with pimozide and chlorpromazine in normal subjects is the lack of effects on sleep. This seems to imply that changes in sleep induced by drugs influencing the catecholaminergic system are not being caused by changes in dopaminergic activity. It seems more likely that they are related to changes in norepinephrine, or result from secondary changes in other neurotransmitters. L-DOPA, for instance, may cause reduction of brain serotonin concentration in rats (Everett and Borcherding, 1970).

Effects on REM Sleep

In general, changes in catecholaminergic activity seem to affect REM sleep in the opposite direction compared to changes in serotonergic activity. Inhibition of tyrosine hydroxylase with AMPT, which may decrease functional levels of norepinephrine, usually has led to increases in REM sleep (Table 2-5). Interpretation of conflicting studies suggests route of administration may be an important factor. Hartmann and Bridwell (1970), for instance, found that AMPT increased REM sleep in rats when given orally, but decreased REM sleep when administered intraperitoneally.

Human studies of AMPT suggest that tolerance develops to the initial effect of increasing REM sleep, as well as to the initial daytime sedation. Studies to determine if there is tolerance to the effects on REM sleep in animals are not available. Upon discontinuation of AMPT in humans, sleep is disrupted for several nights. As in the case of the serotonergic system, the body seems able to adjust to modified levels of catecholamines, and to undergo a period of readjustment when modifying drugs are discontinued.

Data with L-DOPA has given mixed results; when administered intravenously, REM sleep is suppressed. This seems compatible with the increases in REM sleep observed with AMPT. Use of oral L-DOPA in normal subjects has resulted in no change, decreased and even increased REM sleep. Variables that might influence these results include dose, time of administration, duration of administration, and

TABLE 2-5. Effects of Alpha-Methyl-Paratyrosine on Sleep

Study	Animal	NREM	REM	Dosage (mg/kg)
Marantz and Rechtschaffen, 1967	Rat	0	0	150 (1)
Marantz et al., 1968	Rat	0	0	75 (1)
Torda, 1968	Rat	↑	↓	240
Weitzman et al., 1969	Monkey	↑	↓	110–260 (1)
Branchey and Kissin, 1970	Rat	↓	0	200
Hartmann and Bridwell, 1970	Rat	0	↑	50–75 (oral)
		0	↓	75 (intrapertioneal)
Iskander and Kaebling, 1970	Cat	↑	↓	320 (1)
King and Jewett, 1971	Cat	trend ↑	↓	3.125–400
Wyatt et al., 1971a	Man	0	↑	29–43
Hendricksen et al., 1972	Cat	↑	↑	150 (I.V. over 24 hr)
Stern and Morgane, 1972	Cat	0	↑	75
Vaughan et al., 1972	Man	trend ↓	trend ↑	43

use of peripheral decarboxylase inhibitors. Another problem is that the mechanism by which L-DOPA has its effects is unclear. It is known that administration of L-DOPA increases brain dopamine levels (Everett and Borcherding, 1970) and turnover of norepinephrine (Wurtman and Romero, 1972). It may, however, also reduce brain serotonin concentrations in the rat (Everett and Borcherding, 1970) and turnover of brain serotonin in humans (Goodwin, Dunner, and Gershon, 1971).

Cholinergic System

Less information is available about the role of the cholinergic system on human sleep. Available data suggests that it is facilitative to REM sleep. Atropine and scopolamine suppress REM sleep; it is increased by anticholinesterases. These findings seem consistent with results of animal studies, in which systemic administration of atropine (Jouvet, 1969) and intraventricular administration of hemicholinium-3 (Hazra, 1970) reduce REM sleep. Acetylcholine is known to be released from the cerebral cortex of cats at a higher rate during REM as compared with slow-wave sleep (Jasper and Tessier, 1971). Physostigmine induces REM sleep in the pontine cat (Jouvet, 1969). Similarly, Sitaram et al. (1976) have found that intravenous physostigmine can induce episodes of REM sleep in humans without influencing total REM sleep for the night or length of the first REM period. This seems to suggest that cholinergic systems are related to initiation, rather than duration, of REM sleep episodes.

Histaminergic System

Little is known about the role of the histaminergic system in sleep. It has been reported that histamine is found in the venous blood of waking animals, and produces waking when transferred to other animals. Peripheral histamine receptor blockers produce sleep; as these drugs have multiple actions, the mechanism of their sedative effect is not clear. Our studies with the histamine precursor, L-histidine, showed no alterations in sleep.

Interaction between Transmitters

A variety of inconsistencies and unpredicted responses to drugs have been presented here. We have attempted to reconcile differences and find common trends, by noting that responses to drugs may be dependent on dose, duration, and route of administration. Another factor that may aid in the understanding of the effects of drugs on sleep is consideration of interaction between neurotransmitters. It has been observed, for instance, that in some cases cholinesterase inhibiters may not only raise levels of acetylcholine, but also lead to increases in serotonin and decreases in norepinephrine (Karczmar, 1975). Similarly, anatomic or chemical destruction of serotonergic terminals in the raphe nuclei may lead to increased activity of tyrosine hydroxylase, necessary for the synthesis of norepinephrine (Renaud et al., 1975). Thus, it is clear that neurotransmitters cannot be studied in isolation; an understanding of their effects must include recognition of their actions on other transmitters. Finally, it should be remembered that, for all their complexity, the serotonergic, adrenergic, and cholinergic systems make up less than 1% of the synaptic connections in the brain. It seems likely that a more complete understanding of the regulation of sleep will await knowledge of other neurotransmitter systems.

SUMMARY

Human studies involving serotinin precursors and synthesis inhibitors suggest that, within limits, serotonin concentrations are directly correlated with amounts of REM sleep. Rapid decreases in serotonin, induced by high doses of PCPA in animals or discontinuation of 5-HTP or phenelzine in man, may result in a syndrome of insomnia and hyperactivity. One hypothesis that seems to account for a great deal of data is that serotonergic systems are involved in confining phasic events to REM sleep.

In contrast to serotonin, it appears likely that levels of norepinephrine are inversely related to amounts of REM sleep. Drugs blocking dopaminergic receptors appear to have relatively little effect on sleep of normal humans. The body seems able to adapt to pharmacologic manipulation of serotonin and norepinephrine, and to go through a withdrawal period of readjustment when modifying drugs are discontinued.

A cholinesterase inhibitor, which increases cholinergic activity, can induce periods of REM sleep. It seems likely that cholinergic mechanisms are involved in the initiation of REM sleep and waking episodes. A precursor of histamine seems to have little effect on the sleep of normal or narcoleptic humans.

Our understanding of the control mechanisms of sleep is at best very limited. Several areas of research may be of some help. Apparent differences between human and animal studies might be further explored by performing animal studies with the low, chronic doses that have often been employed with humans. A further understanding of the interaction between neurotransmitters may well be of importance. Finally, it seems likely that other neurotransmitters besides serotonin, norepinephrine, and acetylcholine may play a role in the regulation of sleep.

Neuroendocrinology and Sleep

It has become clear that the anterior pituitary hormones are secreted in a pulsatile manner, and that their rhythms bear some relationship to sleep. The nature of this relationship varies with the hormone. Some appear to be associated with a specific electroencephalographic stage of sleep, others to the REM-nonREM cycle or the sleep–waking cycle. In some cases, the nature of the relationship varies with age. The association of secretion to sleep may be statistically significant yet account for only a portion of the variance of plasma levels of the hormone. Other influences that may act simultaneously on secretion include an ill-defined "biological clock," the light–dark cycle, and the effect of pulsatile secretion of other hormones.

Several types of studies need to be done in order to characterize the relation of a hormone—or any physiological event—to sleep. These include:

1. Twenty-four hour studies with repeated blood sampling in order to determine if a circadian and/or ultradian rhythm occurs. It seems clear that the frequency of sampling must not be substantially longer than the biological half-life of the hormone in question. Experience with the gonadotropins emphasizes the need to do such studies in subjects of all ages.

2. Studies of delayed sleep onset and reversed sleep–waking cycle. The function of these is to determine if the secretion is related specifically to sleep or to the time of day (circadian secretion), or to both.

3. Studies of secretion under conditions of constant lighting and of

secretion in blind subjects, to determine if secretion is related to the light–dark cycle.

4. Studies of sleep deprivation and modified sleep–wake cycles (e.g., 3 hours, 33 hours). These have the benefit of determining if secretion is related to the sleep–waking cycle. A disadvantage is that drastic changes in sleep cycle length may distort percentages of various sleep stages.

5. Analyses relating hormone levels to specific sleep stages. A basic characterization may be made by determining what percentage of the variance in hormone levels is accounted for by the presence of a particular sleep stage.

6. Determination of whether sleep-related secretion of a hormone may be regulated by a second sleep-related system. There is, for example, some preliminary evidence that sleep-related secretion of testosterone may be influenced by sleep-related secretion of prolactin (PRL).

7. Pharmacologic manipulation of sleep-related secretion. This provides indirect data on the types of neural pathways that may regulate sleep-related secretion. The actions of a drug must be assessed in terms of the effects on sleep-related secretion as well as secretion during pharmacologic provocative stimulation tests. As will be seen later in the discussion of growth hormone, the same drug may have differing effects on these two types of secretion.

8. Studies to determine what effects administration of the hormone has on the occurrence of the sleep stages. A similar approach is to study sleep in animals in whom the endocrine gland has been removed, and in patients with diseases of over- and undersecretion. The drawback of the latter type of study is that there is always some question as to whether any abnormalities in sleep are due to the modified levels of hormone, or to any lesions of the CNS that may have also produced the endocrine disease.

Data from these types of studies are necessary for the most basic characterization of the relation of a hormone's secretion to sleep. Before the results of these investigations are described, a brief review of the major endocrinologic systems is in order.

BASIC CONCEPTS IN NEUROENDOCRINOLOGY

This discussion will center on the pituitary and pineal glands, which are anatomically contiguous with, and physiologically intimately involved with, the central nervous system. The pituitary gland is a small structure that rests in the *sella turcica*, a cavity in the sphenoid bone of the skull. It is attached by the pituitary stalk to the ventral surface of the diencephalon, just posterior to the optic chiasm. It is divided into the adenohypophysis (or anterior pituitary) and neurohypophysis (or posterior pituitary). The anterior pituitary is known to release the following protein hormones: growth hormone (GH), adrenocorticotropic hormone (ACTH), prolactin (PRL), thyroid-stimulating hormone (TSH), luteinizing hormone (LH), follicle-stimulating hormone (FSH), and melanocyte-stimulating hormone (MSH). These hormones may have direct effects on nonendocrine tissues, as in the case of GH and PRL, or may stimulate the release of hormones from endocrine glands elsewhere in the body, as in the case of ACTH, TSH, LH, and FSH (Fig. 3-1). The posterior pituitary secretes two hormones, vasopressin (or antidiuretic hormone) and oxytocin.

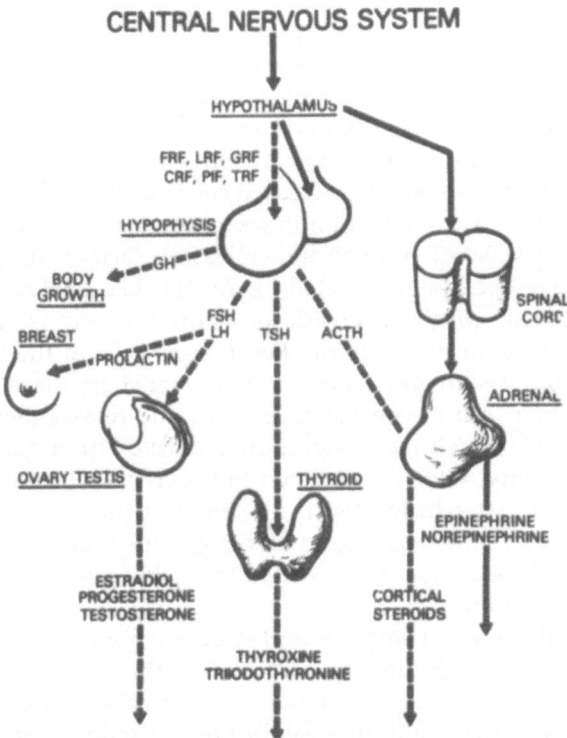

FIGURE 3-1. Schematic representation of pituitary function. (Adapted from Morgan, 1973. Reprinted by permission.)

Anterior pituitary secretion is thought to be regulated by two types of mechanisms. The first of these is *open loop* control, which refers to regulation of the anterior pituitary by stimulation from the central nervous system. This is mediated by releasing or inhibiting factors that are carried from the hypothalamus to the pituitary by portal blood vessels. Seven such substances have been identified: somatotropin-releasing factor, somatotropin-inhibiting factor (somatostatin), cortico-tropin-releasing factor, prolactin-releasing factor, prolactin-inhibiting factor, thyrotropin-releasing hormone, and luteinizing hormone-releasing hormone. Neural pathways in the hypothalamus are thought to be mediated by the biogenic amines, particularly serotonin, norepi-nephrine, and dopamine. These substances are also thought to be involved in the pathways that regulate the sleep stages (see chap. 2). As this chapter progresses, it will be seen that many of the drugs that influence secretion of anterior pituitary hormones (as well as the sleep stages) are thought to do so by stimulating or inhibiting these path-ways. Other mechanisms of drug action might include direct effects on the pituitary.

The second type of control of anterior pituitary secretion is the *closed loop* mechanism, regulation by a negative feedback system sensi-tive to the levels of a circulating hormone. When ACTH is released, for instance, there is a resultant rise in cortisol, which has been secreted in turn by the adrenal cortex. The increased cortisol affects the pituitary in such a way as to cause a reduction in secretion of ACTH, and may also influence the release of corticotropin-releasing factor. Negative feed-back loops have been demonstrated for ACTH, LH, FSH, and TSH.

The posterior pituitary gland, or neurohypophysis, is derived embryologically from nerve tissue. Peptidergic cells in the hypothala-mus synthesize vasopressin and oxytocin, transport these hormones down their fibers into the neurohypophysis, and release them into the blood. The signal to release vasopressin is derived from cells sensitive to blood osmolality, which are located in the hypothalamus, and from cells sensitive to stretch, located in the right atrium of the heart and elsewhere. These latter cells send fibers to the brain via the vagal nerves. Oxytocin secretion is stimulated by suckling and stimulation of the cervix and vagina.

The pineal gland is a small conical structure lying on the dorsum of the diencephalon, projecting backward over the tectum of the mid-brain. In lower vertebrates it contains cells that are directly sensitive to light. In humans this is not the case, but the secretion of its hormone, melatonin, is influenced by the amount of lighting via neural pathways from the retina. The pineal gland is bathed in CSF, and it is not clear whether melatonin is released into the blood, the CSF, or both. As will be discussed later, melatonin is of particular interest because of hypotheses that it may be released by the pineal gland to influence directly other parts of the CNS, possibly by an effect on amounts of serotonin.

The structure and actions of each hormone are summarized at the beginning of the sections on the relationship of each hormone to sleep phenomena. Detailed discussions of these endocrine systems are provided by Daughaday (1974) and Wurtman and Cardinali (1974).

GROWTH HORMONE

We are entering the second decade since the pattern of growth hormone (GH) secretion was first associated with sleep. This relationship has now been described in more detail than is available for any other anterior pituitary hormone. The nature of the hypothalamic control mechanisms of secretion and the relation of this phenomenon to psychiatric illness are less well understood.

GH has a variety of known functions. It stimulates growth of long bones whose epiphyses have not closed, as well as endochondral bone and cartilage. It influences growth of nearly all soft tissues and organs, although various tissues differ greatly in their sensitivity to its effects. Many of these actions may be mediated by release from the liver and possibly the kidney of a second group of substances, the somatomedins (Daughaday, 1975).

GH has been reported to modify glucose, protein, and lipid metabolism; its secretion in turn is altered by changes in blood levels of these three major metabolic groups (Brown and Reichlin, 1972). Decreases in plasma-free fatty acids, induced by nicotinic acid, for instance, result in increased blood GH (Irie et al., 1967), and the infusion of several amino acids is followed by increased GH secretion (Knopf et al., 1965). Of particular interest is the relation of GH to blood levels of glucose. It has been reported that hypoglycemia induced by insulin injection results in increased secretion of GH (Roth et al., 1963; Brown and Reichlin, 1972). This action seems to be specifically related to hypoglycemia, rather than other actions of insulin, as GH secretion is increased by other causes of low blood glucose; e.g., hypoglycemia associated with certain mesenchymal tumors with low levels of endogenous insulin present (Roth et al., 1963). Oral glucose ingestion results in decreased GH, whereas fasting results in increased secretion (Glick et al., 1965).

Among the earliest observations on GH secretion at night is a report by Hunter, Friend, and Strong (1966). They took hourly measurements of GH by day, and up to three measurements at night in nine humans. There was an elevation of GH at night, but it was thought to be a response to not having eaten for some hours. Quabbe, Schilling, and Helge (1966), studying fasting human subjects, noted peaks of GH occurring several times throughout the night that were not associated with blood glucose levels. Although they did not have the benefit of EEG monitoring, they suggested that the peaks of GH were related to the "deeper" periods of sleep. The relation of a GH peak to sleep onset was carefully demonstrated by Takahashi, Kipnis, and Daughaday (1968). In seven out of eight human subjects a plasma GH peak (13–72 ng/ml occurred during the first 90 minutes of sleep and lasted 1.5–3.5 hours (Fig. 3-2). If sleep onset was delayed, the GH peak was also delayed. If the subjects were awakened for two to three hours and then slept, another GH peak occurred. Smaller peaks occurred throughout the night, and seemed to be related to stages 3 and 4; 43% of the peaks were during these stages, even though they comprised only 15% of total sleep time in this study. The GH secretion was not related to plasma levels of glucose, insulin, or cortisol.

The pattern of GH secretion over the 24-hour period varies greatly with age. In the first few weeks of life, plasma GH levels show no difference between sleep or waking, and no difference between "quiet" and "active" sleep (Shaywitz et al., 1971). After the third month of life, waking values drop considerably and are significantly less than levels during sleep (Vigneri and D'Agata, 1971). It is at about this same time that "quiet" sleep, which is thought to be analogous to the adult slow-wave sleep, comes to dominate the infant's sleep cycle (Stern et al., 1969). Prepubertal children secrete GH during sleep but little during the waking state (Finkelstein et al., 1972; Illig et al., 1971). During adolescence, sleep-related secretion increases greatly as does daytime secretion. Young adults have sleep-related secretion somewhat less than

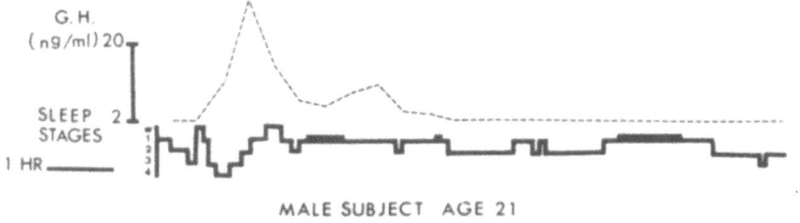

FIGURE 3-2.   Sleep-related growth hormone secretion in a normal young adult.

adolescents, and in the elderly sleep-related secretion is greatly decreased (Finkelstein et al., 1972; Carlson et al., 1972). It has been speculated that this decreased secretion in the elderly is related to their decreased amounts of slow-wave sleep (Rubin et al., 1974).

It seems clear that secretion of GH is closely related to sleep and does not have an independent circadian rhythm. One of the best demonstrations of this was performed by Sassin et al. (1969). They found that a 12-hour reversal of the sleep–waking cycle was followed immediately by reversal of the pattern of GH secretion, which remained related to slow-wave sleep. The exact nature of this relationship has yet to be precisely defined, however. As mentioned above, Takahashi et al. (1968) originally noted that a disproportionate amount of secretion occurred during slow-wave sleep. The problem, of course, is that there is normally a high percentage of slow-wave sleep in the first two hours of sleep, so that it seemed possible that the GH peak was related to sleep onset or to early sleep, and not to slow-wave sleep *per se*. There are several ways to help resolve this problem. One approach is to examine GH peaks that occur late in sleep, when slow-wave sleep is relatively uncommon. Sassin et al. (1969) divided sleep late at night into slow-wave and nonslow-wave cycles. The found that slow-wave cycles contained the majority of peaks, and that those occurring during slow-wave cycles were higher than those that did not. Using a somewhat similar principle, Karacan et al. (1975) examined 29 normal young men who slept for two hours in either the morning or the late afternoon. The morning naps contained relatively more REM sleep and less slow-wave sleep than the afternoon naps. It was found that GH secretion was greater during the sleep in the afternoon. Thus, it seems likely that GH secretion is not associated with sleep onset *per se*, but rather is in some sense related to slow-wave sleep.

The association of GH secretion with slow-wave sleep has been further defined by a variety of studies. Pawel, Sassin, and Weitzman (1972) took plasma samples every four minutes during the first 90 minutes of sleep, and found that delta activity (although not necessarily stage-3 sleep using 30-second epochs) always preceded GH release. Karacan et al. (1971) found that partial slow-wave sleep deprivation resulted in decreased GH secretion shortly after sleep onset. Generally slow-wave sleep preceded GH secretion, but in some cases peaks occurred that had not been preceded by slow-wave sleep. Conversely, episodes of slow-wave sleep frequently occur unaccompanied by peaks of GH secretion (Takahashi et al., 1968). Flurazepam, which decreases slow-wave sleep, has been reported to have no effect on GH secretion (Rubin et al., 1973b). Medroxyprogesterone acetate and free fatty acid infusions can decrease GH secretion without influencing slow-wave sleep (Lucke and Glick, 1971b; Lipman et al., 1972). Weitzman et al. (1974) approached the problem by manipulation of the sleep–waking cycle. They allowed normal subjects to sleep for eight one-hour periods over each 24-hour period. It was found that GH secretion was related to those episodes in which there was more than 36 minutes of sleep. There was no relation between GH secretion and duration of slow-wave sleep during these episodes. The authors suggested that GH secretion is related, not to duration, but to onset of slow-wave sleep. Such a premise might explain why Othmer et al. (1974a) found no relationship between total amounts of slow-wave sleep in the first four hours of sleep and amount of GH secretion, or why GH secretion remains normal even though total slow-wave sleep was reduced following administration of flurazepam (Rubin et al., 1973b).

It is also possible that GH secretion may be influenced by amounts of slow-wave sleep during periods of sleep prior to the one being studied. Othmer et al. (1974b) studied GH secretion during morning naps. GH secretion was not related to amount of slow-wave sleep during the nap or to amounts of GH secretion the previous night. It was found, however, that the subjects with the most secretion during the morning nap were those who had had the least stage 3 sleep the previous night. It would perhaps be worthwhile to pursue the hypothesis that GH secretion is determined not only by the sleep stage present at the time of secretion, but also by the pattern of sleep stages over the previous 24-hour period.

The relationship, if any, between GH secretion and REM sleep is not clear. Studies of GH secretion during REM sleep deprivation have found either no change (Honda et al., 1969) or increased (Daughaday, Othmer, and Kipnis, 1969) GH secretion. One tentative implication worthy of further study might be that REM sleep prevents secretion of GH-releasing factor (see Takahashi, 1974).

Although sleep stages may be related to onset of specific peaks of GH secretion, there is some evidence that the total amount of GH secretion may be relatively constant. In the Weitzman et al. (1974) study, total 24-hour secretion remained the same although the pattern and times of sleep were drastically changed. In an Arctic environment with extremes of daylight and darkness, sleep-related GH secretion was found to be the same during all four seasons (Weitzman et al., 1975). There is some evidence that patterns of secretion differ greatly between individuals but that the pattern of a given individual is relatively constant (Takahashi, 1974; Takahashi et al., 1968). It has been suggested that traits with this combination of qualities are most suited for genetic studies, and the opportunity clearly seems to be here for such work.

The control of GH secretion may be studied by determining the effects of drugs on GH response to various standard stimuli or on GH secretion during sleep. Perhaps the most common provocative agents are insulin, arginine, and L-DOPA. Data comparing GH responses to these provocative agents have been provided in several studies (Lin and Tucci, 1974; Lucke, Hoeffken, and Morgner, 1974; Weldon et al., 1973). In terms of consistency of response, sleep-related secretion would seem to be the same or slightly better than pharmacologic stimulation tests. Of the five subjects examined by Lucke et al. (1974), three had comparable values with all tests; one had a low response to arginine and L-DOPA but a normal response to sleep and insulin. Another subject had low values with sleep, but also had subnormal responses to arginine and L-DOPA. Among the pharmacologic stimuli, L-DOPA seemed to have the highest incidence of "false negatives." Analysis of the data of Underwood et al. (1971) shows that of 13 normal children who slept well, nine had good responses to both insulin and sleep. Three had peak responses of <5 ng/ml to insulin but >5 ng/ml during sleep. Only one subject had <5 ng/ml during sleep but >5 ng/ml with insulin testing. Mace, Gotlin, and Beck (1972), drawing a single sample of blood 90 minutes after sleep onset, found that all of 46 normal children tested had levels >7 ng/ml; they compared this response with studies that report comparable levels of GH in only 70–90% of subjects receiving insulin or arginine provocative tests. A study by Lin and Tucci (1974), in which a sample was taken "1 to 2 hours after the apparent onset of nocturnal sleep" showed a relatively low percentage of GH peaks; such data points to the importance of serial blood sampling while monitoring with a sleep EEG.

An adrenergic system has been thought to be related to the control of GH secretion in response to pharmacologic provocative tests. Evidence for this position has been derived from human studies showing decreased GH response to insulin after administration of the alpha adrenergic blocker phentolamine (Blackard and Heidingsfelder, 1968) and increased response after the beta adrenergic blocker propanolol (Abramson et al., 1966). Although serotonin was found to have no effect on GH release after intraventricular injection in rats (Mueller et al., 1970), two human studies have reported that serotonin receptor blockers inhibit the GH response to insulin (Bivens, Lebovitz, and Feldman, 1973; Mendelson et al., 1975a).

Growth hormone secretion during sleep may not be influenced by agents that modify the response to daytime provocative tests (Table 3-1). Thus, phentolamine and propanolol, discussed above, have been reported to have no effect on nocturnal secretion (Lucke and Glick, 1971a). Other agents such as medroxyprogesterone (Lucke and Glick, 1971b) and free fatty acids (Lipman et al., 1972), which suppress GH response to insulin have the same effect during sleep. Alternatively, the serotonin receptor blocker methysergide has been reported to decrease GH response to insulin, but increase sleep-related secretion (Mendelson et al., 1975b). Thus, effects of drugs on GH secretion during insulin provocative tests do not seem to be predictive of effects on sleep-related secretion. It seems possible, then, that inferences drawn from pharmacologic stimulation tests may lead to erroneous conclusions regarding physiologic control of GH secretion. This problem will become more clear in the following discussion of GH secretion in patients with short stature.

TABLE 3-1. Effects of Substances on Sleep-Related GH Secretion in Humans

Drug	Authors	Effect on sleep-related secretion	Effect on insulin-stimulated secretion
Amylobarbital	Ogunremi et al., 1973	→ [c]	—
Chlordrazepoxide	Takahashi et al., 1968	→	—
Chlorpromazine	Takahashi et al., 1968	→ [a]	↓
Clomiphene	Perlow et al., 1972	↓	↓
Diphenylhydantoin	Takahashi et al., 1968	→	—
Free fatty acids	Lipman et al., 1972	↓	↓
Glucose	Lucke and Glick, 1971a	↓(>350 mg%)	↓
Hydrocortisone	Krieger et al., 1972	→	↓
Imipramine	Takahashi et al., 1968	↓	—
Isocarbozazid	Takahashi et al., 1968	→	—
Medroxyprogesterone	Lucke and Glick, 1971b	↓	↓
Methscopolamine	Mendelson et al., 1976	↓	—
Methysergide	Mendelson et al., 1975b	↑	↓
Phenobarbital	Takahashi et al., 1968	→	—
Phentolamine	Lucke and Glick, 1971a	→	↓
Prednisolone	Illig et al., 1971	↓	—
Propanolol	Lucke and Glick, 1971a	→	↑
Tryptophan	Murri et al., 1973	[b] →	—

[a] Dosage was 30 mg, substantially less than amounts used in conjunction with ITT by Sherman et al., 1971.
[b] Schizophrenic patients.
[c] Increase reported during withdrawal.

Sleep-Related GH Secretion in Disease States

There are several studies available that compare sleep-related secretion and pharmacologic provocative tests in children with short stature (Eastman and Lazarus, 1973; Mace et al., 1972; Underwood et al., 1971; Ilig et al., 1971). Generally, children with constitutional short stature or histories of prolonged corticosteroid treatment for asthma, who have good GH responses to insulin tests, also have comparable sleep-related GH peaks. Patients with short stature related to hypopituitarism that is idiopathic or due to space-occupying lesions usually have decreased secretion during both tests. On the other hand, there are cases where insulin provocative tests give ambiguous results (Underwood et al., 1971). Tanner et al. (1971), for instance, describe a patient whose growth rate following treatment with GH clearly indicated a GH deficiency, but had normal secretion during an insulin tolerance test. One might speculate that the sleep-related secretion in such a patient would be decreased. There are in fact some documented cases of this phenomenon. Eastman and Lazarus (1973) describe an abnormally short patient with a history of surgery for a craniopharyngioma who had a normal response to arginine (20.4 mg/ml), a significant but blunted response to insulin (7.4 mg/ml) and poor response to sleep (4.0 mg/ml). Similarly, Howse et al. (1974) describe two children with clinical GH deficiency who have normal responses to insulin but low sleep-related responses. Another example of dissociation of these two GH responses was seen in a patient following surgery for removal of an adrenal adenoma (Krieger and Glick, 1974). Insulin-induced GH secretion, which had been decreased prior to surgery, returned to normal in four months. Sleep-related GH secretion, however, remained abnormally low until eight months after surgery. It seems possible, then, as Eastman and Lazarus (1973) and Tanner et al. (1971) speculate, that some patients may respond normally to pharmacologic stimuli yet may be incapable of producing normal quantities of GH on a regular basis. This possibility seems well worth pursuing by systematic studies.

There is evidence that there may be reversible GH deficiencies in children with disturbed home environments. These children with "psychosocial dwarfism" may grow at unusually slow rates at home, and show subnormal GH responses to insulin there, yet return to normal when removed from their usual environments and placed in the hospital (Krieger and Mellinger, 1971). Subjective sleep reports have related periods of slow growth to disturbed sleep, and periods of more rapid growth with normal sleep (Wolff and Money, 1973). Data on sleep-related GH secretion in these children is not available.

Studies of sleep-related secretion of GH in acromegalics have been performed by Carlson *et al.* (1972), Sassin, Hellman, and Weitzman (1972b), and Cryer and Daughaday (1969). In general, the findings were high, fluctuating levels throughout sleep, with no peak associated with sleep onset or slow-wave sleep. Cryer and Daughaday (1969) reported slightly lower levels during sleep than waking. Sassin *et al.* (1972b), in a study in which values were plotted as percentage of the 24-hour secretion, found highest levels from midnight to 10:00 A.M. Values often rose before sleep onset, and continued to be high briefly after the end of sleep. A single patient, however, clearly had a peak associated with sleep-onset. The authors speculated that the eosinophilic adenoma present in this disease is not completely autonomous, and that loss of hypothalamic control may be involved in the pathogenesis of acromegaly. It is also interesting that in acromegalics, in contrast to normal subjects, GH secretion is suppressed by L-DOPA (Lucke *et al.*, 1974; Liuzzi *et al.*, 1972).

Sleep-related GH secretion and percentage slow-wave sleep are decreased in treated (remission five months to two years) and untreated patients with Cushing's disease as well as some patients with "eucorticoid" hypothalamic tumors (Krieger and Glick, 1974). On the other hand, nocturnal GH secretion that was decreased in a patient with an adrenal adenoma returned to normal eight months after corrective surgery. These data have been taken to imply a neural dysfunction in Cushing's syndrome, as well as some direct effect of excess cortisol on GH release. Administration of hydrocortisone for one night (Krieger *et al.*, 1972) and prednisone for two weeks (Stiel, Island, and Liddle, 1970) or two years (Krieger and Glick, 1974) did not modify sleep-related GH secretion. It seems likely that studies involving multiple doses, infusions at different times of day, and differing durations of infusion will be needed to characterize the relationship of corticosteroids to GH secretion.

Because of the relation of GH secretion to slow-wave sleep, and reports of increases in slow-wave sleep in patients with hyperthyroidism, the secretion of GH in this illness is of interest. Dunleavy *et al.* (1974) reported that in two adult patients, nocturnal GH secretion was higher than might be expected, and that it decreased along with total slow-wave sleep after treatment with carbimazole.

Sleep-related GH secretion in schizophrenics was examined by Vigneri *et al.* (1974). Three chronic and one acute schizophrenic had normal daytime levels and normal responses on insulin tolerance tests. During sleep, the three chronic patients had constant levels throughout the night, with no relationship to sleep onset or any sleep stage. The acute schizophrenic had one peak at sleep onset and one late at night, with no apparent relation to slow-wave sleep. These findings were thought to be associated with the decreased amounts of slow-wave sleep found in schizophrenics. A study by Murri et al. (1973) of four chronic schizophrenics showed no consistent rises during sleep, and noted that administration of tryptophan did not change the amount or pattern of secretion.

There is little available data on sleep-related GH secretion in depression. Several studies suggest that depressed patients have decreased GH responses during insulin provocative tests, however (Mueller, Heninger, and McDonald, 1969; Sachar et al., 1973; Gruen et al., 1975).

There is some evidence that sleep-related secretion of GH is disturbed in dry alcoholics. Othmer et al. (1972) found in eight alcoholics that slow-wave sleep and GH secretion were abnormally low in the first two hours of sleep. Elevations of GH secretion occurred at irregular intervals without a clear relation to slow-wave sleep. When the patients drank alcohol, slow-wave sleep during the first two hours increased, but there was no noticeable change in GH secretion. It might be speculated that these effects are related to modification of biogenic amine metabolism by alcohol, which is discussed at length in chapter 6.

Effects of Injections of GH on Sleep

A large part of this chapter has been devoted to the effects of various compounds or manipulations of sleep stages on GH secretion. Conversely, there is some evidence that administration of GH may modify the sleep stages. Vogel et al. (1972) administered GH to human GH-deficient dwarfs (who were reported to have unusually high amounts of slow-wave sleep), and found a further increase in slow-wave sleep. This seemed to militate against a hypothesis that GH release is stimulated by slow-wave sleep and then in turn by negative feedback causes decreases in this sleep stage. Several studies (Stern et al., 1975; Stern, Jalowiec, and Morgane, 1974; Drucker-Colin et al., 1975), have reported that injections of GH may increase REM sleep in a dose-dependent manner in the cat and rat. They speculated that this supports the view that secretion of GH during slow-wave sleep may help trigger subsequent REM sleep episodes. The hypothesis that GH may in fact be involved in the regulation of sleep stages seems to be worth pursuing.

THE PITUITARY–ADRENAL AXIS

It has been known for some time that cortisol, secreted in response to adrenocorticotropic hormone (ACTH) from the pituitary, possesses a circadian cycle. Blood cortisol levels are lowest in the early hours of sleep (1:00–3:00 A.M.) and highest toward 4:00–8:00 A.M. the next morning (Hellman et al., 1970a; Weitzman et al., 1971). Hellman et al. (1970a) have provided evidence that cortisol is secreted in multiple discrete episodes, whose total time may be only 6¼ hours out of 24, and that the rest of the time the adrenals may be quiescent. Over half of the 24-hour secretion occurs during sleep.

As radioimmunoassays for ACTH itself became available, it became clear that, as expected, it is lowest in the few hours before and just after sleep onset, increases after three to five hours of sleep, and is at its highest shortly after awakening (Liddle, 1974; Gallagher et al., 1973; Berson and Yalow, 1968). Individual episodes of ACTH secretion are closely related to episodes of cortisol secretion, which tend to occur about 10 minutes after the initiation of the former (Gallagher et al., 1973).

ACTH secretion is thought to be primarily affected by a biological clock and by various physiologic stresses, presumably via CNS mechanisms (an open loop system) and by closed loop negative feedback from levels of glucocorticoids (Reichlin, 1974; Rubin, 1975). The episodic nature of the secretion, the acute responses to various stresses, and the disruption of ACTH secretion following deafferentation (removal of nerve pathways) of the medial ventral hypothalamus (Halasz, 1969) emphasize the importance of neural regulation of ACTH secretion. This is accomplished via a corticotropin-releasing factor (CRF) from the hypothalamus. Release of CRF may be stimulated by cholinergic neurons and inhibited by noradrenergic neurons (Liddle, 1974; Van Loon, 1973).

One interesting quality of the closed system of negative feedback from circulating corticosteroids is that its importance relative to the neurologic system may vary during the day in a cyclic manner. Ceresa et al. (1969) found that although maximum intravenous doses of dexamethasone could cause decreases in urinary 17-hydroxycorticosteroids when given at any time, submaximal doses could only do this from

4:00–8:00 A.M.. There is some evidence that adrenal sensitivity to ACTH does not change over the 24-hour day (McDonald et al., 1969).

Relation to Sleep–Waking Cycle

The diurnal rhythm of ACTH and corticosteroid secretion is much less closely tied to the sleep–waking cycle than is GH secretion. A urinary 17-hydroxycorticosteroid diurnal rhythm persists despite 205 hours of sleep deprivation (Poland et al., 1972). Altering the sleep–waking cycle for one day by greatly lengthening or shortening sleep time has no effect on the diurnal plasma cortisol cycle; after chronic changes to 19- or 33-hour sleep–waking cycles, or reversal of the 24-hour cycle by 180°, the cortisol cycle adjusts to the new sleep cycle after one to two weeks (Weitzman et al., 1968a; Orth, Island, and Liddle, 1967). Weitzman et al. (1974) put subjects on three-hour sleep–waking cycles (one hour sleep followed by two hours waking) for 10 days. The circadian rhythm of cortisol persisted, but superimposed on it was an ultradian rhythm in which plasma cortisol was lowest during sleep periods and highest in the first hour after waking. These phenomena are associated with sleep and not with the light–dark cycle. Krieger, Kruezer, and Rizzo (1969) showed that the plasma 11-hydroxycorticosteroid rhythm persisted in humans who were kept under constant lighting for 21 days. Although blind subjects show some irregularities in corticosteroid rhythm, they retain the quality of having increases at the end of sleep and beginning of waking (Bodenheimer, Winter, and Faiman, 1973; Krieger and Rizzo, 1971).

The relation of corticosteroids to specific sleep stages is complicated by the very loose association with the sleep–waking cycle described above, and by its half-life of about 68 minutes (Hellman et al., 1970a), which is relatively long compared to the various EEG events that are measured. It is possible that studies relating ACTH to sleep stage will be more helpful, as the polypeptide has a half-life of only about 10 minutes (Liddle, 1974). Since plasma cortisol levels are normally highest after several hours of sleep, it has been speculated that there is a relationship of cortisol secretion to episodes of REM sleep, which are highest at that time. Mandell and Mandell (1969) reported that all 14 episodes of REM in four normal subjects were associated with elevations of urinary 17-hydroxycorticosteroids. Perhaps one of the most careful studies of plasma cortisol levels and sleep stages was provided by Hellman et al. (1970a). In one subject they found that all three peaks of plasma cortisol occurring in sleep were in juxtaposition to REM episodes, as were four out of five in a second subject. Rubin, Kales, and Clark (1969), monitoring sleep stages and urinary 17-hydroxycortico-steroids in subjects who received glutethimide, found that secretion was related more closely to phasic events (eye movement density) rather than to percentage of REM sleep. Since glucocorticoids tend to increase hepatic gluconeogenesis, it has been speculated that the function of increased glucocorticoid secretion during REM sleep is to prepare nutrients for use by the brain (Mandell and Mandell, 1969).

REM sleep and cortisol secretion can, however, clearly be disso-ciated, as in the 12-hour sleep-waking cycle reversal studies (Weitzman *et al.*, 1968a) where for several days there were multiple episodes of REM sleep during the daytime with little cortisol secretion. During the study of three-hour sleep–waking cycles described above (Weitzman *et al.*, 1974), total 24-hour plasma cortisol secretion was unchanged, although total amount of REM sleep was reduced by almost half. The relation of cortisol secretion to REM sleep is, then, clearly not yet well defined.

Another adrenal steroid, aldosterone, may be secreted in relation to REM sleep (Rubin *et al.*, 1975b). Because it is important in the regulation of renal function, it is discussed in the section of this chapter dealing with antidiuretic hormone.

Sleep-Related Cortisol Secretion in Disease States

The circadian rhythm of cortisol secretion appears to remain intact in a variety of disease states. Cortisol secretion in Cushing's syndrome has been studied by Hellman *et al.* (1970b) and Krieger and Gewirtz (1974). In the former study a patient with idiopathic Cushing's syn-drome with adrenal hyperplasia was found to have episodic secretion, with retention of a diurnal rhythm whose low point occurred early in sleep. Secretion was remarkably like normal except for the larger quan-tities of cortisol involved. The authors suggested that if cortisol secre-tion should be found to be constant in patients with autonomous adrenal tumors, then serial sampling of cortisol might be helpful in distinguishing idiopathic Cushings from that related to neoplasms. Krieger and Gewirtz (1974) measured ACTH and cortisol secretion in a patient with the latter condition, although sampling was done only every three hours. There was in fact a loss of the circadian pattern. In addition there was a loss of ACTH, cortisol, or growth hormone response to hypoglycemia or Pitressin administration. These endocrine responses to hypoglycemia and Pitressin returned 3½ months after surgical removal of the tumor. In contrast, the circadian rhythm of

ACTH did not return until seven months after surgery. The authors suggested that these differing time courses for recovery imply the existence of separate mechanisms governing response to pharmacologic provocation tests and circadian rhythmicity. (It will be recalled from earlier in this chapter that the issue of multiple CNS control mechanisms has also been raised regarding growth hormone.) As in idiopathic Cushing's syndrome, there is also evidence that plasma ACTH retains its diurnal rhythm in cortisol-deficient patients with Addison's syndrome (Graber et al., 1965).

Gallagher (1971) and Perlow et al. (1971) described cortisol patterns in narcoleptic patients. The patient in the former study had a history of cataplectic attacks, but all sleep episodes documented with the EEG were slow-wave sleep. In the latter study, three patients, all of whom had secondary symptoms of narcolepsy, had daytime sleep attacks of REM sleep and nocturnal sleep-onset REM. In both cases the 24-hour cortisol secretory patterns were in fact normal. Gallagher (1971) also reported on a patient with parkinsonism, whose cortisol secretory pattern remained normal, including decreased secretion early in sleep. Treatment with L-DOPA, which ameliorated the motor symptoms of parkinsonism, did not change the pattern of cortisol secretion. This might be taken to imply that in this one patient L-DOPA in amounts sufficient to alter function in striatal dopaminergic neurons may not alter whatever hypothalamic pathways control corticotropin-releasing factor secretion.

A variety of studies have been performed on cortisol secretion in depressed patients (Fullerton et al., 1968a, 1968b; Doig et al., 1966; McClure, 1966; and Bridges and Jones, 1966). The general direction of the findings is an increase in the degree of diurnal variation of plasma cortisol, with either the 6:00 A.M. "high" point or the entire mean cortisol value higher than controls. These findings should be taken in the context of sleep stage disturbances (which often include multiple awakenings, and decreased total sleep time, REM sleep and slow-wave sleep), which are discussed in chapter 7. There is some tendency to change toward normal upon recovery, although some studies (Bridges and Jones, 1966) found absolute levels to be actually lower in recovered patients than in controls. Doig et al. (1966) noted that in seven out of ten depressed patients, the highest peak occurred at 3:00 A.M., but on recovery moved to the more normal 6:00 A.M. Similarly, the nadir of serum cortisol levels has been reported to occur three hours earlier in depressed patients than controls (Fullerton et al., 1968a, 1968b). McClure (1966), citing studies in which ACTH treatments were associated with wakefulness, suggests that the increased plasma cortisol in depressed patients may be responsible for their early morning awakenings.

Effects of ACTH and Cortisol on the Sleep Stages

Adrenal corticosteroids have been shown to influence various mea-sures of neural activity, such as nerve conduction velocity (Henkin *et al.*, 1963) and thresholds for smell (Henkin and Bartter, 1966) and hearing (Henkin and Daly, 1968). They are thought to have effects on the metabolism of the monoamines (Maas and Mednieks, 1971; Grelak *et al.*, 1970; Green and Curzon, 1968), which in turn are thought to be related to control of the sleep stages (Wyatt, 1972). Thus, there was some basis for the expectation that subjects receiving exogenous corti-costeroids and patients with excessive endogenous adrenal activity might have disturbances in sleep stage regulation.

Krieger and Gewirtz (1974), whose study of Cushing's syndrome is mentioned above, observed that their patients had virtually no slow-wave sleep, a reduction in REM periods, and an increase in stage 1 sleep. This pattern did not return to normal until 16 months after surgical removal of the adenoma. These findings regarding slow-wave sleep seem to agree with data by Gillin *et al.* (1974a) on sleep in patients with adrenal insufficiency. They found that during the baseline period in which they were receiving replacement therapy, slow-wave sleep was slightly higher than that of normal controls. When replacement therapy was discontinued, slow-wave sleep increased markedly. Simi-larly, when cortisol secretion was decreased in normal subjects follow-ing administration of metyrapone (SU 4885) there was an increase in slow-wave sleep.

Gillin *et al.* (1974b) found that infusions of ACTH begun at 8:00 A.M. or 3:00 P.M., but not at 11:30 P.M., resulted in decreased REM sleep. As this effect was more marked in normal volunteers than in Addisonian patients, an implication would seem to be that changes in human sleep induced by ACTH are probably mediated by secretion of adrenocortical steroids. The REM suppressive effect seemed to require four hours of infusion and to persist for at least 12 hours. Thus, the effects of REM would seem to last some time after the levels of infused ACTH and resulting adrenocortical steroids had probably returned to normal. Amounts of slow-wave sleep also decreased after infusions of ACTH at 8:00 A.M.

Gillin *et al.* (1972a) have observed that single oral doses of 60 mg prednisone given to normal volunteers resulted in decreased REM sleep time and increased REM sleep latency, with no change in slow-wave sleep. These changes may only reflect acute responses, as there is some evidence that asthmatic patients chronically receiving prednisone have sleep patterns similar to those not receiving it (Kales *et al.*, 1968). As Gillin *et al.* (1972a) pointed out, extrapolations from an acute study on normal subjects can be only tentatively applied to the pathophysiology of disease states; nonetheless, their data are consistent with the notion that some changes in sleep in patients with major psychiatric illnesses may partly be secondary to stress-related secretion of corticosteroids.

It is clear that the presence of circulating corticosteroids is not needed for the existence of REM sleep. Jouvet (1965b), for instance, reported that complete removal of the hypothalamus and hypophysis in the pontine cat is still compatible with the appearance of REM sleep. Although circulating steroids would have left the body in a few hours, REM sleep continued to appear (although in declining amounts) until death on the sixth or seventh day. Injections of ACTH and posterior pituitary extract could restore periodicity of REM sleep in these animals. Thus, although REM sleep can clearly occur in the absence of corticosteroids, it seems possible that secretion of corticosteroids may have some modulating effect on its appearance.

Other evidence of a possible modulating role of corticosteroids on the maintenance of the sleep cycles comes from the work of Johnson and Sawyer (1971). They placed rats on a one-hour light–dark cycle, and found that although REM sleep began to appear in a one-hour ultradian rhythm, the basic circadian rhythm persisted. Most of the total 24-hour REM sleep still occurred in what had formerly been the daylight hours. Following adrenalectomy, however, the circadian distribution of REM sleep disappeared. Administration of cortisol in the late afternoon established a new circadian rhythm out of phase with the original one. They speculated that cortisol may be released by stress or exposure to drugs, resulting in REM sleep, which in turn might have the function of encouraging biochemical syntheses to repair the nervous system (Oswald, 1970). Since REM sleep in humans has been reported to be decreased by pharmacologic doses of prednisone (Gillin *et al.*, 1972a) or ACTH (Gillin *et al.*, 1974b), and to be decreased in patients with adrenal adenomas (Krieger and Gewirtz, 1974), the observation in this study of increased REM sleep after administration of cortisol, as well as the hypotheses derived from the observation, must await further work for confirmation. Interpretation of this study is also made more difficult by the authors use of cortisol, which in the rat is not a major glucocorticoid. (Corticosterone plays the more important role in rats.)

PROLACTIN

Prolactin (PRL) is a single-chain polypeptide that participates in the initiation and maintenance of lactation, has some metabolic effects in many ways similar to GH in animal studies, and may be related to some animal behavioral responses such as nesting behavior in birds (Daughaday, 1974). Neurotransmittors that may control hypothalamic regulation of PRL secretion are reviewed by Meites (1973). There is fairly good evidence that catecholamines inhibit release of PRL (Meites et al., 1972). Similarly, increased release of Prolactin Inhibiting Factor from the hypothalamus results from giving drugs that increase hypothalamic catecholamine activity (Kamberi, Mical, and Porter, 1971a). Some recent evidence suggests that the inhibiting factor is in fact dopamine (Shaar and Clemens, 1974). Studies on the serotonergic system are less clear. Although Coppola (1971) and Talwalker, Ratner, and Meites (1963) were unable to find a role for serotonin in prolactin release, Kamberi, Mical, and Porter (1971b) demonstrated that intraventricular injection of serotonin resulted in increased plasma prolactin in rats, as did intraperitoneal injection of 5-HTP. Perhaps consistent with the possibility that a serotonergic system is involved in PRL release are drug studies showing that ergot derivatives such as ergocornine, ergonovine, and LSD inhibit prolactin release in several species (Meites and Clemens, 1972). There is some evidence that this is due to both a direct effect on the anterior pituitary and an effect on hypothalamic release of Prolactin Inhibiting Factor (Meites, 1973). MacIndoe and Turkington (1973) observed that intravenous infusion of L-tryptophan is associated with a rise in serum prolactin in humans, and that this effect was decreased by pretreatment with methysergide. There is no known long-loop hormonal negative feedback in the control of PRL secretion (Turkington, 1972).

Sassin et al. (1972a) demonstrated that prolactin possesses a diurnal rhythm. There is an initial peak 60–90 minutes after sleep onset, with subsequent peaks resulting in maximal levels at 5:00–7:00 A.M. During the hour after awakening the levels begin to drop, reaching a nadir from about 10:00 A.M. to noon. Studies of modifying the hours of sleep over the 24-hour day demonstrated an immediate shift to the new hours of sleep (Sassin et al., 1973). In this sense PRL secretion is more similar to that of GH, rather than to ACTH, which, as described earlier, seems to have some stability as a true circadian rhythm in addition to some relationship to sleep.

PRL secretion in nonpregnant women appears to be the same (Sassin et al., 1972a) or slightly higher (Nokin et al., 1972) than that of men, and both sexes possess a similar diurnal rhythm. PRL levels rise during pregnancy. Although a study in which blood samples were drawn every four hours suggested that the circadian rhythm of PRL is no longer present during pregnancy (Nokin et al., 1972), a study with sampling every 20 minutes found this rhythm to be intact (Boyar et al., 1975).

Unlike GH, PRL secretion does not seem to be related to a specific sleep stage. Sassin et al. (1972a) found no gross relationship, although no detailed analysis was made. Parker, Rossman, and Vanderlaan (1974) found that although secretory peaks did not occur with specific stages, PRL levels were found to be decreased during REM sleep and increased during the nonREM sleep following REM episodes. This study, however, was composed of 58 recordings performed on 14 subjects. Since there seem to be large differences between individuals, the repeated use of some subjects (up to 11 times) may have had an influence on the results. Mendelson et al. (1975b) were unable to confirm the REM-nonREM secretory pattern that Parker, Rossman, and Vanderlaan (1974) had described.

Relation of PRL Secretion to Other Hormones

The initial rise of PRL after sleep onset often coincides with the rise of GH, but peak values occur some 40 minutes after GH (Sassin et al., 1972a). Although there is, then, some temporal relationship in initial sleep-related secretion, there are often cases when PRL is released with no changes in GH. This is particularly true late in sleep, where overall values of PRL are increasing, but GH release becomes infrequent (Sassin et al., 1973). Rubin et al. (1975a) have reported a positive correlation between PRL and testosterone levels.

Effects of Drugs on Sleep-Related Prolactin Secretion

There are several studies available on the effects of drugs on acute daytime secretion of PRL. These include observations that phenothiazines, tricyclic antidepressants, reserpine and methyldopa increase (Turkington, 1972), and L-DOPA decreases (Kleinberg, Noel, and Frantz, 1971) daytime secretion in humans. In contrast, at the time of this writing there is almost no data on effects of drugs on sleep-related PRL secretion as ascertained by multiple frequent samplings. Kales et al. (1975) reported that thioridazine increased the total nightly secretion of PRL in two subjects; the interpretation of what mechanisms are involved is hampered by the multiple neurochemical effects of phenothiazines, which include adrenolytic and anticholinergic actions. Mendelson et al. (1975b) reported that the serotonin-receptor blocker methysergide greatly decreased sleep-related PRL secretion. An implication might be that serotonergic pathways may stimulate sleep-related PRL secretion.

FOLLICLE-STIMULATING HORMONE AND LUTEINIZING HORMONE

Follicle-stimulating hormone (FSH) and luteinizing hormone (LH) are glycoproteins, somewhat similar in structure to TSH and human chorionic gonadotropin. FSH is related to follicular development and spermatogenesis in the testis; LH is synergistic with FSH in stimulating maturation of the follicle, is involved in ovulation and maintenance of the corpus luteum of the ovary and in the production of androgens by Leydig cells of the testis (Bardin, 1973). LH release from the pituitary is stimulated by LH-releasing hormone (LRH), a decapeptide from the hypothalamus. LRH is also known to stimulate release of FSH. It seems likely at this time that there is in fact only this one releasing hormone for both gonadotropins. Since circulating levels of LH and FSH may be quite different, it has been speculated that pituitary content or sensitivity to LRH may vary at different times. There is some evidence that noradrenergic and dopaminergic neuronal systems may be involved in control of LRH release (Coppola, 1971; Franchimont, 1971). Release of LRH may also be modified by a negative closed loop feedback system sensitive to circulating estrogen levels (Reichlin, 1974).

Relation of LH and FSH Secretion to Sleep

Analysis of the relation of gonadotropins to sleep is in many ways a study of ontogeny of endocrine function. Prepubertal children of both sexes and adult men are thought to show no consistent relationship between LH secretion and the sleep–waking cycle (Rubin et al., 1975a; Boyar et al., 1974; Rubin et al., 1973a; De Lacerda et al., 1973; Boyar et al., 1972a; Boyar et al., 1972b). In contrast, pubertal boys and girls have been found to have increases in LH during sleep (Boyar et al., 1974); Kapen et al., 1974; Boyar et al., 1972a). When these authors examined LH secretion after experimental delayed sleep onset in their pubertal subjects, LH secretion was also delayed and retained its relation to sleep. In sleep reversal studies, LH secretion also reversed itself to retain a relationship to daytime sleeping, but it was noticed that there was still some cyclic increase during nocturnal waking (Boyar et al.,

1974; Kapen et al., 1974). It has been speculated that the nocturnal increases in LH, which may reach levels two to four times greater than during waking, may be responsible for the Leydig cell stimulation and increasing chorionic gonadotropin responsiveness that occur during puberty.

As described above, LH secretion seems to have no relation to sleep in adult men. In adult women, Alford et al. (1973a) found increases of LH and FSH in the morning compared to the evening, and Kapen et al. (1973) reported decreases in LH in the first few hours of sleep. In contrast, Naftolin et al. (1973) found no relationship of LH or FSH to sleep in adult women. There is, of course, in women a monthly cycle of "basal" LH levels, probably due to variation in the magnitude of ultradian secretory pulses, which is reflected in waking (Yen et al., 1972) and sleep (Naftolin et al., 1973) studies.

It is not clear whether FSH possesses a diurnal rhythm in adults. Bodenheimer et al. (1973) reported a cycle with its high point at 8:00 A.M. in a study in which plasma was sampled every few hours in normal and blind men. Studies with sampling every 20 or 30 minutes in men and women failed to show a circadian or ultradian rhythm (Rubin et al., 1973a; Naftolin, 1973; Rubin et al., 1972).

Boyar et al. (1972a), studying the increases in LH secretion during sleep in puberty, reported that LH levels varied in an ultradian manner, with cycles of 75–100 minutes. They noted that this is approximately the periodicity of the nonREM-REM cycle, and pointed out that increases in LH usually began in nonREM sleep whereas decreases tended to occur in close proximity to REM sleep episodes. Most of the studies of LH and FSH in adults that found no relation to the sleep–waking cycle also found no relationship to specific sleep stages (Naftolin et al., 1973; Alford et al., 1973a; Kapen et al., 1973; Boyar et al., 1972b). The one exception is a study of adult men by Rubin et al. (1973a) that found that although there was no circadian or ultradian rhythm of LH or FSH, there was a small but significant association of increases in LH with REM sleep. This is consistent with the observation by Clemens et al. (1972) of increases in LH during REM sleep in rats.

Relation of Testosterone Secretion to Sleep

As with LH, testosterone seems to increase during sleep in pubertal subjects (Judd et al., 1974; Boyar et al., 1974). The latter study included a delayed sleep onset experiment in one subject in which testosterone remained related to sleep, and a sleep–waking reversal study, in which testosterone continued to be related to sleep in a more intimate manner than was the case with LH. Evans *et al.* (1971a) also noted a reversal of diurnal testosterone secretion with sleep–waking reversal in one subject.

It is not clear whether the relation of testosterone to sleep holds true in adults also. Most studies have reported a diurnal rhythm in which levels are highest late in sleep, on which a fluctuating pattern may be superimposed (Rubin *et al.*, 1975a; Schiavi *et al.*, 1974; De Lacerda *et al.*, 1973; Piro *et al.*, 1973; Rose *et al.*, 1972; Evans *et al.*, 1971a and 1971b). Other studies found no diurnal pattern (Boyar *et al.*, 1974; Alford *et al.*, 1973a). In terms of relationship to individual sleep stages, the results of the adult studies have also been varied. Evans *et al.* (1971a, 1971b), using a largely impressionistic approach, noted increases in testosterone either during or just before REM sleep. Roff-warg *et al.* (1974) found some evidence of peaks around the nonREM-REM junction and found that testosterone tended to rise just before this time. They noted, however, that these trends accounted for only a small part of the total variance, and suggested that any relation to REM sleep may be a relatively weak time-linked association. Schiavi *et al.* (1974) did not find a relation to REM sleep, but did observe that testosterone levels were lowest during slow-wave sleep. They pointed out that this could be coincidental, since the diurnal rhythm of testosterone was such that testosterone was lower early in sleep, which is when slow-wave sleep is most heavily concentrated.

The control of nocturnal episodic testosterone secretion during puberty seems to be related and in response to LH secretion (Boyar *et al.*, 1974). As described above, however, some of the data in adults could be interpreted as showing a sleep-related diurnal rhythm of testosterone but not of LH. Thus, one might have to look at other mechanisms besides LH secretion for the control of a diurnal rhythm of testosterone. Rubin *et al.* (1975a) found some positive relation of PRL and testosterone levels, and suggested that PRL may play a role in the regulation of nocturnal testosterone secretion. The secretion of testosterone, as well as LH and FSH, has been reported to be unchanged in blind men (Bodenheimer *et al.*, 1973), suggesting that the light–dark cycle does not have a role in the regulation of these hormones. Although there is some conflicting data, it may well be that this is also the case with cortisol and GH release (Weitzmann *et al.*, 1972).

Effects of Sex Hormones on Sleep

One indirect indication of the relation of sex hormones to sleep is the examination of sleep changes during the menstrual cycle in humans. Ho (1972) examined three women at three different times: premenstrually, when there was high progesterone and estrogen levels; during the menses, when these were both low; and early in the cycle, when there was low progesterone and rising estrogen. The only parameter that varied significantly was slow-wave sleep, which was decreased premenstrually. Similar results at a corresponding time of cycle were found on three women taking oral contraceptives. Other measures, including amounts of REM sleep, did not vary. Kapen et al. (1972) examined four women on days 5–28 of the cycle. The findings were generally negative, except for a single subject who had a large increase in REM sleep time on the 18th day of the cycle, when there was a marked increase in LH.

A variety of animal studies on effects of sex hormones on sleep have been performed. Colvin (1969) reported decreases in REM sleep following estrogen administration. Branchey, Branchey, and Nadler (1971b) reported decreases in REM when estrogen was given to ovarectomized female rats, and that both REM and nonREM decreased when progesterone was given in addition. This effect did not occur in males (Branchey, Branchey, and Nadler, 1971a). An interesting sexual dimorphism was observed: Males who had been castrated since birth responded similarly to ovarectomized females, but these hormones had no effect on the sleep of males castrated in adulthood (Branchey, Branchey, and Nadler, 1973). Sawyer (1969) summarizes a series of studies from his laboratory elaborating on the observation that coitus in female rabbits stimulated slow-wave sleep, followed by "hippocampal overactivity." Although administration of steroids has been associated with changes in sleep, he points out that in physiological doses none of the gonadal or adrenal steroids are specific sleep-inducing hormones. They may, however, play a role in reactivity of neurons, as reflected in changing thresholds of electrically stimulated sleep.

It is possible that testosterone plays a role in reported sex differences in response to hypnotic effects of barbiturates (Kato, Chiesara, and Frontino, 1962; Dundee, 1954). Effects of exogenous testosterone on barbiturate sensitivity may vary with duration of pretreatment with testosterone. This may reflect an effect on induction of enzymes for barbiturate metabolism, as well as a possible true synergistic effect (Gessner and Gessner, 1973).

Sleep-Related Secretion in Disease States

Studies of nocturnal secretory patterns have been done in various disease states. Cerone et al. (1975) found no unusual pattern in the episodic release of LH and FSH in an uncontrolled study of chronic schizophrenics. In contrast, nocturnal secretion of LH and FSH in patients with anorexia nervosa is less than that of normal controls (Kalucy et al., 1975). Patients with the Chiari-Frommel syndrome, which involves postpartum amenorrhea and galactorrhea, may have unusually low nocturnal LH secretion (Kapen et al., 1975). Children with idiopathic precocious puberty and congenital adrenal hyperplasia with precocious puberty have been reported to have the episodic LH release and sleep-related increases seen in normal adolescents (Boyar et al., 1973). This observation seems generally analogous to the finding of intact cyclic secretion of cortisol in idiopathic Cushing's syndrome with adrenal hyperplasia, which has been described previously.

THYROID-STIMULATING HORMONE

Thyroid-Stimulating Hormone (TSH) is a glycoprotein, which stimulates the growth and vascularity of the thyroid gland, and increases iodotyrosine and iodothyronine formation and tri-iodothyronine (T_3) release. Release of TSH is thought to be controlled by negative feedback exerted by circulating levels of thyroid hormones, and by Thyrotropin-Releasing Hormone (TRH) from the hypothalamus (Daughaday, 1974). A noradrenergic system may be involved in release of TRH (Reichlin, 1974). In addition to its effect on TSH, TRH may also stimulate prolactin secretion (Reichlin, 1974).

Although some studies have failed to show diurnal variation in TSH release (Hershman and Pittman, 1971; Webster, Guansing, and Paice, 1972), there is a large body of evidence suggesting that a diurnal rhythm is in fact present (Weeke, 1973; Patel, Alford, and Burger, 1972; Alford et al., 1973b; Vanhaelst et al., 1973 and 1972; Nicoloff, Fisher, and Appleman, 1970). Although the time of increases and maximum values vary in each study, the tendency is to report increases in TSH sometime prior to sleep onset (8:00–11:00 P.M.) Peak values are reported to occur anywhere from 10:00 P.M.–3:00 A.M. (Alford et al., 1973b) to 4:00 A.M.–6:00 A.M. (Vanhaelst et al., 1972). In general, the sleep-related increase in TSH levels above baseline is relatively small, compared to GH, PRL, and ACTH.

In addition to a diurnal rhythm, TSH, like GH, ACTH, and PRL, seems to be released episodically with an ultradian rhythm of one to three hours (Alford et al., 1973b; Vanhaelst et al., 1972 and 1973; Weeke, 1973; and Patel et al., 1972).

Regulatory mechanisms of the diurnal rhythm of TSH are not well understood. It has been observed that administration of maintenance doses of hydrocortisone to Addisonian patients, and pharmacologic doses of glucocorticoids to normal subjects results in suppression of TSH secretion (Patel et al., 1974; Nicoloff, Fisher, and Appleman, 1970). This has led these authors to speculate that rhythmic glucocorticoid secretion may play a role in physiologic control of release of TSH. Since peak levels of TSH occur during sleep, it seems possible that to some degree it is related to the sleep–waking cycle.

TSH Secretion and Sleep

As described above, several studies have indicated that there is a general temporal relation of TSH secretion to sleep, although the initial cyclic increases may occur in the hours immediately before nocturnal sleep onset. Another indication of a relationship to sleep was provided by Patel et al. (1972), who noted that when three subjects took daytime naps, there were increases in TSH in two cases. One approach that would help clarify this association would be to study the effects of reversing the sleep–waking cycle, to determine if TSH secretion would also reverse itself.

The only available data on direct EEG monitoring of sleep during plasma sampling for TSH comes from the work of Alford et al. (1973b). In overnight studies on four adults they found some positive correlations between TSH levels and wakefulness and slow-wave sleep and negative correlations with non-slow wave sleep and REM sleep. The authors believed these findings to be due to large differences between subjects and believed there to be no temporal relationship between TSH levels and specific sleep stages. Johns et al. (1975) measured the Free Thyroxin Index (FTI) from plasma samples taken from normal subjects just before sleeping, after awakening, and in the middle of the day. They found that the FTI taken just before sleep varied directly with the amount of subsequent delta sleep, and inversely with the amount of REM. The authors suggested that the relation of thyroid function to sleep is indirect, possibly mediated by effects of the general metabolic rate on biogenic amine metabolism.

Sleep in Hyper- and Hypothyroidism

The relation of thyroid function to delta sleep observed by Johns et al. (1975) is consistent with the findings of Dunleavy et al. (1974) that patients with hyperthyroidism have increased delta and decreased REM sleep. Conversely, delta sleep has been reported to be decreased in hypothyroid adults (Kales et al., 1967a). After treatment, amounts of delta sleep returned to normal. Studies of hypothyroid infants (Schulte and Parmelee, 1970; Schultz et al., 1968) have reported decreased amounts of sleep spindles, a finding thought to represent a lack of normal CNS maturation.

CNS Actions of TRH

It seems likely that Thyrotropin Releasing Hormone (TRH) itself may also have direct CNS effects. Breese et al. (1974) and Prange et al. (1974) showed that in mice TRH reduces the sleeping time and hypothermic effects produced by ethanol and pentobarbital. As these effects were not produced by T_3, it seems possible that they were in fact due to TRH. There is also some evidence that TRH may be useful in the treatment of depression (Prange et al., 1972; Kastin et al., 1972). There is as yet no data available on the effects of TRH on sleep monitored by electroencephalography.

ANTIDIURETIC HORMONE

Antidiuretic hormone (ADH) is a pentapeptide ring closed by an S–S bridge, with a tripeptide side chain. As described earlier, it is secreted from the posterior pituitary gland in response to changes in blood osmolality and volume. Its main action is to increase the permeability to water and urea of tubule cells in the collecting ducts in the kidney, resulting in increased retention of water, and a more concentrated urine.

Another hormone important in regulation of kidney function is aldosterone. This is a steroid secreted by the adrenal gland, which results in increased reabsorption of sodium, and hence water, by the kidneys. Its secretion is thought to be related to changes in renal blood perfusion due to variation of blood pressure and volume. Decreased perfusion results in release of the substance renin from the kidney, which converts a circulating substrate to angiotensin. This in turn stimulates aldosterone release. The ultimate effect of aldosterone is thought to be an isosmotic decrease in urinary volume, whereas ADH decreases volume but results in a more concentrated urine.

Urine output decreases at night, during which perhaps one-third of the 24-hour volume is excreted (Brod, 1973). This is probably a result of a complex group of factors including decreased glomerular filtration and increased reabsorption of water (Brod, 1973), a circadian rhythm of renin release (Leaf and Liddle, 1974), and other factors. In addition, there is some evidence in favor of sleep-related ultradian changes in urine volume and osmolality.

ADH SECRETION DURING SLEEP

Mandell *et al.* (1966) and Mandell and Mandell (1969) reported that in seven urological patients, the urine volume decreased, and osmolarity increased in association with episodes of REM sleep. They speculated that this was due to periodic secretion of ADH from the posterior pituitary during REM sleep. Bailey, Jenner, and Wheeler (1971) similarly found that urinary sodium, potassium, and chloride increased during REM sleep. In the former study, urinary 17-hydroxycorticosteroid secretion was increased during REM sleep; in the latter, no relationship to sleep states was found. Neither study, however, provided formal statistical analyses of these phenomena. With the more recent development of a radioimmunoassay for ADH, it has become possible to do direct blood determinations of ADH levels, rather than to gather indirect data by studying urine osmolality. Rubin *et al.* (1975b), employing such an assay, found that ADH, like the anterior pituitary hormones, is secreted in a pulsatile manner. There was, however, no relationship to specific sleep states. Interestingly, aldosterone was found to be increased during REM sleep.

Effects of ADH on Sleep

Faure (1962) demonstrated that injections of large amounts of ADH resulted in increases in REM sleep in rabbits. Similarly, Jouvet (1965b) found that hyperosmolarity induced by water deprivation or infusion of hypertonic saline—which presumably caused an increase in ADH release—resulted in increased duration and frequency of REM sleep episodes. Conversely, hypo-osmolarity of the blood, induced by ingestion of large volumes of water and small amounts of exogenous ADH, resulted in suppression of REM sleep. There may be, as Mandell and Mandell (1969) suggested, a relationship between neural mechanisms controlling ADH release and those that regulate REM sleep. Whether this represents a normal physiological system, or is only an observation that occurs under unphysiological laboratory-induced conditions, is not clear.

MELATONIN

All of the hormones discussed previously in this chapter have been products of the pituitary gland or one of its target organs. Another area of interest in the study of neuroendocrinology and sleep is the role of melatonin, which is released from the pineal gland.

Melatonin (5-methoxy-N-acetyltryptamine) is a serotonin derivative synthesized mainly in the pineal gland in mammals. It causes contractions of the melanophores in the skin of fish and frogs. In rats it lowers levels of LH (Fraschini, Collu, and Martini, 1971). This seems to fit well with data from early-morning blood samples in humans, which suggests that melatonin levels are lowest at the time of ovulation and highest during menstrual bleeding (Wetterberg et al., 1976). An implication of this is that low melatonin levels may be a permissive factor for ovulation. Increased levels of melatonin may be involved in the early-morning rise of PRL (Ronnekiev, Krulich, and McCann, 1973). Administration of melatonin to humans has been reported to result in decreased GH secretion during an insulin tolerance test (Smythe and Lazarus, 1974).

The rate-limiting step in synthesis of melatonin is its acetylation, catalyzed by serotonin N-acetyltransferase. In the rat the activity of this enzyme and pineal concentrations of melatonin itself possess a circadian rhythm with highest levels at night; the precursor, serotonin, has a reciprocal rhythm in which the highest level is at midday (Axelrod, 1974). Two human studies of melatonin in urine suggest a similar circadian rhythm (Lynch et al., 1975; Pelham et al., 1973).

In the rat, the circadian pattern of synthesis of melatonin is maintained by circadian discharges of the noradrenergic sympathetic fibers that innervate the pineal and stimulate receptors. The basic rhythm appears to rely on a biological clock located in or near the suprachiasmatic nucleus of the hypothalamus. The clock itself is modulated by the light–dark cycle, in such a manner that light results in decreased sympathetic discharge and, consequently, low levels of serotonin N-acetyltransferase activity (Axelrod, 1974). In a rat study, enzyme activity increased an hour after the onset of darkness at 6:00 P.M. (Deguchi and Axelrod, 1972). This effect was prevented by keeping lights on after this time. On the other hand, darkness during the daytime did not result in increased activity. The implication seems to be that both darkness and the night setting of the biological clock are necessary for melatonin synthesis in the pineal.

Effects of Melatonin on Sleep

Marczynski *et al.* (1964) observed that direct application of melatonin to the preoptic region of the hypothalamus in cats induced behavioral and EEG-documented sleep. On the basis of this and previous studies with serotonin and norepinephrine, they suggested that the preoptic region possesses at least two types of autonomic nervous system receptors concerned with the regulation of sleep, sensitive to norepinephrine and tryptamine. It was speculated that melatonin may play a neurohumoral role in such a control mechanism of wakefulness and sleep. Two studies of administration of melatonin to humans have reported that it has sleep-inducing effects (Cramer *et al.*, 1974; Anton-Tay, Diaz, and Fernandez-Guardiola, 1971). The latter study suggested an increase in REM sleep but did not present quantified data; Cramer *et al.* (1974) found no change in total duration of any sleep stage, but in another study found increased REM sleep during afternoon sleep (Reinhard *et al.*, 1974).

It could be speculated that changes in amounts of REM sleep induced by melatonin might be mediated by its effects on serotonergic activity. Cramer *et al.* (1974) reported that in their human subjects, urinary 5-HIAA was reduced following melatonin administration, and suggested that melatonin may inhibit serotonin metabolism. This would seem to agree well with observations of increased serotonin in the midbrain of rats after melatonin administration (Anton-Tay *et al.*, 1968), although increased serotonin concentrations could be achieved in a variety of ways (e.g., inhibiting release, enhancing re-uptake, etc.). In view of the possibility that serotonergic systems may be involved in the regulation of REM sleep (see chap. 2) the potential role of melatonin in regulation of sleep may be a promising area for further work.

SUMMARY

The anterior pituitary hormones ACTH, GH, PRL, TSH, and LH are secreted in a pulsatile manner, each with its own relationship to some aspect of the sleep–waking or REM-nonREM cycle. They are regulated by a combination of open loop control mechanisms mediated by releasing or inhibiting factors from the hypothalamus, and (in the cases of ACTH, TSH, FSH, and LH) a closed loop negative feedback system responsive to circulating hormone levels. Hypothalamic pathways in the open loop system may be mediated by the putative neurotransmitters norepinephrine, dopamine, and serotonin, which have also been implicated in the control mechanisms of the sleep stages. In the case of GH, it is possible that the neural mechanisms that control sleep-related secretion may differ from those regulating secretion in response to pharmacologic provocative tests.

The relation of some hormones (GH, LH) to sleep may vary with the ontological level of development. In some cases (LH, cortisol) the relation to sleep persists even in the presence of some diseases of oversecretion. Tentative data regarding GH, cortisol, and the pineal hormone melatonin suggest the possibility that endocrine secretion may participate in the regulation of the sleep stages.

Narcolepsy and Diseases of Excessive Sleep

Sleep may be produced by excessive direct or indirect debility; but such sleep is not salutary or refreshing, but what is termed morbid.—*Thomas Ball, 1796*

Narcolepsy is often considered to be an illness of excessive sleep; more precisely, it is a disorder manifested by brief, inappropriate episodes of sleep, often in association with other "auxiliary" symptoms. Sleep attacks have been described by a number of 19th-century physicians, among whom the best known is Westphal (1877). Gelineau in 1880 gave the name *narcolepsy* to a disturbance "characterized by an imperative need to sleep of sudden onset and short duration, recurring at more or less close intervals." As Zarcone (1973) points out, characters with symptoms suggestive of narcolepsy have appeared in many famous works of fiction, including Eliot's *Silas Marner*, Poe's "The Premature Burial" and Melville's *Moby Dick*.

DEFINITION

Yoss and Daly (1957, 1960a, 1960b) considered narcolepsy as being composed of a primary symptom—inappropriate attacks of sleep—to which may be added three auxiliary symptoms: cataplexy, hypnogogic hallucinations, and sleep paralysis. Another feature—disturbed nocturnal sleep—has been emphasized by some authors. The clinical manifestations of each of these symptoms will be described in turn.

Sleep Attacks

These are brief episodes (about 15 minutes) of sleep that occur at any time of day. Some patients recognize that such an attack is imminent; others describe them as occurring without warning. They are usually thought of as irresistible, although some patients seem able to prevent their occurrence by concentrating on staying awake. These episodes may tend to occur during times of boredom or after meals, but they can also appear when least expected: during sexual intercourse, while engaged in a sports event, and so on. After these brief episodes of sleep, the patient may awaken completely refreshed. In many patients there seems to be a refractory period of one to several hours before the next attack.

Cataplexy

This is a sudden loss of tone in the major striated muscles of the body, which may last from perhaps 30 seconds to 15–30 minutes. Loss of muscle tone may be only partial, resulting in "buckling" of the knees or sagging of the head, or may be more generalized, resulting in complete collapse. Cataplectic attacks (like sleep attacks) often result in injury to the patient. During these episodes, the patient remains conscious. Interestingly enough, the extraocular muscles are not affected; a patient experiencing a cataplectic attack can roll his eyes on command. In contrast to sleep attacks, cataplectic episodes typically occur at moments of increased emotion. Thus, patients may report having cataplexy in response to getting angry at a naughty child, hearing a funny joke, seeing a particularly exciting scene in a movie, and so on. Cataplexy, incidentally, should be distinguished from *catalepsy*, the waxy rigidity of the muscles seen in catatonic schizophrenia.

Sleep Paralysis

These are episodes of paralysis of the striated musculature occurring in the transition period between wakefulness and sleep. The subject is fully conscious, and may experience extreme anxiety or fear. Sleep paralysis at the onset of a nap was well described by a patient of Edward Binns, a physician writing in the 1850s about what he termed "day-mares":

> During the intensely hot summer of 1825, I experienced an attack of this affection. Immediately after dining, I threw myself on my back upon a sofa, and, before I was aware, was seized with difficult respiration, extreme dread, and utter incapability of motion or speech. I could neither move nor

cry, while the breath came from my chest in broken and suffocating parox-
ysms. During all this time I was perfectly awake; I saw the light glaring in at
the windows in broad sultry streams; I felt the intense heat of the day
pervading my frame; and heard distinctly the different noises in the street,
and even the ticking of my own watch, which I had placed on the cushion
beside me; I had, at the same time, the consciousness of flies buzzing
around, and settling with annoying pertinacity on my face. During the
whole fit, judgment was never for a moment suspended. I felt assured that I
labored under incubus. I even endeavored to reason myself out of the feeling
of dread which filled my mind, and longed, with insufferable ardour, for
some one to open the door, and dissolve the spell which bound me in its
fetters. The fit did not continue above five minutes: by degrees I recovered
the use of sense and motion; and, as soon as they were so far restored as to
enable me to call out and move my limbs, it wore insensibly away.

Episodes of sleep paralysis are often accompanied by hypogogic
hallucinations. A common experience is to perceive a frightening object
or person sitting on one's chest. Schenck (1969) has commented that
this experience may be the basis of Henry Fuseli's famous painting, *The
Nightmare,* in which such a situation takes place (Fig. 4-1). The woman

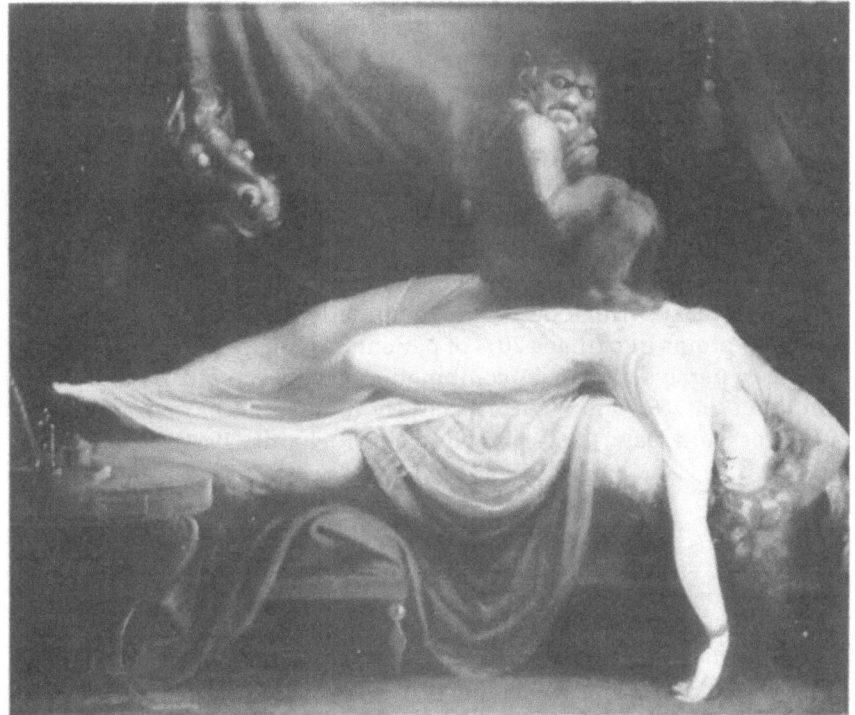

FIGURE 4-1. *The Nightmare,* by Henry Fuseli (English, 1741–1825). Courtesy of the
Detroit Institute of Arts.

pictured appears to be terrified of a demonic figure crouching on her chest, but is unable to move.

The duration of episodes of sleep paralysis is usually a few seconds, but it can be up to 20 minutes. In contrast to cataplexy, the subject can be easily released from this state by calling his name or touching him. In addition to being part of the narcoleptic tetrad, sleep paralysis has been described as an isolated, benign experience occurring from time to time in nonnarcoleptics (Schenck, 1969).

Hypnogogic and Hypnopompic Hallucinations

These are episodes of auditory, visual, or tactile hallucinations, which occur during the transition between wakefulness and sleep. When these occur at sleep onset they are known as *hypnogogic hallucinations;* those that occur upon awakening in the morning are referred to as *hypnopompic hallucinations.* The general clinical impression is that hypnogogic and hypnopompic hallucinations carry more emotional impact, and have more of a storylike quality than the relatively bland images that often occur in normal persons. These experiences can be extremely frightening to the patient. In the unusual (5%) of cases in which this is the dominant symptom, the patient may be mistakenly diagnosed as schizophrenic.

The symptoms of narcolepsy may start at different times and occur in varying combinations (Fig. 4-2). Perhaps the most typical pattern is the onset of sleep attacks, with development of other symptoms occurring later. While virtually 100% develop sleep attacks (by definition), only 10% have the complete tetrad. The most common auxiliary symptom is cataplexy, which occurs in combination with sleep attacks and other symptoms in perhaps 70% of patients. Hypnogogic hallucinations and sleep paralysis occur in combination with sleep attacks and other symptoms in 25% and 30% respectively (Sours, 1963; Yoss and Daly, 1957; Yoss and Daly, 1960a; Bowling and Richards, 1961).

NATURAL HISTORY

Symptoms of narcolepsy usually begin in patients between 10–20 years old, 5% of cases may appear prior to 10 years old, and 25% after the age of 20 (Zarcone, 1973). Kessler, Guilleminault, and Dement (1974) found a mean age of onset of 19.4 years. Both sexes are affected approximately equally (Yoss and Daly, 1960a and b). Once the illness develops, it usually lasts for most of one's life, although the clinical im-

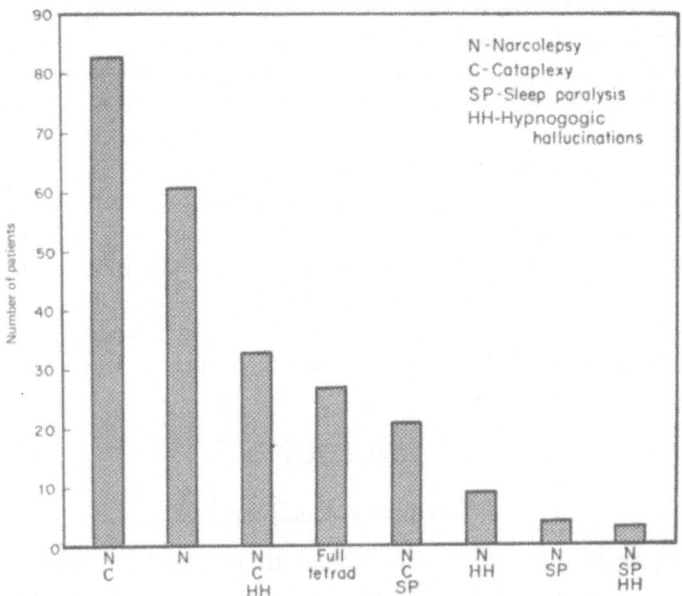

FIGURE 4-2. Frequency of the various combination of symptoms in the narcoleptic tetrad in 241 patients. (From Yoss and Daly, 1957. Reprinted by permission.)

pression is that symptoms decrease in old age. A small proportion of patients may have a course of remissions and exacerbations.

EPIDEMIOLOGY AND GENETICS

The prevalence of persons with episodes of excessive sleepiness was reported to be about 0.02–0.03% in a Yugoslavian study (Bruhova and Roth, 1972). A study in the San Francisco Bay area suggests a prevalence of 0.097% for persons with sleep attacks and cataplexy (Dement, Carskadon, and Ley, 1973a). The latter figure suggests that as many as 100,000 persons in the United States have these symptoms (Guilleminault, Carskadon, and Dement, 1974).

Nevsimalova-Bruhova (1973), examining the first- and second-degree relatives of 64 probands with sleep attacks plus an auxiliary symptom, found various types of sleep disorders in 34.4%. Kessler *et al.* (1974) found that 52% of first- or second-degree relatives of REM narcoleptics had either narcolepsy or a disorder of excessive sleep. The incidence in parents, sibs, or children of probands was 9.2%. Symptoms of narcolepsy itself were found in 2.5%; this familial prevalence would be about 60 times the rate expected in the general population. In both studies there was no evidence of a simple Mendelian mode of transmission. The latter authors suggested that the high incidence of other diseases of excessive sleep (DES) in relatives of narcoleptics implies a single continuous distribution of liability to these disorders with one or more thresholds. Leckman and Gershon (1975) have determined that the data from the Kessler, Guilleminault, and Dement (1974) study are compatible with a two-threshold multifactorial model. The principal implication of this model would be that diseases of excessive sleep and narcolepsy have a common genetic origin, such that narcolepsy is the more severe and less frequent manifestation.

ETIOLOGY

Narcolepsy–Cataplexy

The precise etiology of the narcoleptic syndrome is unknown. A number of possible causes for narcolepsy have been proposed. It has been considered to be an epileptic equivalent (Roth, 1946) and a manifestation of psychodynamic conflicts (Levin, 1959). In 1963, Rechtschaffen et al. suggested that the syndrome of narcolepsy plus auxiliary symptoms may represent a defect in the control of REM sleep. They performed 18 recordings of nocturnal sleep on nine patients with sleep attacks, eight of whom had at least one other symptom. In 11 of the recordings (in seven of the nine patients) it was found that episodes of REM sleep occurred either at sleep onset or within about 11 minutes of sleep onset. This was in marked contrast to the sleep of normal subjects, in whom approximately 90 minutes of nonREM sleep occur prior to the first REM period. The narcoleptic patients did not differ from normal subjects in the total percentage of REM sleep during the night. Their sleep was felt to be disturbed, however, as manifested by an increased number of body movements and decreased amounts of large slow-wave activity.

In 1966, Dement, Rechtschaffen, and Gulevich demonstrated that sleep attacks in patients with this symptom plus cataplexy were also characterized by REM at sleep onset. Subsequent studies showed that recordings of daytime naps of similar patients contain at least some episodes of REM onset sleep. Roth, Bruhova, and Lehovsky (1969), for instance, found REM onset sleep during afternoon naps in 47% of 70 recordings done on 50 patients with narcolepsy plus cataplexy or sleep paralysis. Similarly, Wilson et al. (1973) recorded daytime naps of 49 patients with sleep attacks plus one or more auxiliary symptoms; 90% of the patients had at least one episode of REM onset sleep. Twenty-four or 36 hour recordings of six patients studied by Guilleminault et al. (1973c) showed that the patients fell asleep a total of 55 times, of which 48 were the REM onset type.

It seemed likely, then, that patients with sleep attacks plus one or more auxiliary symptoms were suffering from a disorder of control of REM sleep. Viewed in this way, it could be argued that the auxiliary symptoms of narcolepsy represent the intrusion into wakefulness of the tonic inhibition of muscle tone ordinarily observed in REM sleep (Guilleminault, Smythe, and Dement, 1973e; Dement, Guilleminault, and Mitler, 1973b). Further strength for this viewpoint comes from studies of the H-reflex, which is measured by stimulating an afferent nerve and measuring the resulting muscle contraction. A decreased H-reflex is thought to represent increased descending inhibition on this system. The H-reflex, which is greatly decreased or absent in normal subjects during REM sleep (Hishakawa and Kaneko, 1965), is also decreased during cataplectic attacks (Guilleminault et al., 1973e). Guilleminault et al. (1974) have also pointed out that during cataplectic attacks patients can voluntarily move their extraocular muscles; this, too, seems similar to the situation during REM sleep, in which the major striated muscle groups show decreased tone and yet rapid eye movements occur. Sleep paralysis and hypnogogic hallucinations can also be viewed as episodes of REM-associated events (decreased muscle tone and dreaming) occurring in other states of arousal.

In summary, a great deal of data suggests that the sleep attacks and auxiliary symptoms of narcolepsy represent the intrusion into wakefulness of various physiologic components of REM sleep. There is no clear understanding of the control system that might be disturbed to produce these symptoms.

Secondary Narcolepsy

Some classifications of sleep disorders include a category of secondary narcolepsy (Zarcone, 1973), which refers to narcoleptic symptoms following head trauma, encephalitis, and other CNS pathology. Although reports of excessive sleepiness following these conditions are common, it is not well established that organic lesions can result in symptoms of narcolepsy as we have defined it. Nevsimalova-Bruhova (1973) and Roth and Nevsimalova (1975) refer to 11 such patients with sleep attacks plus auxiliary symptoms ("sleep dissociation"). Detailed analysis of EEG data is not provided, however. Such a condition must be very unusual, if it exists at all. The majority of cases might well be referred to as "excessive daytime sleepiness associated with known organic disease." The use of the term "narcolepsy" in such patients is confusing, and adds little to the understanding of the condition.

OTHER DISORDERS OF EXCESSIVE DAYTIME SLEEP

Independent Narcolepsy or NonREM Narcolepsy

In contrast to patients with sleep attacks plus auxiliary symptoms, patients with sleep attacks alone have generally *not* had REM onset sleep (Hishikawa and Keneko, 1965; Roth *et al.*, 1969). Such patients have been referred to as having *independent narcolepsy, slow-wave sleep narcolepsy* or *hypersomnia.* The general clinical impression is that the description of the sleep attacks in these patients differs from those in patients with sleep attacks plus auxiliary symptoms. In independent narcolepsy the attacks are thought to be of longer duration (Guillemi-nault *et al.*, 1974). There is a common clinical impression that, upon awakening, the patient with independent narcolepsy often continues to feel lethargic. This is in contrast to the refreshed alert state that usually (but not always) follows an attack in a patient with sleep attacks plus auxiliary symptoms. The nocturnal sleep of these patients seems relatively normal (Passouant *et al.*, 1968), in contrast to the disturbed sleep of patients with sleep attacks plus auxiliary symptoms (Rechtschaffen *et al.*, 1963).

Current studies of patients with excessive daytime sleep characterized by nonREM sleep suggests that most have specific definable syndromes. Many have been found to have the *obstructive sleep apnea syndrome;* others have narcolepsy-cataplexy with sleep apnea, or chronic drug dependency. These syndromes will be described in the remainder of this chapter.

It may be that some patients have sleep attacks characterized by nonREM sleep, with neither the auxiliary symptoms of narcolepsy nor other symptoms such as sleep apnea. It seems likely that this is very unusual compared to the bulk of nonREM sleep conditions we are about to describe. Referring to such a state as a form of narcolepsy seems to add little, and confuses it with a well-defined disorder. Thus, it seems more appropriate to consider this state as a nonspecific form of excessive daytime sleepiness, and to reserve the term "narcolepsy" for patients with sleep attacks, auxiliary symptoms (particularly cataplexy), and REM-onset sleep.

Obstructive Sleep Apnea Syndrome

The respiratory rate of normal persons may become irregular during REM sleep, and occasionally during nonREM sleep (Duron, 1972). Pauses in respiration at these times rarely exceed 15 seconds. In some patients, such respiratory irregularities have been noted to be excessively pronounced, and to lead to clinical disturbances of sleep (Guilleminault *et al.*, 1972a). This may occur in several forms. The *obstructive* form has been associated with excessive sleepiness; in one series, approximately half the patients with excessive daytime sleepiness who did not have narcolepsy were found to have this syndrome (Guilleminault *et al.*, 1975a). In physiologic terms, an obstruction of the upper airway prevents air exchange, despite vigorous movements of the chest and diaphragm. This may be due to muscle atonia in the oropharynx and further obstruction by the tongue. Nasal obstruction may also occur (Simmons and Hill, 1974). Tests of pulmonary function during the daytime may be normal. An almost invariable finding in these patients is a history of loud snoring. Treatment of severe and disabling cases consists of tracheostomy, and sometimes submucous nasal resection (Simmons and Hill, 1974).

In the *central* type of sleep apnea, which has been associated with insomnia, diaphragmatic movement may cease for brief periods of time (see chap. 5). In the *mixed* form, features of both obstructive and central sleep apnea are present. Actually, most patients with obstructive apneas may have a brief period in which the diaphragm does not move.

The decreased oxygen saturation during episodes of sleep apnea may be related to the occurrence of the sudden infant death syndrome (Guilleminault, Dement, and Monod, 1973b; Steinschneider, 1972). It has also been speculated that the increased pulmonary arterial pressure and right and left ventricular disorders found in sleep apnea may lead to the development of severe cardiac disease (Guilleminault, Eldridge, and Dement, 1972b). The hypersomnia of obese patients with the Pickwickian syndrome may be a result of sleep apnea (Coccagna *et al.*, 1970).

Narcolepsy with Sleep Apnea

Patients with narcolepsy may also have sleep apneas of the central type (Guilleminault *et al.*, 1972b). Evidence from the Stanford University Sleep Disorders Clinic suggests that sleep apnea clinically complicates narcoleptic symptoms in less than one-tenth of patients with narcolepsy-cataplexy (Guilleminault *et al.*, 1975a). It may be hypothesized that either condition is involved in the etiology of the other, but it seems more likely that both are due to a central defect in the control of sleep and respiration (Guilleminault *et al.*, 1972a).

Hypersomnia with Automatic Behavior

Occasionally patients who complain of excessive nocturnal sleep or daytime sleepiness will describe having had episodes of automatic behavior (Guilleminault, Phillips, and Dement, 1975b). During these episodes, for which they afterward have amnesia, they will carry out inappropriate acts such as putting salt in their coffee or having loud outbursts of speech. Clinical EEGs may show no evidence of seizure activity. Total sleep time for 24 hours may be normal. During waking, however, there are multiple episodes of *microsleep*, associated with decreased performance on psychological testing. Some, but not all, of these patients have decreased slow-wave sleep.

Hypersomnia with Sleep Drunkenness

Some patients with a history of hypersomnia complain that upon awakening in the morning they are disoriented and confused for some time (Roth, Nevsimalova, and Rechtschaffen, 1972). Nocturnal sleep is not disturbed, but is described as excessively "deep." Further descriptions and EEG data will determine whether this unusual condition deserves classification as a discrete symptom complex.

Excessive Daytime Sleepiness Associated with Known Organic Disease

Excessive sleepiness is found in a variety of organic conditions, including brain tumors, hypoglycemia, severe anemia, left ventricular cardiac insufficiency, hypothyroidism, and early stages of narcotic withdrawal. Preliminary work at the Stanford University Sleep Disorders Clinic suggests that a number of patients taking amphetamines chronically may develop long-term daytime drowsiness. Studies of patients with definable organic states leading to hypersomnia generally find that daytime sleep episodes begin with nonREM sleep. Clinically, episodes of daytime sleep in these patients last longer than the sleep attacks of narcolepsy. In contrast to the narcoleptic patient, the patient awakens still feeling fatigued.

Excessive Daytime Sleepiness in Depression

Excessive sleepiness is often seen in patients suffering from depression; sleep disorders in this condition are discussed in detail in chapter 7. Parenthetically, many physicians have the impression that there is a higher incidence of depression among narcoleptics than might be expected by chance. The relationship (if any) between the two disorders is not well understood, but a number of intriguing similarities occur. These include some reports of decreased REM latency in depressed patients, the use of REM deprivation as a treatment for depression (see chapter 7), and the use of tricyclic antidepressants to treat narcolepsy.

DIAGNOSIS

When a patient presents with a complaint of excessive daytime sleepiness, a carefully detailed history is mandatory. Brief periods of sleep that terminate leaving the patient refreshed, the presence of auxiliary symptoms, and disturbed nocturnal sleep strongly suggest narcolepsy. A definitive diagnosis can be made by observing the presence of REM-onset sleep in at least one of several daytime nap EEG recordings. A history of day-long sleepiness, or sleep attacks longer than 30 minutes that leave the patient feeling drowsy suggests one of the other diseases of excessive daytime sleepiness. In this case, the patient should be questioned thoroughly about a history of loud snoring, which suggests an obstructive sleep apnea. A complete diagnosis of the latter condition requires an all-night polygraphic recording that includes measurement of chest expansion, percentage CO_2 expired, and similar measures. This is, of course, generally not available in most clinical settings. Patients should be questioned regarding a history of depression, abuse of stimulants or other drugs, and seizure disorder. It is important to distinguish between sleep attacks and episodes of syncope due to cardiac disorders, orthostatic hypotension, or carotid sinus dysfunction. A physical examination should be performed, and any suggestions or neurologic, metabolic, or endocrine disease should be followed up with appropriate testing. Hypothyroidism in particular should be considered, and a T_4 level determination should be performed if indicated. Hypoglycemia due to tumors of the pancreas may produce episodes of sweating, palpitations, and decreased levels of consciousness. If this is suspected, blood sugar determinations should be performed during prolonged fasting.

PHARMACOTHERAPY OF NARCOLEPSY

Stimulants

Since the first reports of therapy with amphetamine sulfate (Prinzmetal and Bloomberg, 1935) and methylphenidate (Daly and Yoss,

1956), stimulants have been widely used in the treatment of narcolepsy. Dextroamphetamine has been found to be more potent than L-amphetamine (Parkes and Fenton, 1973), though in equipotent doses, both result in decreases in daytime sleepiness. They are relatively ineffective in the treatment of auxiliary symptoms (Parkes and Fenton, 1973; Guilleminault, Carskadon, and Dement, 1974). Complications include abuse, insomnia, and "paradoxical" increased sleepiness in some cases (Guilleminault et al., 1974).

Symptoms of depression may occur when dextroamphetamine is discontinued in narcoleptic patients. Guilleminault et al. (1974) have found that this problem can be alleviated by changing the patient to a tricyclic antidepressant plus methylphenidate, and withdrawing slowly. In this latter procedure, it is recommended to wait at least 24 hours between the last dose of amphetamine and the first dose of antidepressant, in order to avoid a possible toxic interaction effect.

Tricyclic Antidepressants

Imipramine has been found useful in the treatment of the auxiliary symptoms, although it has relatively little effect on the sleep attacks (Akimoto, Honda, and Takahashi, 1960; Guilleminault et al., 1974). Chlorimipramine, which is available only for research in the United States, may be more effective than imipramine (Guilleminault et al., 1974). Shapiro (1975) found that patients treated with it had improvement in auxiliary symptoms within 48 hours, and that most continued to do well after up to 21 months of follow-up. Difficulties with the use of tricyclics include anticholinergic effects such as dry mouth and blurred vision. Impotence develops in many male patients. The REM-suppressing effects of this group of drugs have been cited as evidence that these symptoms are in fact "attacks" of some components of REM sleep.

Monoamine Oxidase Inhibitors

Wyatt et al. (1971b) administered phenelzine (60–90 mg/24 hr) for one year to seven narcoleptic patients who had previously had unsatisfactory responses to more conventional forms of therapy. All seven noted improvement in cataplectic and sleep attacks, although three continued to experience some drowsiness. All reported improvement in their vocational and interpersonal lives. Side effects included hypotension, edema, and impaired sexual function. If medication was discontinued abruptly, depression, anxiety, and sometimes hallucinations were noted. Tapering off the medicine over one to three weeks resulted in reappearance of narcoleptic symptoms without severe psychological disturbances. Polygraphic recordings of patients during treatment showed a decrease in daytime sleep (Fig. 4-3). REM sleep was greatly decreased, for periods of over a year in some cases.

Methysergide

Wyler, Wilkus, and Troùpin (1975) administered the serotonin receptor blocker methysergide (2–4 mg/24 hr) to four patients with narcolepsy and one patient with sleep attacks. All patients had a reduction in sleep attacks comparable to improvement during previous treatment with dextroamphetamine. Cataplexy was less well controlled. Calf muscle claudication was a problem in two patients. Potential use of methysergide with narcoleptics should perhaps await further studies with appropriate controls. Reports of retoperitoneal fibrosis in a small percentage of patients who take methysergide for periods of a year or longer would seem to militate against its long-term use.

Other Pharmacotherapies

In a recent preliminary report, gamma-hydroxy-butyrate (a metabolite of the putative neurotransmitter gamma-aminobutyric acid) was found to reduce daytime sleep attacks, cataplexy, and nocturnal wakefulness in four patients (Broughton and Mamelak, 1975). Trials with

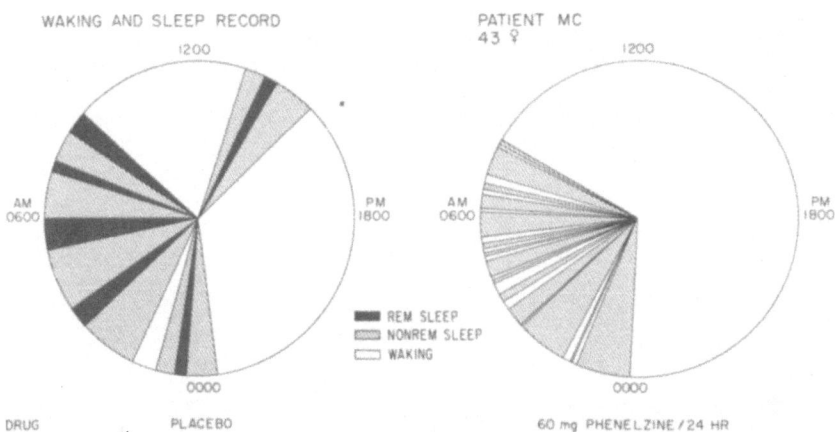

FIGURE 4-3. Effect of phenelzine on 24-hour recordings of a 43-year-old female suffering from overwhelming sleepiness, cataplexy, and sleep paralysis.

amantadine (Ersmark and Lidvall, 1933) and L-DOPA (Gunne, Lidvall, and Widen, 1971) have shown no benefit. Although thyroid extract is frequently given, it is probably of no benefit (Yoss and Daly, 1960a and b).

SUMMARY

Narcolepsy is a condition characterized by sleep attacks plus one or more auxiliary symptoms (cataplexy, hypnogogic hallucinations, and sleep paralysis). Evidence suggests that these symptoms are intrusions of some components of REM sleep into wakefulness. Episodes of excessive daytime sleepiness, without auxiliary symptoms, generally are composed of nonREM sleep. This condition, which is sometimes referred to as "hypersomnia" or "independent narcolepsy," is probably not a single discrete entity, but rather is composed of a variety of conditions. These include the obstructive sleep apnea syndrome, drug abuse, excessive daytime sleepiness with automatic behavior, depression, and a variety of neurologic problems such as brain tumors. Tricyclic antidepressants are effective in treating the auxiliary symptoms of narcolepsy; the stimulants dextroamphetamine and methylphenidate are of benefit in the treatment of sleep attacks. Monoamine oxidase inhibitors may be of use in patients resistant to other forms of therapy.

CHAPTER 5

Clinical Studies of Insomnia

Insomnia can be defined as the subjective feeling that an individual is not sleeping or not getting enough sleep. The important characteristic of insomnia is that it is a symptom, not a sign. The complaint comes from the insomniac himself. It derives from what a person feels, not from observations of him (Kleitman, 1963). "Those who sleep eight hours and believe they need ten consider themselves to be suffering just as much from insomnia as others who cannot get more than four or five hours sleep, but who would be satisfied with six or seven" (Kingman, 1929).

It is clear that there can be discrepancies in what a person thinks his sleep is like and what it is like according to the electroencephalogram (EEG) (Held, Schwartz, and Fischgold, 1959; Schwartz, Guilbaud, and Fischgold, 1963; and Zung, 1968). Patients complaining of insomnia have been examined with EEG techniques. They generally go to sleep quickly, fail to respond to noises, and are oblivious to people in the same room. In the morning, the insomniacs announce they have not closed their eyes all night. Rechtschaffen and Monroe (1969) found that poor sleepers exaggerate the amount of time it takes to fall asleep and once asleep, how long they are able to stay asleep. They also observed that poor sleepers have decreased Rapid Eye Movement (REM) sleep percentage, greater stage 2, more body movements, more changes in sleep stages, greater peripheral vasoconstriction before sleep and during sleep, and a faster heart rate. When awakened from Non-Rapid Eye Movement (nonREM) sleep, insomniacs while in bed claimed they were not sleeping, and remembered that they did more thinking while in bed than did good sleepers. Reichtshaffen concluded his study by saying that even though poor sleepers may be asleep by the EEG, they feel awake and have heightened systemic activity. Thus, the poor sleeper fails to experience whatever restorative benefits sleep has to offer and is uncomfortable.

NORMAL SLEEP

Sheldon (1942), studying behavior in relationship to body type, found endomorphs (fat people who like to eat) enjoy sleep, sleep well, and rarely become insomniacs. Ectomorphs (thin people who are hyper-alert and attentive) dislike going to sleep, but once asleep dislike being awakened. According to Sheldon, the ectomorph becomes an insomniac. Mesomorphs (large-boned, heavy-muscled people who are very athletic) need little sleep and are rarely tired.

Costello and Smith (1963) examined the sleep of medical patients admitted to a hospital and found introverts slept considerably less than extroverts, a finding in agreement with a later study of Tune (1969a). In contrast, Hartmann, Baekeland, and Zwilling (1972) studied volunteers free of overt medical and psychiatric pathology who regularly slept either less than six hours or more than nine hours. The short sleepers were efficient, hardworking, and somewhat hypomanic. The long sleepers were anxious, depressed, or withdrawn. Both groups had the same amount of delta sleep, but the long sleepers had twice as much REM sleep. The authors proposed that the amount of REM sleep is related to personality and life-styles. A similar EEG study by Webb and Agnew (1970) also found long sleepers had more REM sleep. Brewer and Hartmann (1973), using a questionnaire, found that of many life situations, the only one that decreased the sleep need was "when everything was going well."

Tune (1969b), using a questionnaire in a study of 509 volunteer adults, found that the mean duration of sleep declined until age 60, when there was a slight rise. At age 20, the mean duration of sleep was 8.0 hours, while at age 50 it was 7.2 hours. By age 70, however, it had risen to 7.6 hours. Older people chose to go to bed earlier and awaken earlier. The number of nighttime awakenings increased steadily from age 20 to 70, with there being 6.5 times as many awakenings at age 70 as at age 20 (see Fig. 1-8). Johns et al. (1970) found similar results, as did Kahn and Fisher (1969), who used EEG techniques. (A more detailed account of the changes in sleep at different ages is presented in chapter 1.)

McGhie and Russell (1962) questioned 2500 persons in Scotland, representing a cross section of the country. They found that women had less sleep than men. Advancing age again was highly correlated with decreased sleep. However, only the young complained of being tired in the morning, indicating that perhaps older people need less sleep. Feinberg, Koresko, and Heller (1967), using EEG techniques, found that the normal elderly (65 to 96 years) have more wakefulness and sleep interruptions than do the young. The total amount of sleep, however, was different since the elderly spent about 50 minutes more in bed per night. This was also a finding in a study of Kales *et al.* (1967b). In these studies, stage 4 sleep also decreased with age. It should be realized, however, that the amount of sleep normals of any age receive varies greatly from individual to individual.

Weiss, Kasinoff, and Bailey (1962) questioned 100 general medical outpatients, 100 psychiatric clinic outpatients, and 100 healthy persons of similar ages. The psychiatric group had four times the sleep problems as the healthy persons and medical patients. Despite arthritis and other problems that might tend to prevent sleep, the medical patients were no different from the healthy controls. Married persons sleep less than single and, again, increasing age was associated with less sleep.

It should be pointed out that there are individuals who sleep as little as three hours every 24 hours without complaint (Jones and Oswald, 1968). Recently Meddis, Pearson, and Langford (1973), using EEG techniques, confirmed a 70-year-old woman's report that she slept only 52 minutes per 24 hours and was wide awake and happy the rest of the time.

INCIDENCE OF INSOMNIA

In a questionnaire sampling of 1,645 persons, Karacan *et al.* (1973) found 14% often had trouble getting to sleep. Rates were higher as age increased and were higher for women than men. Two percent of the individuals had frequent nightmares. Kales *et al.* (1969a), in a California survey of physicians' patients, found that 38% had been taking hypnotics for one month or more and 54% for one month or less. Tiller (1964), studying 83 healthy office patients of 60 years or over, found that 21% complained of insomnia, slightly higher than the 15% generally given for the population at large.

KINDS OF INSOMNIA

Prior to attempting to describe the kinds of insomnia that can occur, brief mention should be made of the overall problem of sleep disorders. In addition to the subjective feeling of not having enough sleep, which we define as insomnia, a person can walk and talk in his sleep, have rhythmic body rocking, wet the bed, etc. He can also have narcolepsy, hypersomnia, or other forms of daytime sleepiness. Wetting the bed (enuresis) can be disruptive to sleep, but is usually not associated with insomnia. This at times can be treated successfully with tricyclic drugs such as imipramine (Kales *et al.*, 1970a; Maxwell and Seldrup, 1971).

TENTATIVE LIST OF CAUSES OF INSOMNIA

This list of causes of insomnia is not all inclusive. As the study of insomnia progresses, this list will become longer with more logical subdivisions.

I. Psychogenic
   A. Anxiety (Fodor, 1945; Olden, 1942; Rothenberg, 1947; Wexberg, 1949)
      1. Acute
      2. Chronic
   B. Depression (see chap. 7)
      1. Acute
      2. Chronic
   C. Ruminative (Coursey, Buchsbaum, and Frankel, 1975): This form of insomnia can be distinguished from anxiety because of the constant attempt at problem-solving without accompanying tense feelings. This sleep may be associated with excess alpha rhythm in the EEG (Phillips, Mitler, and Dement, 1974).
   D. Sexual Arousal: Unrelieved sexual arousal may make falling asleep difficult in some individuals. Relaxation after orgasm is, however, highly variable (Kinsey *et al.*, 1953). Some people are ready for vigorous exercise or mental activity after orgasm while others are fatigued, particularly at night.
   E. Fear of phenomena associated with sleep
      1. Fear of loss of consciousness
      2. Fear of death during sleep
      3. Fear of content of dreams (Gilman, 1958)
      4. Fear of not sleeping, which can contribute considerably to the problems of individuals already having insomnia
   F. Other psychiatric disturbances: Monroe (1967) and Kales and Cary (1971), for example, found poor sleepers had more psy-

chopathology on the MMPI and Cornell Medical Index than good sleepers. There thus may be a large part of the "normal" population with considerable psychopathology, as has frequently been found in large population surveys. Acute schizophrenics may not sleep for many nights (Kupfer *et al.*, 1970c) and chronic schizophrenics can have markedly reduced sleep (Kaplan *et al.*, 1974).

II. Situational: Includes excess noise (Kramer *et al.*, 1971), bright light, uncomfortable beds, crowded beds, etc. Older individuals seem less adaptable to unusual situations than younger individuals (Lukas, 1972). Monroe (1969) found married couples had less stage 4 and REM sleep when they slept together than when they slept apart. It is not clear, however, if the loss of stage 4 sleep is perceived as insomnia.

III. Alterations of normal activity—rest cycle: This normally occurs with traveling, particularly to different time zones (Nicholson, 1970). It is also common in hospitals. We recently saw a person whose biological clock was very different from his social one. He had an important administrative position that required him to be at work at 7:00 A.M.. He had never been able to fall asleep before 3:00 A.M. and needed eight hours of sleep, which, once he fell asleep, took place naturally. Thus, his biological clock that said, "Go to bed at 3:00 A.M. and get up at 11:00 A.M." was inconsistent with his and most people's social clock.

IV. Dream related

  A. Dream interruption: Awakening from REM periods and having difficulty falling back to sleep (Greenberg, 1967)

  B. Nightmares are associated with arousal, are dreams of mild to moderate intensity and occur during REM sleep. They are much more common than night terrors (Fisher *et al.*, 1970). Night terrors *(pavor nocturnus)* are a combination of panic, attempts to fight or flee while asleep, utterances that may include bloodcurdling screams. They occur during stage 4 sleep. The entire episode lasts only a minute or two and there is usually amnesia for it (Broughton, 1968). Fisher *et al.* (1973) found that 2 to 20 mg of diazepam taken before bed decreased the incidence of night terrors and stage 4 sleep. Hällström (1972) followed cases of night terrors through three generations of a family and suggested they may be hereditary. A chronic form of dream-related sleep disturbance was described (Eitinger, 1964) in a group of 60 Nazi concentration camp survivors. They had sleep disturbances with nightmares persisting for over 15 years. The nightmares were directly related to the concentration camp experiences.

V. Sleep apnea (Gastaut *et al.*, 1969; Lugaresi *et al.*, 1973; Guilleminault, Eldridge, and Dement, 1972b) is a syndrome associated with excessive sleepiness during the day, restlessness at night (insomnia), and apnea (failure to breathe) that may last for 10 seconds or longer. The apnea only occurs during sleep. When awake, the individual may appear to be entirely normal except for his sleepiness. Obstructive sleep apnea has been described in chapter 4. *Central* sleep apnea, which is thought to be produced by a disorder in the nervous system, is characterized by a failure of the diaphragm and accessory muscles to contract for periods up to three minutes. It occurs primarily in males. It may first be seen in children. Since the disorder is so disturbing, considerable psychological changes can accompany it. Patients with sleep apnea can have serious associated cardiopulmonary abnormalities. Sleep apnea can be diagnosed by careful nighttime recording of a patient's sleep using an abdominal strain gauge and nasal thermistors for measuring air flow. Patients with sleep apnea frequently snore and it has been suggested that the placement of a tape recorder in the room of the patient can help in the diagnosis.

VI. Restless legs syndrome is characterized by severe, difficult-to-describe dysesthesia (rather than paresthesia or actual pain) that is felt deep within the legs and rarely in the arms. It is relieved or avoided by leg movement. The syndrome occurs mainly when at rest and produces insomnia because the leg movements prevent falling asleep (Ekbom, 1960; Frankel, Patten, and Gillin, 1974).

VII. Nocturnal myoclonus occurs once an individual is asleep. Jerking occurs in both anterior tibialis muscles in the lower leg corresponding to EEG arousals. It is usually recognized by a bed partner.

VIII. Oversleeping: Staying in bed or sleeping very long periods can lead to a feeling of tiredness and poor sleep. Taub *et al.*, 1971 found that subjects who extended their normal sleep did poorly on vigilance and motor tasks.

IX. Drug related
  A. Acute
    1. Due to stimulants such as caffeine: For example, Karacan, Booth, and Thornby (1973) found that caffeine in amounts equivalent to four cups of coffee taken just before bedtime increased awakenings from sleep in normals.

2. Paradoxical: Stimulant effects (opposite from the drug's usual sedative effects) can occur from drugs such as alcohol, or hypnotics, particularly in the young or elderly.
   B. Chronic
   1. Dependency: Chronic use of hypnotics that initially increase sleep, but when given for a long enough period of time, produce fractured sleep. When this happens, discontinuence of hypnotics must be very gradual in order to avoid withdrawal symptoms.
   2. Withdrawal
      (a) Hypnotics (Kales et al., 1969b)
      (b) Alcohol (Mello and Mendelson, 1970). This is discussed at length in chapter 6.
      (c) Other examples—opiates (Oswald, 1968)
   X. Neurological: An example of this is a patient described by Guilleminault et al. (1973a) who suffered from hyposomnia following an automobile accident. Fischer-Perroudon, Mouret, Jouvet (1973) described a 27-year-old man who had a complaint of muscular fasiculations, distal pains, diarrhea, and insomnia (Choree fibrillaire de Morvan). Despite total lack of sleep, the patient never felt sleepy. Hallucinations were enhanced by tryptophan loading and disappeared with high dosages of 5-hydroxytryptophan (5-HTP), which also restored normal sleep. The implications of this finding on theories of the regulation of sleep are described in chapter 2.
   XI. Secondary to or accompanying a medical illness. The wakening at 2:00 A.M. from the pain of a duodenal ulcer (Dragstedt, 1959; Armstrong et al., 1965) or nocturnal angina (Nowlin et al., 1965; Snyder, 1967) or nocturnal asthma (Kales et al., 1968; Ravenscroft and Hartmann, 1968) are frequent producers of insomnia and are common complaints to the internist.

SLEEP INDUCTION

Synthetic substances for inducing sleep were introduced over a century ago by Liebreich (1869), who reported on chloral hydrate use. In 1883 Cervello introduced paraldehyde because of concern over chloral hydrates' "toxicity." Barbital was introduced in 1903 (Fisher and von Mering), and became the parent for a whole series of barbiturate derivatives. Subsequently, bromides, as well as many other hypnotics, came into use.

The quest for effective but safe hypnotics has persisted. Hypnotics or other medicines that have a hypnotic effect are the most frequently prescribed drugs. There are currently about 50 prescription sedative-hypnotics in the *Physicians' Desk Reference* (PDR) and perhaps an equal number sold as over-the-counter agents in the United States.

Despite the large expenditure in developing effective and safe hypnotics, and the enormous monetary and human expenditure that comes from drug use and abuse, very little has been done to understand the problem of insomnia. Only in the last five years have there been sleep clinics devoted to the study, diagnosis, and treatment of sleep problems. At the same time, the Food and Drug Administration and drug manufacturers have worked to demonstrate that their drugs are both useful and safe.

For the purposes of judging a good hypnotic for widespread use, the following criteria might be used:

1. The drug should be given orally.

2. It must produce a state with as little loss of natural sleep stages as possible. There is currently no evidence that the loss of natural sleep stages in the adult is injurious. Before accepting this as fact, however, more investigation is needed.

3. The hypnotic effect should cease at the desired time without leaving any aftereffects. The individual should awaken refreshed.

4. There should be no side effects.

5. With prolonged use, the drug should continue to be effective; neither tolerance nor physical dependence should develop.

6. Overdoses should neither lead to prolonged sleep nor other dangers, including death.

There is no currently available drug that fits all of these criteria fully, but the following examines some of what we do know about them.

It is rather surprising that many of the first electrophysiological studies of the hypnotics in sleep laboratories were carried out on individuals without insomnia. Although this situation has begun to change, the majority of controlled studies are ones that use either nurses' observations or self-evaluation, usually for only several days, and for the most part, in patients having significant psychiatric and medical illness. While non-EEG observational techniques may not be as reliable as the EEG and certainly do not answer the question of drug induction of normal sleep, they do allow for the gathering of considerable information quickly and with only moderate expense. Subjective questionnaires are particularly useful, since they give an estimate of how the patient felt about his sleep. With questionnaires, at least we know the symptoms are being treated, something the EEG will not tell us.

Alcohol

Probably the most often used hypnotic is alcohol. Despite almost universal experience that alcohol is soporific, we found no double-blind studies demonstrating this in patients with insomnia. While temperate use of alcohol may be useful, chronic alcohol use produces fragmented sleep (Allen et al., 1971; Mello and Mendelson, 1970; Johnson, Burdick, and Smith, 1970; Gross et al., 1973; and Lester et al., 1973), a disturbance known since the time of Galen (Leibowitz, 1967). A comprehensive review of alcohol and sleep is presented in chapter 6.

Benzodiazepines

Tables 5-1 and 5-2 depict the effect of benzodiazepines on the sleep of insomniacs. There are few studies of lorazepam, nitrazepam, and diazepam, but those that were done indicate they are effective hypnotics. Our own clinical experience suggests diazepam 10 mg both decreases sleep latency and increases total sleep when taken for several days. We have no experience with longer administration. In fact, many patients prefer diazepam to flurazepam. Diazepam, however, is not officially recognized as a sleeping medication in the United States.

Flurazepam is the best-studied of the hypnotics. It shortens sleep latency, decreases intermittent awakenings, and increases total sleep. It decreases slow-wave sleep. A 30-mg dose does not seem to decrease the amount or percent of REM sleep, but does decrease the REM density. Chlordiazepoxide is not a good hypnotic.

For some people, the problem of hypnotic hangover is a significant one. When specific attempts to examine this problem were made, they are referred to in the tables. One particularly useful study was done by Harper and Kidera of United Airlines (1972). They gave flurazepam (30 mg) or glutethimide (500 mg) to 30 aviators for two nights. They found in using a flight simulator that there was no deficit in performance 12 hours after taking either drug. When possible, patients who are prescribed hypnotics should take the lowest reasonable dosage (for example, 15 mg flurazepam) on a night when they do not actually expect insomnia and when it is not important that they function at their best the following day, and when someone is available should they need help.

TABLE 5-1. The Effects of Flurazepam on Insomnia

Study	Drug	Dose mg/night	Subjects	Hangover	Feeling fit	Patients studied 1–7 nights					
						SL	SWS	RS	INTA	EMA	TS
Jacobson et al., 1970*	Flurazepam	30	40 hospitalized psychiatric patients	—	—	→	—	—	→	—	↑
Kales et al., 1971b; Allen, Scharf, Kales, 1971a; Bixler, Scharf, Kales, 1973; Kales and Scharf, 1973	Flurazepam	30	Insomniacs	—	—	→	→	→	→	—	↑
Vogel et al., 1971	Flurazepam	15	Insomniacs	—	—	→	→	0	—	—	↑
Bignotti et al., 1972†	Flurazepam	30	20 insomniacs	—	—	←	—	—	←	—	↑
Panaccio and Tetreault, 1972†	Flurazepam	30	61 psychiatric patients with insomnia	—	—	→·→	→·→	—	—	→	↑
Dement et al., 1973c	Flurazepam	15 / 30	4 insomniacs / 4 insomniacs	— / —	— / —	→·→	—	→·→	→·0	— / —	←·←·←
Meyer and Kurland, 1973*	Flurazepam	30	28 medical patients	—	—	—	—	—	—	—	←

Study	Patients studied 7–30 nights						Patients studied greater than 30 nights					
	SL	SWS	RS	INTA	EMA	TS	SL	SWS	RS	INTA	EMA	TS
Jacobson et al., 1970*	—	—	—	—	—	—	—	—	—	—	—	—
Kales et al., 1971b; Allen, Scharf, Kales, 1971a; Bixler, Scharf, Kales, 1973; Kales and Scharf, 1973	→	→	→	→	—	←	—	—	→	—	—	—
Vogel et al., 1971	—	—	—	—	—	—	—	—	—	—	—	—
Bignotti et al., 1972†	—	—	—	—	—	—	—	—	—	—	—	—
Panaccio and Tetreault, 1972†	—	—	—	—	—	—	—	—	—	—	—	—
Dement et al., 1973c	—	—	—	—	—	—	—	—	—	—	—	—
Meyer and Kurland, 1973*	—	—	—	—	—	—	—	—	—	—	—	—

All studies were done with EEG techniques except as noted.
* Nurses' ratings.
†Data about sleep from questionnaire given in A.M.
N.S. = Not stated.
SL = Sleep latency.
SWS = Slow-wave sleep-delta.
RS = REM sleep or some parameter of it.
INT A = Intermittent awakening.
EMA = Early morning awakening.
TS = Total sleep.

TABLE 5-2. The Effects of Benzodiazepines (Not Including Flurazepam) on Insomnia

Study	Drug	Dose mg/night	Subjects	Hangover	Feeling fit
Bordeleau, Charland, and Tetreault, 1970*	Chlordiazepoxide	50	64 psychiatric patients	—	—
Bordeleau, Charland, and Tetreault, 1970*	Nitrazepam	10	64 psychiatric patients	—	—
Bordeleau, Charland, and Tetreault, 1970*	Diazepam	10	64 psychiatric patients	—	—
Globus et al., 1973	Lorazepam	1–5	6 insomniacs	—	—
Kales and Scharf, 1973	Chlordiazepoxide	25–50	Psychiatric patients; insomniacs	—	—

Study	Patients studied 1–7 nights						Patients studied 7–30 nights					
	SL	SWS	RS	INTA	EMA	TS	SL	SWS	RS	INTA	EMA	TS
Bordeleau, Charland, and Tetreault, 1970*	—	—	—	—	—	0	—	—	—	—	—	—
Bordeleau, Charland, and Tetreault, 1970*	—	—	—	—	—	↑	—	—	—	—	—	—
Bordeleau, Charland, and Tetreault, 1970*	—	—	—	—	—	↑	—	—	—	—	—	—
Globus et al., 1973	—	—	—	—	—	—	—	0	0	—	—	↑
Kales and Scharf, 1973	↓	—	—	0	—	0	—	—	—	—	—	—

All studies were done with EEG techniques except as noted.
* Nurses' ratings.
N.S. = Not stated.
SL = Sleep latency.
SWS = Slow-wave sleep = delta.
RS = REM sleep or some parameter of it.
INT A = Intermittent awakening.
EMA = Early morning awakening.
TS = Total sleep.

Mebutamate

One study of mebutamate (Table 5-3) in a psychiatric population indicated it was a good hypnotic when used for periods of a month or greater.

Barbiturates

Until Lasagna's 1956 studies comparing secobarbital, pentobarbital, and phenobarbital in patients with chronic disease and insomnia, clinicians made the analogy from animal studies to man that phenobarbital was the best of the barbiturates for inducing and sustaining sleep. Lasagna's controlled studies, however, found equal dosages of pentobarbital to be better than phenobarbital. From Table 5-4 it can be seen that barbiturates, with the exception of butabarbital (which in one study did not decrease sleep latency) improve all parameters of poor sleep. While the barbiturates produce a hangover, they do not seem to do so more frequently than placebo (Lasagna, 1956).

Chloral Hydrate

Chloral hydrate is recognized clinically as a good hypnotic, but has been studied rarely under controlled conditions (Table 5-3). One disadvantage, however, is that it has a relatively low therapeutic index. The lethal dose is relatively close to the therapeutic dose.

Glutethimide

Glutethimide has been studied in a small number of patients. It does seem to decrease sleep latency, but has questionable effects on total sleep (Table 5-3).

Methaqualone

Methaqualone both decreases sleep latency, intermittent awakenings, and increases total sleep (Table 5-3).

Diphenhydramine

Diphenhydramine is a clinically useful hypnotic. The few controlled studies with insomniacs indicated that it is effective and has rela-

TABLE 5-3. The Effect of Other Drugs on Insomnia

Study	Drug	Dose mg/night	Subjects	Hangover	Feeling fit	Patients studied 1–7 nights					
						SL	SWS	RS	INTA	EMA	TS
Scharf, Allen, and Kales, 1970	Glutethimide	500	4 insomniacs	—	—	→	—	—	0	0	0
Goldstein et al., 1970; Goldstein, Stoltzfus, Smith, 1971	Glutethimide	500	5 insomniacs	—	—	→	0	→	→	—	←
Lelek and Danhauser, 1970	Methaqualone	200	60 insomniacs	—	—	→	—	—	—	—	←
Von Hoffmeister and Koller, 1970†	Methaqualone	250	72 patients	—	—	→	—	—	→	—	←
Goldstein et al., 1970	Methaqualone	300	5 insomniacs	—	—	→	→	0	—	←	—
Goldstein, Stoltzfus and Smith, 1971	Methaqualone	300	5 insomniacs	—	—	→	→	0	—	←	—
Kales, Bixler, and Kales, 1974a	Methaqualone	300	Insomniacs	—	—	→	—	—	—	—	—
Jick et al., 1969†	Chloral hydrate	500	50 hospitalized patients	—	—	—	—	—	—	—	←
Ayd, 1972†	Mebutamate	300 600	180 psychiatric outpatients with insomnia	—	← ←	← ←	—	—	—	—	← ←

Study	Patients studied 7–30 nights						Patients studied greater than 30 nights					
	SL	SWS	RS	INTA	EMA	TS	SL	SWS	RS	INTA	EMA	TS
Scharf, Allen, and Kales, 1970	0	—	—	0	0	0	—	—	—	—	—	—
Goldstein et al., 1970; Goldstein, Stoltzfus, Smith, 1971	—	—	—	—	—	—	—	—	—	—	—	—
Lelek and Danhauser, 1970	—	—	—	—	—	—	—	—	—	—	—	—
Von Hoffmeister and Koller, 1970†	—	—	—	—	—	—	—	—	—	—	—	—
Goldstein et al., 1970	—	—	—	—	—	—	—	—	—	—	—	—
Goldstein, Stoltzfus, and Smith, 1971	—	—	—	—	—	—	—	—	—	—	—	—
Kales, Bixler, and Kales, 1974a	—	—	—	—	—	—	—	—	—	—	—	—
Jick et al., 1969†	←	—	—	—	—	←	→	—	—	—	—	—
Ayd, 1972†	←	—	—	—	—	←	—	—	—	—	—	←

All studies were done with EEG techniques except as noted.
* Nurses' ratings.
† Data about sleep from questionnaire given in A.M.
N.S. = Not stated.
SL = Sleep latency.
SWS = Slow-wave sleep-delta.
RS = REM sleep or some parameter of it.
INT A = Intermittent awakening.
EMA = Early morning awakening.
TS = Total sleep.

TABLE 5-4. The Effects of Barbiturates on Insomnia

Study	Drug	Dose mg/night	Subjects	Hangover	Feeling fit
Lasagna, 1956†	Secobarbital	100	59 hospitalized	↑	—
	Secobarbital	200	patients	↑	—
	Phenobarbital	100	with chronic	↑	—
	Phenobarbital	200	disease and	↑	—
	Pentobarbital	100	insomnia	↑	—
	Pentobarbital	200		↑	—
Hinton, 1963a†*	Cyclobarbital	200	24 psychiatric	—	—
	Hexobarbital	500	patients	—	—
	Quinabarbital	100		—	—
	Quinabarbital	200		—	—
	Pentobarbital	200		—	—
	Phenobarbital	200		—	—
	Nealbarbital	200		—	—
Oswald et al., 1963	Heptabarbital	400	6 patients with melancholia and insomnia	—	—
Feinberg et al., 1969a	Phenobarbital	200	3 schizophrenics and sociopaths	—	—
Jick et al., 1969*	Pentobarbital	100	50 hospitalized patients	—	—
Bordeleau, Charland, Tetreault, 1970*	Seeobarbital	200	64 psychiatric patients	—	—
Stotsky et al., 1971†	Butabarbital	50	53 aged psychiatric	0	↑
	Butabarbital	100	patients with sleep disorders	0	0
Pattison, Allen, 1972*	Secobarbital	100	50 hospitalized	0	—
	Pentobarbital	100	patients with chronic disease & insomnia	0	—
Panaccio and Tetreault, 1972*	Secobarbital	100	6 psychiatric patients with insomnia	—	—
Stewart et al., 1973†*	Amylobarbital	200	100 patients on medical wards with insomnia	0	—
Kales, Bixler, and Kales, 1974a	Secobarbital	100	Insomniacs	—	—

All studies were done with EEG techniques except as noted
* Nurses' ratings.
† Data about sleep from questionnaire given in A.M.
N.S = Not stated
SL = Sleep latency.
SWS = Slow-wave sleep = delta.
RS = REM sleep or some parameter of it.
INT A = Intermittent awakening.
EMA = Early morning awakening.
TS = Total sleep.

Patients studied 1–7 nights						Patients studied 7–30 nights					
SL	SWS	RS	INTA	EMA	TS	SL	SWS	RS	INTA	EMA	TS
↓	—	—	↓	—	↑	—	—	—	—	—	—
↓	—	—	↓	—	↑	—	—	—	—	—	—
↓	—	—	↓	—	↑	—	—	—	—	—	—
↓	—	—	↓	—	↑	—	—	—	—	—	—
↓	—	—	↓	—	↑	—	—	—	—	—	—
↓	—	—	↓	—	↑	—	—	—	—	—	—
0	—	—	—	—	↑	—	—	—	—	—	—
0	—	—	—	—	↑	—	—	—	—	—	—
0	—	—	—	—	↑	—	—	—	—	—	—
0	—	—	—	—	⏐	—	—	—	—	—	—
0	—	—	—	—	↑	—	—	—	—	—	—
0	—	—	—	—	↑	—	—	—	—	—	—
0	—	—	—	—	↑	—	—	—	—	—	—
—	—	↓	↓	↓	↑	—	—	—	—	—	—
—	—	↓	↓	—	↑	—	—	—	—	—	—
—	—	—	—	—	↑	—	—	—	—	—	—
—	—	—	—	—	↑	—	—	—	—	—	—
0	—	—	↓	—	↑	↓	—	—	↓	—	↑
0	—	—	↓	—	↑	↓	—	—	↓	—	↑
↓	—	—	0	—	↑	—	—	—	—	—	—
↓	—	—	↓	—	↑	—	—	—	—	—	—
—	—	—	—	—	↑	—	—	—	—	—	—
↓	—	—	↓	—	↑	—	—	—	—	—	—
↓	—	—	↓	—	↑	0	0	—	—	0	0

tively few adverse effects. Long-term studies have not been done (Table 5-5).

L-Tryptophan

L-Tryptophan is not marketed as a hypnotic, but is included here because there are a number of reports that it increases total sleep in insomniacs. Because it is a substance that is ingested in our food, it has advantages over conventional drugs. It is hard to imagine, for example, someone becoming allergic to it. Large dosages produce nausea and vomiting that would decrease the likelihood of an overdose (Table 5-6). Implications of observations with L-tryptophan on theories of sleep regulation are discussed in chapter 2.

Electrosleep

Electrosleep or cerebral electrotherapy was designed by Giliarorsky (1958) to enhance or induce natural sleep. As it is currently used, however, cerebral electrotherapy is given during the daytime for a number of days. Its effects are supposed to last for many nights thereafter.

Weiss (1973), using double-blind procedures, found electrosleep given for 24 days decreased sleep latency in patients with insomnia. As used in a study by Frankel, Buchbinder, and Snyder, 1973 (a 15- or 100-Hz square wave of 1-second duration) direct current was applied from the eyes to the mastoid for 45 minutes, for 30 weekdays. This study, using good controls, found no effect in 17 patients with chronic primary insomnia.

AN APPROACH TO PATIENTS WHO COMPLAIN OF INSOMNIA

The examination of a person complaining of insomnia is no different from that a physician would use for any other patient. Careful attention is paid to the sleep history, the onset of the insomnia, how it is perceived, what has been tried in the past, and what success there has been. Referring letters or calls to past physicians and paramedical professionals are most important. The importance of a review of systems with emphasis on any psychological difficulties and drug use (including alcohol) cannot be overemphasized. Naturally, a complete

TABLE 5-5. The Effects of Antihistamines on Insomnia

Study	Drug	Dose mg/night	Subjects	Hangover	Feeling fit	SL	SWS	RS	INTA	EMA	TS
Jick et al., 1969†	Diphenhydramine	50	50 hospitalized patients	—	—	—	—	—	—	—	↑
Teutsch et al., 1975*	Diphenhydramine	50	159 hospitalized patients	—	—	↓	—	—	—	—	↑
	Methapyrilene	50	159 hospitalized patients								
Vogel et al., 1975a	Diphenhydramine	50	6 insomniacs	—	—	↓	—	↓	↓	—	↑

All studies were done with EEG techniques except as noted.
* Nurses' ratings.
† Data about sleep from questionnaire given in A.M.
SL = Sleep latency.
SWS = Slow-wave sleep = delta.
RS = REM sleep or some parameter of it.
INT A = Intermittent awakening.
EMA = Early morning awakening.
TS = Total sleep.

TABLE 5-6. The Effects of L-Tryptophan on Insomnia

Study	Drug	Dose mg/night	Subjects	Hangover	Feeling fit	Patients studied 1–7 nights					
						SL	SWS	RS	INTA	EMA	TS
Cazzulo et al., 1969	L-tryptophan	N.S.	6 depressed patients with insomnia	—	—	0	—	—	0	—	↑
Wyatt et al., 1970a	L-tryptophan	7,500	7 patients with insomnia; 2 with history of depression	0	—	0	0	0	→	→	↑
Hartmann, Chung, and Chien, 1971*	L-tryptophan	2,000	14 chronic schizophrenics with insomnia	0	↑	0	—	—	0	—	0
		3,000		0	↑	0	—	—	0	—	0
		4,000		0	↑	→	—	—	→	—	↑
		5,000		0	↑	→	—	—	→	—	↑
Makipour, Iber, and Hartmann, 1972*	L-tryptophan	5,000	29 chronic schizophrenics	0	0	→	—	—	—	—	↑
Brezinova, Loudon, and Oswald, 1972	L-tryptophan	7,500	6 patients during withdrawal from known hypnotics	—	—	0	—	—	—	—	—

All studies were done with EEG techniques except as noted.
* Nurses' ratings.
N.S. = Not stated.
SL = Sleep latency.
SWS = Slow-wave sleep = delta.
RS = REM sleep or some parameter of it.
INT A = Intermittent awakening.
EMA = Early morning awakening.
TS = Total sleep.

physical examination including testing of neurological functions should be performed. If the diagnosis can be made, a treatment program can be tried. If the diagnosis is in doubt or any adequate treatment program cannot be found, we suggest a referral to one of the several sleep clinics usually associated with major university medical centers.

CHAPTER 6

Alcohol, Alcoholism, and the Problem of Dependence

Investigators of both sleep physiology and alcoholism share several common interests. Ethanol ingestion affects the EEG sleep stages. It may also modify the metabolism of the biogenic amines, which are thought to play an important role in the regulation of sleep (see chaps. 1 and 2). Finally, there is some evidence to suggest that a disorder of sleep stage regulation may be involved in the withdrawal syndromes that occur when the chronic ingestion of ethanol is discontinued.

Each of the above areas will be discussed in this chapter, in terms of knowledge gained from animal studies, effects of ethanol on sleep of normal humans, and effects in patients with alcohol addiction.

ANIMAL STUDIES

Ethanol and the Sleep EEG of Animals

One of the earliest animal studies on the effects of ethanol on sleep was performed by Yules *et al.* (1966b). They found that oral administration of 1.0 gm/kg produced a small but significant (8–14%) decrease in REM sleep time during seven-hour recordings of cats. This effect, which was most pronounced during the first half of the night, was due to decreases in the mean duration of REM sleep episodes, with no systematic changes in number of episodes or REM latency. During successive nights of administration, percentage REM time rose until it returned to normal on the fourth night. As will be seen later in this chapter, the decrease in percentage REM due to shortened mean duration of episodes, with a return to baseline values on subsequent nights, is consistent with data obtained from normal humans.

Two studies have examined the problem of whether the sleep EEG effects of ethanol are dose related. Branchey, Begleiter, and Kissin (1970) administered acute intraperitoneal injections of 0.5 or 1.5 gm/kg ethanol to 12 chronically implanted rats, and an EEG was recorded for 24 hours. It was found that nonREM sleep was increased at both doses, particularly in the first few hours after injection. At the lower dose, the percentage of REM sleep was unchanged, but after 1.5 gm/kg of ethanol, it decreased during the first six hours. Mendelson and Hill (1976) administered ethanol in doses of 1.1, 1.5, 2.0, and 2.5 gm/kg intraperitoneally to groups of six rats each, and performed seven-hour EEG recordings. As doses of ethanol increased, percentage of nonREM sleep progressively increased, and percentage REM sleep decreased. These effects were seen most strongly in the first 3.5 hours of recording. The number of awakenings did not change in a systematic manner in the recordings as a whole. They did, however, increase with higher doses of ethanol during the second 3.5-hour period. Interestingly, the percentage of sleep in the total recording was unchanged. As will be seen later, this lack of effect on total sleep time is a common observation in studies of normal humans.

Gitlow *et al.* (1973) stressed the possibility that ethanol may produce effects on the sleep EEG long after administration has been discontinued. They gave a total dose of 4–9 gm/kg of ethanol orally to rats daily for 4–6 weeks. The animals were then housed and fed normally for 6–8 months. When new recordings were performed, there were no changes in total minutes of REM sleep or number of REM sleep episodes, compared to saline-fed controls. On the other hand, the post-ethanol rats responded quite differently from controls when a test dose of 4 gm/kg of ethanol was given. After ethanol, both groups had a reduction in total minutes of REM sleep and the number of REM sleep episodes. In the group that had received ethanol several months earlier, however, this effect was much more pronounced. Thus, there was a persistent abnormal REM sleep response to ethanol months after chronic administration had been discontinued.

Ethanol and Behavioral Measures of Sleep

In addition to the EEG studies, behavioral observations of sleep have provided some interesting insights. It has been shown that mice can be selectively bred to develop strains that differ in length of behaviorally defined sleep in response to acute injections of ethanol (Heston et al., 1974; Randall and Lester, 1974; Camjanovich and MacInnes, 1973). Camjanovich and MacInnes (1973) concluded that differences in blood alcohol clearance accounted for difference in sleep time; on the other hand, Heston et al. (1974) found no difference in clearance rates between long-sleeping and short-sleeping strains, and concluded that the differences in sleep time were related to differing CNS sensitivities to alcohol. Randall and Lester (1974) found that strains that differ in sleep time after ethanol had similar sleep time in response to phenobarbital. Thus, the hypnotic effect of ethanol in a strain seemed to be specific to that agent, and not generalized to other sedatives.

Ethanol and Possible Neurotransmitters

Ethanol-induced sleep time may be influenced by pharmacologic manipulation of biogenic amine levels. Pretreatment with the catecholamine synthesis inhibitor alpha-methyl-p-tyrosine (Figure 2-8) enhances the ethanol sleep time response (Erickson and Matchett, 1974), and this effect is decreased by administration of L-DOPA (Blum et al., 1972). Parachlorophenylalanine, which decreases serotonin synthesis (Figure 2-1) has been reported to have either no effect (Blum et al., 1972) or produce an increase (Erickson and Matchett, 1974) in sleep time. Although the serotonin precursors tryptophan and 5-hydroxytryptophan (Figure 2-1) have been reported to have no effect on ethanol sleep time (Blum et al., 1972), serotonin itself has been reported to increase it (Merritt and Geller, 1973).

Changes in the cholinergic system may also influence ethanol-induced sleep time. It is shortened by administration of physostigmine, which increases cholinergic activity (Ericson and Burnam, 1971).

It can be seen, then, that changes in biogenic amines and acetylcholine in the CNS may influence the hypnotic effect of ethanol; conversely, ethanol itself may produce changes in levels of CNS biogenic amines. Experimental data has been generally thought to fall into two categories: that alcohol acts similarly to the MAO inhibitors, or that it acts similarly to reserpine (Williams and Salamy, 1972). Perhaps consistent with the first hypothesis are a variety of studies showing that ethanol administration is related to decreased formation of 5-HIAA, the product of oxidative metabolism of serotonin (Feldstein, 1973; Davis et al., 1967a; Rosenfeld, 1960). The former two authors suggested that ethanol causes a shift in serotonin metabolism away from the oxidative route in favor of reductive metabolism, resulting in formation of 5-hydroxytryptophol. The tryptophols, derived from serotonin metabolism that has been altered by ethanol, may induce sleep (Feldstein et al., 1970). It has been speculated that ethanol might also act directly on whatever hypothesized receptors interact with the tryptophols to produce sedation (Williams and Salamy, 1972). A similar change in the metabolism of norepinephrine has been reported in studies of metabolites in urine of humans: There was a shift away from the usual excretory product (3-methoxy-4-hydroxy-mandelic acid) in favor of 3-methoxy-5-hydroxyphenylglycol (Davis et al., 1967b). More recent studies of brain tissue in rats, however, failed to show this shift from an oxidative to a reductive pathway (Karoum, Wyatt, and Majchrowicz, 1976).

The second hypothesis—that ethanol acts in a manner similar to reserpine—receives support from a variety of studies. Gursey and Olson (1961) reported that acute intravenous injection of ethanol results in lowered brainstem serotonin and norepinephrine in the rabbit. Pscheidt, Issekuty, and Himwich (1961) did not observe a decrease in serotonin after acute treatment, but did report decreases in serotonin and norepinephrine after five daily injections of ethanol. In contrast, serotonin levels have been reported to be increased by acute doses in mice (Erickson and Matchett, 1974) and rats (Palaic et al., 1971). Studies of acute versus chronic administration have been inconsistent. Palaic et al. (1971) found that the increased serotonin in rats during acute treatment was followed by decreased levels after chronic administration. On the other hand, Kuriyama, Rauscher, and Sze (1971) found exactly the opposite pattern in mice. Other studies have failed to show any effect on monoamines (Efron and Gerson, 1963; Haggendal and Lindqvist, 1961). Thus, it appears that differences in species, techniques, dosage, and other factors have resulted in a complex and inconsistent series of reports on the effects of ethanol on amines. Until the data appear more consistent, the reserpine model (like the MAO inhibition model) must be considered a very tentative and incomplete view on the mechanism of the biochemical action of ethanol.

Davis and Walsh (1970) and Davis (1973) have suggested that one effect of ethanol on biogenic amine metabolism may help explain the development of dependence and cross-dependence with other drugs. She has noted that ethanol (via its metabolite acetaldehyde), chloral hydrate, and barbiturates may modify catecholamine metabolism to produce tetrahydroisoquinoline alkaloids. It has been speculated that these compounds, which are intermediates in the biosynthesis of morphinelike substances, may play a role in the pharmacologic effects shared by these drugs. This hypothesis has been challenged on a number of grounds, however (e.g., see Halushka and Hoffman, 1970) and is best considered very speculative at this time.

Animal Studies of Spontaneous Ethanol Selection

Studies of spontaneous ethanol selection in animals show some interesting similarities to the studies of sleep and biogenic amines that we have just reviewed. Randall and Lester (1974) found that strains of mice that had the least sedative response to ethanol had higher rates of spontaneous selection. It also seems that pharmacologic manipulation of biogenic amine levels, which may modify ethanol-induced sleep time, will also cause changes in spontaneous ethanol selection (Hill, 1974; Hill and Goldstein, 1974; Geller et al., 1973). Studies of this type may also help explain conflicting reports on effects of ethanol on biogenic amines. Ahtee and Erikkson (1973) bred rats according to their tendency to select ethanol, until they developed one strain that preferred to drink a 10% solution rather than water, and one that did not. They found that ethanol consumption had differing effects on serotonin levels in the two strains: It increased serotonin content in the ethanol-preferring group, but caused no change in the other group. Thus, ethanol affects different strains differently in terms of actions on both sleep time and levels of serotonin.

ETHANOL IN NORMAL HUMAN SUBJECTS

The effects of acute ethanol ingestion on sleep in normal humans have been reviewed by Williams and Salamy (1972) and Freemon (1972). Six such experiments are outlined in Table 6-1. There is generally a sedative effect, demonstrated more consistently by decreased sleep latency rather than changes in total sleep time. There is good agreement in the observations of decreased REM sleep in the first half of the night. This may occur even when ethanol consumption has been some hours before sleep so that blood levels at sleep onset are only 50 mg% (Yules, Lippmann, and Freedman, 1967), below the levels at which inebriation is evident (Mirsky et al., 1941). Sometimes evidence of the initial REM sleep suppression is "washed out" by increased amounts of REM sleep in the second half of the night. Thus, in some studies (Gresham et al., 1963; Yules, Freedman, and Chandler, 1966b; Yules et al., 1967) there is a decrease in REM for the whole night, whereas in others (Williams and Salamy, 1972) total REM sleep is unchanged. The biphasic effect of REM

TABLE 6-1. Effects of Ethanol on Sleep of Normal Subjects

Author	Subjects	Dose	Duration of administration (days)	Sleep stages on first night of administration			Sleep stages on subsequent nights of administration			Sleep stages during withdrawal			Comment
				% REM	% SWS	% Waking	% REM	% SWS	% Waking	% REM	% SWS	% Waking	
Gresham et al. (1963)	7	1 gm/kg	5	→	—	—	—	—	—	—	—	—	
Yules et al (1966a)	3	1 gm/kg	5	→	↑	↑	←	↑	—	←	↑	↑	
Yules et al. (1967)	4	1 gm/kg	3	→	← (stage 4)		↑			←	→ (stage 4)	↑	Administered 4 hr before sleep
Knowles et al. (1968)	1	3.5 oz 6 0 oz	27	→	—	↑	↑	—	↑	←	—	↑	
Williams and Salamy (1972)	6	.87 gm/kg	3	→	↑		←	↑	↑	↑	↑	↑	
Rundell et al. (1972)	7	.9 gm/kg	3	→	↑	↑	↑	↑	←	↑	↑	↑	
Williams and Salamy (1972)	10	.87 gm/kg	1	→	←	→				↑	↑	↑	
Rundell et al (1972)	10	.9 gm/kg	1	→	↑	↑				↑	↑	↑	

sleep has been thought of as a "partial drug withdrawal" phenomenon. As evidence to support this view, it has been pointed out that ethanol is cleared from the blood in a linear manner at about 10–20 mg% per hour in both waking and sleeping subjects (Knowles, Laverty, and Kuechler, 1968; Williams and Salamy, 1972). Thus, a blood level of 80 mg% seen in many of these studies would be at least half-gone after the first four hours of an eight-hour sleep study. It follows then that with a higher initial dose REM sleep may be suppressed for a longer period of time. Knowles et al. (1968), in one of the rare multiple dose studies, demonstrated such a dose-related phenomenon. When they administered 3.5 oz of ethanol to a subject, the familiar pattern of initial decreases in REM sleep followed by later increases occurred; at a high dose (6 oz), REM sleep was clearly suppressed for the whole night. It should also be noted that the biphasic effect on REM sleep is not at all unique to ethanol studies, and has been reported with short-acting hypnotics (Kales et al., 1969b).

Decreased percentages of REM sleep following ethanol administration in normal subjects seem to be largely due to decreased mean duration of REM sleep episodes rather than due to changes in periodicity (Yules, Freedman, and Chandler, 1966b; Williams and Salamy, 1972; Rundell et al., 1972); a single study (Rundell et al., 1972) also reported a small but significant decrease in REM-to-REM periodicity during repeated administration. Data on "compensatory" increases in other stages during the period of decreased REM sleep have been varied. Yules et al. (1967), found increases in stage 2 in subjects who had received ethanol immediately before sleep, and increases in stages 2 and 4 in subjects who drank four hours before sleep. Williams and Salamy (1972) noted a tendency for slow-wave sleep to increase during the decreased REM sleep, but this effect did not reach statistical significance.

When ethanol is administered chronically to normal subjects, REM sleep gradually returns to normal (Yules et al., 1967) or slightly above normal (Yules et al., 1966b; Williams and Salamy, 1972) levels (Fig. 6-1). Upon withdrawal, there may be an initial "rebound" increase in REM sleep above baseline levels (Yules et al., 1966b; Yules et al., 1967; Knowles et al., 1968) that lasts a few days. This finding has not been constant, however, and was not observed during withdrawal in normal subjects in at least two studies (Williams and Salamy, 1972; Rundell et al., 1972). The rebound phenomenon, in which total REM sleep time during withdrawal may be greater than the amount "lost" during ethanol administration (Yules et al., 1966b), has been the basis of two ideas seen throughout the literature on ethanol and sleep. The first is that ethanol

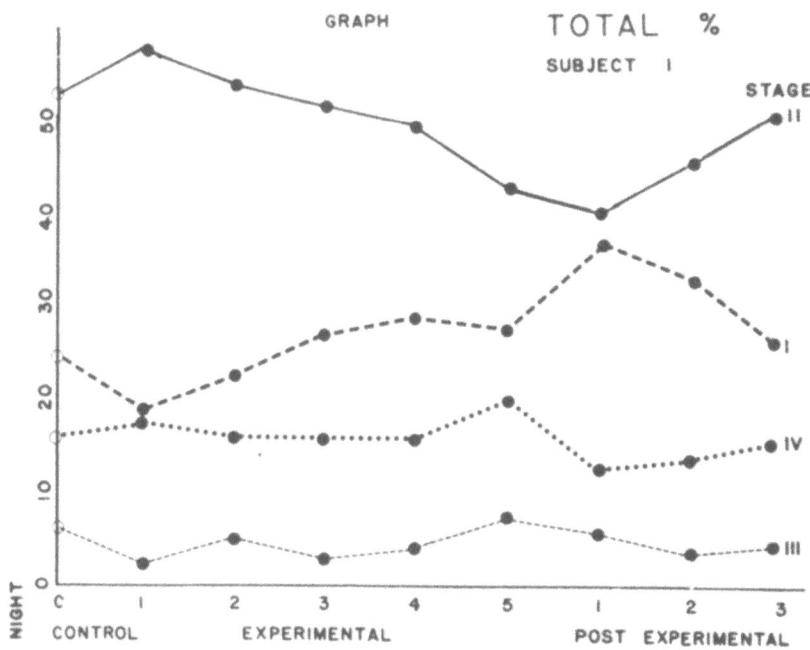

FIGURE 6-1. Effect of ethanol (1gm/kg) taken 15 minutes before retiring on seven-hour sleep EEG recordings. Subjects were three normal adult males. (From Yules, Freedman, and Chandler, 1966b.)

may produce a "self-sustaining disregulation" of control of sleep stages, which may persist long after the drug itself is no longer present (Yules *et al.*, 1966b; Yules *et al.*, 1967). The second is that the rebound phenomena may be characteristic of drugs of addiction (Oswald, 1969a; Kales *et al.*, 1969a). (This latter concept has been derived from studies of a variety of agents, which also includes morphine, barbiturates, and amphetamines.)

In analyzing data accumulated from the studies of ethanol in normal subjects, several methodological points should be considered. The first is that although changes in sleep due to ethanol may well be dose related, there has been very little EEG work that carefully evaluates the dose-response relationship. It should also be noted that interpretation of sleep studies has been greatly complicated by the rapid clearance of ethanol from the blood. One approach that might be of help would be to follow the sleep EEG in subjects with relatively constant blood levels maintained by continuous infusion. A final difficulty is that studies on normal subjects usually involve administration of a single dose of ethanol each day. In contrast, studies of chronic alcoholics usually are designed so that the patient receives a cumulative dose of ethanol given over many hours. The rationale for the latter design is that it more closely simulates the normal drinking pattern of the patient. The result of these different methods of administration is that comparisons of available studies on normal subjects with those on alcoholics must be made with great caution.

EFFECTS OF ETHANOL ON CHRONIC ALCOHOLICS

Sleep in "Dry" Alcoholics

Data on the sleep of chronic alcoholics are summarized in Table 6-2. Lester et al. (1973) provided one of the few studies in which alcoholics were directly compared with age-matched controls. It was found that alcoholics who had been abstinent for at least three weeks had more stage 1 and REM sleep, and less stage 3 sleep than controls. Younger alcoholic subjects (24–39 years old) had less stage 4; this difference was not observed among older alcoholics, presumably because the older control subjects displayed the decreased stage 4 that is usually observed in normal aging (Feinberg and Carlson, 1968). The increased amount of REM sleep in the alcoholics was related to increased periodicity of REM cycles, rather than to longer duration of REM episodes. The sleep of the alcoholics appeared to be disturbed, as reflected by an increased number of arousals and more changes of sleep stages.

The decreased slow-wave sleep and increased number of stage changes in the sleep of alcoholics have been seen after as long as one or two years of abstinence (Adamson and Burdick, 1973). Wagman and Allen (1974) found that 200 weeks of abstinence were required for complete recovery of slow-wave sleep (defined as 18% of total sleep). Significant variables in slow-wave sleep recovery included age and logarithm of duration of abstinence. Gross et al. (1973), who observed decreased slow-wave sleep during acute withdrawal, have suggested that the return of slow-wave sleep to normal may be used as an indication of physiologic recovery.

Smith, Johnson, and Burdick (1971) have suggested that the disturbed sleep pattern, with decreased slow-wave sleep, seen in alcoholics is similar to that of the elderly. They also provided data from psychological testing in which alcoholics produced scores that might be expected of patients with senility or diffuse cortical damage. However, a recent review of intellectual deficits reported in alcoholics supports

TABLE 6-2. Effects of Ethanol on Sleep of Chronic Alcoholics

Author	Subjects	Dose	Duration of administration (days)	Sleep stages when drinking compared to abstinence			Sleep stages during withdrawal compared to abstinence			Comment
				% REM	% SWS	% Awake	% REM	% SWS	% Awake	
A. Studies with data on abstinence, drinking, and withdrawal										
Greenberg and Perlman (1967)	3	.4–2.1 oz of 4 hr	4–10	↓	—	—	↑	—	—	Behavioral data only
Mello and Mendelson (1970)	12	4.4 oz	14–32	—	—	↓	—	—	↑	
Gross et al. (1973)	4	3.1 gm/kg	15	↓	↑	↓	↑	→	↑	
Lester et al. (1973)	17	150 MG%† at HS	2	↓	↑	↓	↑	← (Stage 3)	↑	Changes in 1st half of night
Wolin and Mello (1973)	14	50–300 MG%†	12	↓ in 36%	—	—	↑ in 29%	—	—	Data estimated from graphs of individual pts.
B. Studies comparing sleep during drinking with withdrawal										
Johnson et al. (1970)	14	150 MG%†	2				↑	↑	↑	Decreased intermittent waking
Allen et al. (1971b)	6	8 oz	3–7				↓	↑	↓	
C. Studies comparing abstinent alcoholics with normal values			*Duration of abstinence*				*Sleep stages compared to normal values*			
Adamson and Burdick (1973)	10		1–2 yr				↑	→	↑	Uncontrolled
Lester et al. (1973)	17		3 wks minimum				↑	→	↑	
D. Studies comparing sleep during acute withdrawal to normal values			*Duration since drinking (days)*				*Sleep stages compared to normal values*			
Gross et al. (1966)	4		0–4				↑	→	↓	Uncontrolled
Greenberg and Perlman (1967)	14		0				↑	—	↓	Uncontrolled

* Method of presentation of dosage varies in different studies. When sufficient information was provided, this was converted to gm/kg; otherwise, it is listed as presented in the papers.
† Blood alcohol concentration.

that few are observed, that they are subtle, and may be reversible (Goodwin and Hill, 1975).

Lester *et al.* (1973) have observed that the increased REM sleep periodicity, disruption of REM-sleep episodes, and decreased slow-wave sleep seen in alcoholics are similar to the effects produced by reserpine (Coulter *et al.*, 1971). This is particularly interesting in view of previously mentioned work suggesting that ethanol may have biochemical effects similar to those of reserpine (Williams and Salamy, 1972).

Response to Ethanol

Although the sleep of abstinent alcoholics is very different from that of normals, both groups have at least some similarities in their response to ethanol. There is a decrease in sleep latency and percentage REM sleep, and an increase in slow-wave sleep. Lester *et al.* (1973) noted that ethanol administration in alcoholics decreased the inter-REM interval. This was reported in one study of normals (Rundell *et al.*, 1972), but most evidence has been that normal subjects respond to ethanol with decreases in mean REM period duration. Mello and Mendelson (1970) observed that the distribution of behaviorally defined sleep over the 24-hour day changes when alcoholics spontaneously consume ethanol. They found that ethanol consumption resulted in a tendency to sleep in a series of relatively brief episodes, although total sleep time for the 24 hours might be increased.

Sleep during Acute Withdrawal

During acute withdrawal, REM sleep may increase. Johnson *et al.* (1970) found this to be due to an increased number of REM periods and shorter inter-REM intervals, with no change in mean duration of REM intervals, with no change in mean duration of REM episodes compared to measurements during drinking. Allen *et al.* (1971b) have provided data suggesting that there is first an initial decrease in REM followed by an increase. This might be taken to imply that there is an oscillating system, rather than a simple rebound in response to previously decreased REM. As mentioned earlier, a decreased percentage of slow-wave sleep seems to occur in alcoholics during acute withdrawal (Gross *et al.*, 1973) as well as during chronic abstinence.

Psychotic episodes during alcohol withdrawal are associated with increases in the number of REM-sleep episodes and large increases in percentage REM sleep. In some cases REM sleep may make up over 90% of sleep time (Greenberg and Perlman, 1967). Waking hallucinations

142

CHAPTER SIX

may occur during this time with a predominant alpha rhythm and active rapid eye movements (Gross et al., 1966). Greenberg and Perlman (1967) found that this elevation and fragmentation was similar in kind, but quantitatively greater in alcoholics who developed delirium tremens than in those who developed nonpsychotic abstinence syndromes.* Wolin and Mello (1973) reported that although the relationship of REM rebound to hallucinations during withdrawal was not inevitable in all subjects, there was at least some positive relation. In a group of five subjects who developed hallucinations, three had rebounds; of six subjects who had vivid dreaming only, one had a rebound; of three subjects who had no change in dreaming, there were no rebounds.

ISSUES RAISED BY OBSERVATIONS OF THE REM SLEEP REBOUND

Reports of increased REM sleep during ethanol withdrawal syndromes have led to hypotheses that this phenomenon is etiologically related to the development of hallucinations during ethanol withdrawal and to a basic mechanism of drug dependence. These hypotheses will be discussed in turn.

The REM intrusion hypothesis, which has been reviewed by Vogel (1968), suggests that hallucinations in fact represent intrusions of REM sleep into the waking state. This notion was anticipated by Lasegue, who in 1881 wrote a paper entitled "Alcoholic Delirium is not a Delirium, but is a Dream." A similar concept has been invoked in studies of schizophrenia as well, and is discussed in chapter 7. Several possibilities exist: It may be that hallucinations during alcohol withdrawal do in fact represent the intrusion of REM sleep into waking, there may be no relationship between the two states, or finally both increased REM sleep and hallucinations may be reflections of some more basic phenomenon. An effective hypothesis would have to be consistent with observations of hallucinations in alcoholics when REM sleep is normal (Wolin and Mello, 1973) and of REM rebound in both alcoholics (Wolin and Mello, 1973) and normal subjects (Yules et al., 1966b) who have no evidence of psychosis. As mentioned earlier, it may be that there is a quantitative difference in REM sleep between those who develop hallu-

* It is not clear in this paper whether the amount of REM sleep is higher in those patients with hallucinations only, or in those with the complete syndrome of delirium tremens. The latter state is usually thought to include not only hallucinations, but also disorientation and autonomic changes.

cinations and those who do not. An alternative is that an additional, as yet unknown, change in CNS function must also be present if hallucinations are to occur. Feinberg (1969a) has speculated that impairment of the mechanisms that govern stage 4 sleep may be the second factor. Clearly, the relation of increases in REM sleep to the occurrence of hallucinations is not a simple one, and has yet to be elucidated.

A second unanswered question, somewhat different from the problem of whether the REM rebound is a cause of hallucinations during drug withdrawal, is whether the effects of ethanol on REM sleep are intimately related to the development of dependence. Oswald (1969a) and Kales *et al.* (1969a) pointed out that this pattern—initial REM suppression during administration, later return to normal, and a large increase upon withdrawal—is seen not only with ethanol but also with a variety of drugs generally considered to be addicting, such as amphetamines, morphine, and barbiturates. On the other hand, it has been suggested that psychoactive drugs not generally considered to be addictive, such as lithium and chlorpromazine, acutely suppress REM sleep but have little or no rebound upon withdrawal.

As in the problem of hallucinations, the relation between changes in REM sleep and the addictive process could be formulated in several ways. REM suppression and withdrawal rebound could be involved in the etiology of dependence. Alternatively, these changes may be a reflection of the process, an example of tolerance and dependence in a particular physiologic system. Finally, of course, the two processes may be unrelated. In evaluating these alternatives, several points should be made. First of all, since the time that this relationship was first formulated, a number of contrary observations have been reported. It appears that an increase in REM sleep does not always occur during withdrawal from addicting substances. Feinberg *et al.* (1974a), for instance, found that several barbiturates given to normal volunteers for five to eight days did not result in a withdrawal REM rebound. Wolin and Mello (1973) found that some alcoholics with signs of clinical withdrawal did not have increased REM sleep. There are also reports in which there was no REM sleep suppression during drug administration, but increases occurred after discontinuation. This has been seen in several subjects receiving amphetamines (Feinberg *et al.*, 1974b) and in a subject receiving the antihistamine chlorpheniramine maleate (Kales *et al.*, 1969). Thus, the association of drugs of addiction with a REM-sleep rebound upon withdrawal is less constant than was originally supposed. A second problem is that a variety of studies (e.g., Yules *et al.*, 1966b) have described tolerance to the REM-suppressing effects of ethanol, and withdrawal rebound, after only a few days of administration of moderate doses to normal volunteers. This is a very different time course from the development of clinical tolerance and dependence. Finally, by selectively awakening subjects, one can produce REM suppression and later rebound. Although this was initially thought to produce psychotic changes, it appears that this probably has little harmful effect on humans and certainly does not produce changes in mental status similar to drug withdrawal syndromes (Vogel, 1968; see chap. 1).

EXPERIMENTAL THERAPIES

Traditional therapy for alcohol withdrawal includes use of minor tranquilizers, nutrition, and hydration if indicated (Greenblatt and Greenblatt, 1972; Kaim and Klett, 1972). There is some evidence that drugs such as chlordiazepoxide that have cross-tolerance to alcohol can help prevent occurrence of delirium tremens (Kaim, Klett, and Roth-feld, 1969). In treatment of those patients who do develop delirium tremens, there may be little difference in outcome between patients treated with drugs that have a cross-tolerance and those that do not, such as the phenothiazines (Kaim, 1974). Interestingly enough, none of these compounds seems to decrease the duration of delirium tremens to less than the three days described in untreated patients of the last century (Ware, 1841).

Observations from biochemical and sleep studies such as those outlined in this chapter have led to new approaches that are currently under investigation. Those mentioned here are of interest in that they were derived from observations on the metabolism of alcohol and its effects on sleep.

Bates (1972), noting reports of decreased total sleep time in alcoholics and studies showing psychotic states resulting from sleep deprivation (see chap. 1), has provided data on the efficacy of "sleep therapy" during alcohol withdrawal. Thirty-two subjects who showed hallucinations during withdrawal were given continuous infusions of pentobarbital, producing sleep for 12–24 hours. This may have reduced the duration of psychotic withdrawal phenomena to about 30 hours, which appears to be shorter than is expected on the basis of some other studies (Figurelli, 1958; Lundquist, 1961; Kaim and Klett, 1972).* Further evalu-

---

* Actually, most studies give data on the duration of delirium tremens, without providing definitions of this state. As noted earlier, it is usually thought to include hallucinations, disorientation, and autonomic changes. The Bates paper apparently refers to the duration of hallucinations only, in patients with delirium tremens. Thus, it is somewhat difficult to compare this data with that of other studies.

ation of this approach by controlled studies will be needed to determine accurately the efficacy of this approach. It would also seem important to evaluate the possible hazards of aspiration during sleeping, an issue that has been raised regarding sleep therapies for other conditions. A second issue is whether the possible benefits of this treatment are in fact related to correcting a state of sleep deprivation, as the author suggests, or whether they are due to some other mechanism. Among other things, this study could just be viewed as a therapy using large doses of a cross-tolerant drug already known to be of use in treatment of withdrawal.

One experimental approach to the treatment of alcohol withdrawal has been the administration of NAD (nicotinamide-adenine dinucleotide-nadide). This is a cofactor active in such reactions as the metabolism of ethanol by oxidation to acetaldehyde and the subsequent oxidation of the latter to acetic acid (Caldwell and Sever, 1974). Although initial results had suggested that NAD might be of benefit, a 10-day trial of 3 gm daily was found to produce no difference from controls in measures of sleep or clinical tests (Smith, Johnson, and Burdick, 1971).

Another therapeutic approach has been the administration of 5-hydroxytryptophan (5-HTP), a precursor of serotonin (see Fig. 2-1). Zarcone and Hoddes (1975), reasoning that alcohol may create an imbalance of serotonergic sleep mechanisms, gave 300 mg of 5-HTP for four nights to 12 alcoholics who had been abstinent for at least 23 days. They found that there was no change in total amount of REM sleep. However, the fragmentation of REM sleep periods (e.g., the interruption of REM sleep periods by brief episodes of other stages), which is characteristic of alcoholics, was greatly decreased. This would seem to support the hypothesis that at least some of the sleep disturbances in alcoholics are related to abnormalities of serotonergic control mechanisms. Whether correction of these sleep disturbances by agents such as 5-HTP will lead to changes in the clinical course of alcoholism is, of course, as yet unknown.

SUMMARY

Ethanol ingestion influences the occurrence of the sleep stages. This may be attributable to its possible effects on the metabolism of the biogenic amines. Acutely, ethanol given to normal subjects causes decreases in percentage of REM sleep, largely due to decreased mean duration of REM episodes. Whether this effect occurs in only the first half of the night or all night may be related to the dose of ethanol given. When chronic alcoholics are "dry," they have disturbed sleep characterized by multiple awakenings, normal to mildly increased REM sleep, and decreased slow-wave sleep. These disturbances have been likened to the sleep of the elderly, and to subjects treated with reserpine. When alcoholics drink, percentage REM sleep decreases while slow-wave sleep increases. The large increases in REM sleep that occur during ethanol withdrawal have been related by some authors to the development of hallucinations, and to the process of dependence itself. At the present state of knowledge it is not clear whether sleep stage changes have an etiologic relationship to these phenomena or, conversely, whether they are secondary reflections of them. Knowledge from sleep studies has, however, provided new approaches to treating alcoholism.

Affective Disorders and Schizophrenia

Long before the discovery of REM sleep, many observers of human behavior had suggested that there is an interrelationship between sleep and mental illness. The English neurologist Hughlings Jackson wrote, "Find out about dreams and you will find out about insanity." Likewise Jung predicted, "Let the dreamer walk about and act like one awakened, and we have the clinical picture of dementia praecox." And, Freud, after a long review of the postulated relationships between sleep and insanity wrote, "We shall be working towards an explanation of the psychoses while we are endeavoring to throw light on some of the mystery of dreams." To paraphrase Frederick Snyder's graceful expression of these views, "Troubled minds have troubled sleep, and troubled sleep causes troubled minds."

The reasons for this theorizing are not hard to find. The mentally ill do indeed sleep poorly. This is particularly true of depressed persons, but also includes, at times, patients with schizophrenia, mania, and alcoholism. In light of the traditional notion that sleep serves a restorative function, it was entirely reasonable to suppose that prolonged sleep disturbance might contribute to mental illness, or even cause it. Shakespeare expressed this view of sleep when he wrote, "Sleep that knits up the ravelled sleave of care, the death of each day's life, sore labours bath, balm of hurt minds." Moreover, the daytime hallucinations of the psychotic have always been intriguingly similar to the nighttime hallucinations experienced by everyone in dreams. This similarity suggested that hallucinations might result from the appearance of the dreaming process during waking life. Furthermore, since the biogenic amines may play an important role in the regulation of the sleep and waking states (see chap. 1) and have been implicated in pathophysiological theories of depression and schizophrenia, many investigators hoped that sleep alterations might reflect the biochemical mechanisms involved in mental illness.

Following the discovery of REM sleep in 1953, Dement, Snyder, Vogel, Feinberg, Hawkins, Mendels, Oswald, and others made pioneering studies of sleep in the mentally ill. As we shall see, early studies did not establish any specific abnormalities of sleep correlated with specific mental disorders. Earlier findings did, however, raise intriguing possibilities. Indeed, some evidence, to be presented in this chapter, even indicates that deliberate disturbance of sleep by total sleep deprivation, selective REM deprivation, or drugs may alleviate depression. This chapter will review the findings of sleep studies in affective disorders and schizophrenia, as other chapters have focused on sleep in alcoholism (chap. 6) and sleep disorders (chaps. 4 and 5).

BASIC DEFINITIONS

Affective Disorders

The term *affective disorders* refers to depression and mania. They are characterized by low mood and euphoria, respectively. Depression may be associated with feelings of worthlessness and helplessness, suicidal thoughts, anxiety, guilt, and poor concentration. Many depressed patients also complain of somatic disturbances, such as headache, constipation, rapid heart rate, and shortness of breath. They may experience loss of appetite with weight loss, fatigue, and loss of interest in usual activities, including sex.

In contrast, manic patients are typically euphoric and hyperactive and digress rapidly from one idea to another *(flight of ideas)*. They may also be irritable and show, at times, symptoms also seen in schizophrenia such as hallucinations, delusions of grandeur, and ideas of passivity (the false conviction that external forces control one's mind or body).

Various subclassifications for affective disorders have been proposed. *Unipolar* patients experience depression only, whereas *bipolar* patients (manic-depressive patients in older terminology) suffer discrete episodes of mania and depression. Depressive disorders are called *primary* if they occur in individuals who have had no previous psychiatric disorder other than affective disorder, and *secondary* if they occur in patients with other psychiatric disorders such as schizophrenia, alcoholism, drug addiction, and so on. Affective disorders may also be called *reactive* or *endogenous*. The former are considered to be milder, more often the direct result of precipitating events or stress, and less responsive to drug therapy than the latter. Endogenous depressions presumably are caused by a biochemical abnormality in the individual. Affective disorders may also be considered *nonpsychotic* or *psychotic*, the latter usually signifying severe delusions or hallucinations or loss of ability to function.

An individual may suffer from an affective disorder only once during his lifetime, recurrently or continuously. The age mean of onset is usually near thirty for bipolar illness and near forty for unipolar illness. Bipolar illness is more common among the relatives of bipolar patients than among the relatives of unipolar patients.

Several types of drugs are commonly used to treat affective disorders. Tricyclic antidepressants include imipramine (Tofranil), desipramine (Norpramine), and amitriptyline (Elavil), while the monoamine oxidase inhibitor antidepressants include phenelzine (Nardil), tranylcypromine (Parnate), and pargyline (Eutonyl). Lithium salts are often used in bipolar patients, for management of manic episodes and as a prophylaxis against both depression and mania. Lithium salts may also have antidepressant properties in some unipolar patients. In addition, electroshock therapy (ECT) may be used for suicidal or psychotically depressed patients.

Schizophrenia

Schizophrenia is usually a chronic disorder, characterized at times by a disturbance in thinking, delusions, and hallucinations in a clear sensorium. The reasoning of such a patient may lack normal goal directedness and the usual association between ideas *(loosening of associations)*. Subjective feelings may be shallow, blunted, or inappropriate; physical movements odd, bizarre, or extremely few in number (catatonia).

Common schizophrenic delusions include those of persecution and control ("others are controlling my mind or reading my thoughts"), as well as feelings that bizarre bodily changes have occurred ("a snake is eating up my insides"). Auditory hallucinations are common.

The subclassifications of schizophrenia are controversial and confusing. Patients with a poor prognosis are generally labeled as chronic, process, or nonremitting, while good prognostic patients are described as schizophreniform, schizoaffective, reactive, or remitting. Patients with a good prognosis usually display more prominent changes in mood, particularly depression, and appear more confused, perplexed, and disoriented than patients with a poor prognosis. The diagnosis of schizophrenia is usually first made when the patient is in his teens or early twenties, and rarely after the age of forty. Schizophrenia is more common among the relatives of schizophrenics than among the relatives of normals or psychiatric controls. Schizophreniform illness may or may not be a type of schizophrenia; some genetic evidence suggests that it may be an atypical manifestation of affective disorder.

Among the drugs used to treat schizophrenia are the phenothiazine derivatives such as chlorpromazine (Thorazine), thioridazine (Mellaril), and trifluoperazine (Stelazine) and butyrophenone derivatives such as haloperidol (Haldol). Pimozide, clozapine, and sulpiride are effective neuroleptics that are used in Europe but that are not currently available in the United States. Although reserpine (Serpesil) is an effective neuroleptic and was commonly used during the 1950s, it is not frequently used now because it is less effective than the other drugs and has more side effects.

While the etiology of the affective disorders and schizophrenia remains obscure, biological models are pursued more avidly than they once were. This is because genetic factors have been established in both. Somatic treatment but not psychotherapy has been shown in controlled studies to significantly speed recovery and forestall future recurrences, and biological research is, in many respects, easier than psychosocial research.

STUDIES OF SLEEP IN DEPRESSED PATIENTS

Comparative Studies

The first polygraphic study of the sleep of depressed patients was made by Diaz-Guerrero, Gottlieb, and Knott (1946). They studied six manic depressed patients, depressed type, all under the age of 40. None of the patients had received drugs or electroshock treatment. Realizing that sleep on the first night in the laboratory might not be representative (later to be called the *first night effect*), the authors allowed one adaptation night and presented only the data of the second night. They summarized the results as follows: "The disturbed sleep of patients with manic-depressive psychosis, depressed type, is not only characterized by difficulty in falling asleep and/or by early or frequent awakenings, but by both a greater proportion of sleep which is light and more frequent oscillations from one level of sleep to another than normally occurs." Since their study occurred before the discovery of REM sleep, it is not possible to directly compare their results with later studies.

Despite its limitations, the study of Diaz-Guerrero and associates accurately anticipated the major findings of modern sleep studies in depression. As can be seen in Table 7-1, most studies indicate that the sleep of depressed patients is short, fragmented, and shallow. Sleep is frequently interrupted by wakenings and changes in sleep state. With additional studies, however, it became clear that not all depressed patients sleep alike, that these sleep disturbances do not necessarily distinguish depression from other clinical conditions, and that sleep disturbance may not occur in all depressed patients.

Although total time spent asleep was reported to be low in depressed patients as compared with normals (Diaz-Guerrero et al., 1946; Green and Stajduher, 1966; Oswald et al., 1963; Mendels and Hawkins, 1967a and b, 1968; Kupfer and Foster, 1975; Kupfer, 1976; Castelloti and Pittaluga, 1966; Snyder, 1968, 1972a and b; Gianelli, Penati, Pietropolli-Charmet, 1968; Hauri and Hawkins, 1973; Muratorio and Maggini, 1967; Muratorio, Maggini, and Murri, 1967; Muratorio, Maggini, and Marcacci, 1968a), this was by no means an invariant finding (Zung, Wilson, and Dodson, 1964; Kupfer and Foster, 1972; Hajnšek et al., 1973; Hartmann, 1968a). Based on a questionnaire administered to outpatients in a lithium clinic, Detre et al. (1972) reported that unipolar depressed patients slept less than bipolar depressed patients, some of whom actually described increased sleep rather than insomnia while depressed. Likewise, Michaelis and Hofmann (1973) found that about 9% of endogenously depressed patients told of hypersomnia rather than insomnia.

Kupfer et al. (1972) compared the EEG sleep patterns of hyposomniac patients with those of hypersomniac bipolar patients. They found that the hypersomniac patients slept longer and more efficiently (they slept a greater proportion of the time spent in bed) and had more nonREM sleep and stage 2 than the hyposomniac patients. Hypersomnia, however, is not exclusively associated with bipolar illness since some unipolar patients may show either no change in sleep or hypersomnia (Kupfer and Foster, 1975; Hauri and Hawkins, 1973). For example, Hauri and Hawkins found completely normal EEG sleep records in three unipolar depressed, somewhat hysterical women, aged 40–45.

TABLE 7-1. EEG Sleep Studies of Patients with Affective Disorder

Authors	Type	No.	Total sleep (min)	REM sleep	Delta	REM latency (min)	Comments
Diaz-Guerrero et al., 1946	Manic-depressive, depressed	6	342	—	1.6%	—	Increased state changes. Delta = high voltage, slow-wave activity ("random").
Oswald et al. 1963	Endogenous or manic-depression						Depressed patients exhibited more wakefulness.
	depressed	6	—	20.6%	E8.0%	—	
	Controls	6	—	23.3%	5.6%ᵃ	—	
Zung et al., 1964	Depressed	8	420	—	E9%	—	Stage A 26.6%, B 20.2, C 20.5, D 23.1. Decreased auditory arousal threshold in depression.
Gresham et al., 1965	Mildly depressed	19	423	19.9%	7.7%	—	Wakefulness increased.
Green and Stajduher, 1966	46-year-old manic psychotic depression	1	243 to 273	20.5% to 20.6%	0	47	Two-night study.
Castelloti and Pittaluga, 1966	Depressed	7	255	14.5%			Depressed wake more frequently and longer.
	Controls	7	360	18.3%			
Mendels and Hawkins, 1967a	Depressed	21	328	19.1%	20%	—	Increased number of awake and early morning awakening in depressed patients.
	Controls	15	414	24.6%ᵃ	34%ᵇ	—	

Study	Group	n					Comments
Snyder, 1972a	Nonpsychotic	12	~285	70 min	low	~60	Values estimated from figures. Increased variability in nonpsychotic and psychotic groups.
	Psychotic	12	~200	55	low	~40	
	Normals	12	~310	80		~75	
Hartmann, 1968a	Manic-depressive	6	383	25.9	IV39 min	63	
Mendels and Hawkins, 1968	Neurotic	17	350	85 min	IV24 min	—	Differences in age and severity of depression did not account for sleep differences. Psychotics differed significantly from neurotics in total sleep, REM, and delta.
	Controls	15	415[c]	107[a]	81[b]	—	
	Psychotic	4	216	33 min	1 min	—	
	Controls	6	411[b]	102[b]	83[b]	—	
Gianelli et al., 1968	Endogenous	—	210	10%	—	—	Endogenous depressives take longer to fall asleep and wake up earlier. Schizophrenics sleep more like normals than do depressed patients.
	Reactive	—	360	—	—	—	
	Involutional	—	390	18%	—	—	
	Normals	—	180	—	—	—	
Lowy et al., 1971	Severe depression	6	238	14.2%	IV6.8%	118	Prior to treatment.
Kupfer and Foster, 1972	Mild to moderate	19	392	86 min	22 min	50	REM latency was negatively correlated with severity.
	Severe or psychotic	16		82 min	16 min	18[c]	
Kupfer et al., 1972	Hypersomniac (no drugs)	5	486	109 min	38 min	54	Hypersomnia is common in bipolar patients.
	Hypersomniac (lithium)	5	509	95	47	142	
	Hyposomniac	7	349	75	32	62	
Hajnšek et al., 1973	Depressed	10	466	44 min	E53 min	231	Patients showed increased wakefulness and took longer to fall asleep and to reach deep stages of sleep.
	Controls	20	441	92	75	105	

continued

TABLE 7-1 (continued)

Authors	Type	No.	Total sleep (min)	REM sleep	Delta	REM latency (min)	Comments
Hauri and Hawkins, 1973	"Psychogenic"	5	394	100 min	73 min	—	
	"Biogenic"	5	331	89	26ᵃ	—	
Kupfer and Foster, 1975	Psychotic depression	9	262	51 min	4 min	36	Psychotic depression shows more wakefulness.
	Schizo-affective	6	346	81ᵃ	18ᵃ	32	
	Nonpsychotic depression (unipolar and bipolar)						Hyposomniacs had sleep continuity disorder; hypersomniacs did not.
	"Hyposomniac"	16	350	—	22 min	40	
	"Hypersomniac"	9	450	—	17	43	
Kupfer, 1976	Primary depression	18	298	21.1%	1.9%	39	No difference in total sleep, wakefulness, delta sleep, or sleep efficiency.
	Secondary	11	336	21.1%	5.7%	71ᵇ	

ᵃ p < .05
ᵇ p < .01
ᶜ p < .001

Kupfer and Foster (1975) suggested that insomnia is usually seen in agitated depressed patients, while hypersomnia is associated with loss of energy. Hyposomnia and hypersomnia in depressed patients may also be associated with weight loss and weight gain. In a questionnaire study of 375 consecutive referrals to a psychiatric outpatient clinic, Stonehill and Crisp (1973) found that weight loss was associated with reduced duration of sleep, more broken sleep, and earlier waking. Weight gain was associated with longer duration of sleep, unbroken sleep, and a later waking time in the morning.

Even the weather has been blamed for the disturbed sleep of depressed patients. Faust and Hole (1972) reported that Swiss depressed patients, in comparison with schizophrenics, alcoholics, and neurotics, were particularly likely to be irritable and to sleep restlessly with a cold front or *Föhn*.

When insomnia has been reported in depression, it has more frequently resulted from increased awakenings during the sleep period than from either difficulty in falling asleep or early morning awakenings. For example, Muratorio and Maggini (1967) found that depressed patients showed more arousals and changes of sleep state during each discrete state of sleep than normals. Not only were depressed patients aroused spontaneously out of each stage of sleep, but they showed a heightened arousal response (i.e., lower threshold) to auditory stimuli during each stage of sleep (Zung *et al.*, 1964). With drug treatment, however, the arousal response to auditory stimuli became normal.

Kupfer, Foster, and Detre (1973) compared the EEG sleep patterns of depressed patients with sleep fragmentation to those without sleep fragmentation. The former exhibited significantly more total sleep, nonREM sleep, and REM sleep. Interestingly, however, both efficient and inefficient sleepers showed the other stigma of depression, low amounts of delta sleep, and short REM latencies.

Confirming the early report of Diaz-Guerrero *et al.* (1946) nearly all subsequent studies have shown that high-voltage, slow-wave EEG activity is reduced in depressed patients, whether it is measured as stage E (the older method of scoring sleep records) or as stage 4 (the new criteria) (see Table 7-1): In contrast, however, Oswald *et al.* (1963) reported that depressed patients had significantly more stage E than normal controls; interpretation is complicated, however, by the use of barbiturates on some nights.

As far as REM sleep is concerned, no consistent changes in total minutes or percentage of total sleep have been found in patients with affective disorders. Rather, the major finding may be the increased variability of REM sleep, with patients showing low, normal, or even high amounts. This variability is particularly striking in the more severe depressions. Much the same can be said for REM latency, a measure of the elapsed time from sleep onset to the beginning of the first REM period. Kupfer and Foster (1972, 1975; Kupfer, 1976) have particularly emphasized that the short REM latency is a psychological marker for depression, and that the more severe the depression, the shorter the REM latency. Kupfer (1976) also found the REM latency to be short in patients with primary depression but normal or near normal in patients with secondary depression. While some investigators have also shown that the REM latency is short in depressed patients (Green and Stajduher, 1966; Hartmann, 1968a; Hawkins and Mendels, 1966; Hartmann, Verdone, and Snyder, 1966), other investigators have found both short and long REM latencies (Snyder, 1972a; Lowy, Cleghorn, McClure, 1971; Mendels and Hawkins, 1971a) or even very long REM latencies (Lowy et al., 1971; Mendels and Hawkins, 1971a; Hajnšek et al., 1973).

Because of the marked variability of total sleep, REM sleep, and REM latency described in depressed patients, various investigators have attempted to compare the sleep of different subgroups of patients with the hope of determining whether or not sleep disturbance is associated with particular subgroups of patients. The disturbance of total sleep has tended to be greater in the more severely depressed patients (Snyder, 1972b; Gianelli et al., 1968; Mendels and Hawkins, 1968), but this correlation has often not been statistically significant when measured by conventional rating scales of depression (Mendels and Hawkins, 1968; Kupfer and Foster, 1972). Likewise, sleep loss was reported to be greater in *biogenic* as compared with *psychogenic* depressives (Hauri and Hawkins, 1973) or in *primary* as compared with *secondary* depressives (Kupfer, 1976). Although psychogenic depressed patients showed significantly more delta sleep than did biogenic depressives, both primary and secondary depressives had the same low levels of delta sleep (Kupfer, 1976).

In examining the *endogenous–reactive* dichotomy, Giannelli et al. (1968) suggested that endogenously depressed patients took longer to fall asleep, woke up earlier, and slept less than reactive patients. Two nonpolygraphic sleep studies have also compared the sleep of these two types of depressed patients. Haider (1968) found that endogenously depressed patients reported significantly more early morning awakening than reactively depressed patients. Hinton (1963b), however, found no difference in any sleep parameter between endogenous and reactive patients, based on measured nurses' observations of sleep and an apparatus that measured body motility.

When the comparison has been between *psychotically* and *nonpsychotically* depressed patients, some of the most striking and significant findings have emerged. The psychotic patients almost invariably sleep fitfully for brief periods at any one stretch. They may fall directly from wakefulness into REM sleep without any intervening nonREM sleep and they may show unusually high amounts of eye movement activity during REM sleep (so-called *REM storms*).

Typical records from a normal woman, a nonpsychotic unipolar depressed woman, and a psychotically depressed woman are shown in Fig. 7-1. None of these three middle-aged women had any delta sleep, as would be expected because of their ages. The REM latency was short in both depressed patients, particularly in the psychotically depressed woman. Both also showed frequent awakenings and arousals from sleep, again more so in the psychotic patient than in the neurotic, although the normal subject, like many older people, had one arousal as well. As this figure illustrates, the sleep patterns of depressed patients

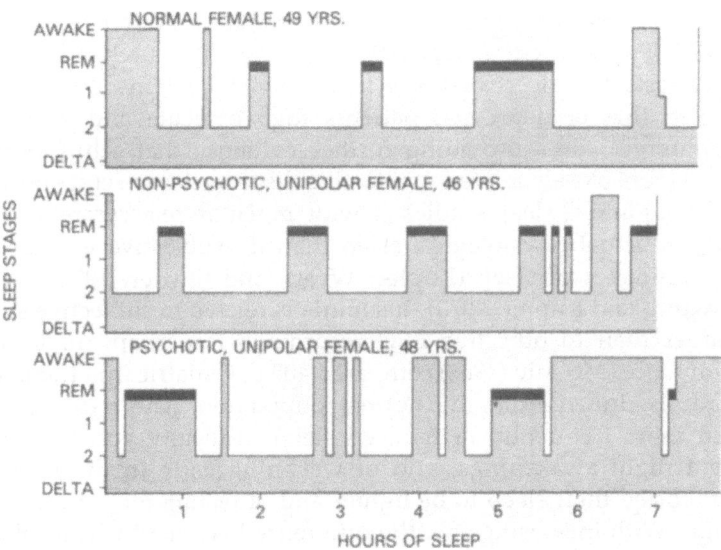

FIGURE 7-1. All-night polygraphic sleep records from three women: a normal control, a nonpsychotically depressed, unipolar patient, and a psychotic depressed, unipolar patient, all matched for age (Gillin and Snyder, unpublished data).

are, in some ways, exaggerated versions of those of normal aging, and those of psychotically depressed patients are exaggerations of those of nonpsychotically depressed patients. In passing, it is interesting to note that the sleep of chronic alcoholics also resembles that of the elderly (see chap. 6).

Mendels and Hawkins (1968) showed that psychotically depressed patients had less total sleep, delta sleep, and REM sleep in comparison not only with normal controls but with neurotically (nonpsychotic) depressed patients. Their data also indicated that the presence of psychotic features (e.g., delusions) was more important than either age or severity of illness (as measured by the Beck Depressive Inventory) in determining the degree of sleep disturbance. Snyder (1972) and Muratorio et al. (1967) have also documented the stark contrast of psychotic and nonpsychotic patients. Snyder (1972) emphasized the variability of number of rapid eye movements, amount of REM sleep, and REM latency in psychotic patients. Based both on nurses' observations of sleep and subjective estimates of sleep by patients, Naylor and LePoidevin (1972) reported that psychotically depressed patients slept less than neurotically depressed patients. In a comparison of psychotic depressives and schizoaffective patients, Kupfer and Foster (1975) found that the former tended to sleep less and exhibited significantly less REM sleep and delta sleep and more wakefulness than the latter. Nevertheless, the sleep of the schizoaffective patients more closely resembled that of depressed patients than of acute and borderline schizophrenics, thus providing further evidence that schizoaffective illness is more closely related to affective disorders than schizophrenia.

Although EEG sleep studies provide much more accurate information about actual physiological sleep than do subjective estimates or nurses' estimates of sleep (Kupfer, Wyatt, and Snyder, 1970a; Weiss, McPartland, and Kupfer, 1973), insomnia is related to subjective suffering rather than to objective EEG recordings (see chap. 5). Using a questionnaire, McGhie (1966) compared 400 psychiatric inpatients with 2500 adults drawn from the normal population. The patients complained more frequently of reduced sleep, difficulty going to sleep, frequent night awakenings, and of wakening early in the morning. They reported their sleep to be lighter and of feeling more tired in the morning. With increasing age, the difference between the control population and the psychiatric patients tended to diminish because of increasing sleep disturbance in the normal population. In view of the importance attached to sleep disturbance in depression, it was somewhat surprising that the questionnaire revealed only one statistically significant difference between the depressed and nondepressed psychiatric patients, and this was not a striking difference. Fifty-one percent of the depressed patients reported morning tiredness, while only 38% of the nondepressed patients did. Both groups reported equal amounts of early morning awakening.

As the cross-sectional studies demonstrated, sleep disturbance in depression is common but not invariant, pervasive but not discrete, exaggerated with psychosis but not with most other measures of severity. We turn now to review the longitudinal studies in which the same patient was studied over time, thus allowing us to gain some insight into the long-term suffering of these patients and the changes in sleep as they recover.

Longitudinal Studies of Depressed Patients

In early studies, Gresham, Agnew, and Williams (1965) and Mendels and Hawkins (1967b) compared the sleep patterns of depressed hospitalized patients on admission and at follow-up prior to discharge. In both studies, total sleep time, REM sleep time, and delta sleep were increased at discharge as compared with admission. Mendels and Hawkins (1967b), however, who studied 23 patients a mean of 47 days after the initial study, reported that recovered patients still exhibited abnormal sleep patterns: more drowsy time, more wakefulness, and less stage 4 than normal controls. Gresham and his colleagues, who studied only four patients, reported that the sleep of the recovered patients was quite similar to that of controls.

In two other early longitudinal studies, polygraphic sleep recordings of depressed patients were made about once a week. Green and Stajduher (1966) studied a 46-year-old psychotically depressed man. Prior to ECT, total sleep time and stage 4 were low, the REM latency was unusually short, and REM percentage was normal (20.5%). Following the first three ECT treatments, REM percentages increased briefly to 35.9%. These data imply that he was in a state of REM deprivation before treatment, that his *REM pressure* was high, but a REM rebound was prevented from occurring because of his illness. With the initiation of treatment, REM compensation occurred. As he gradually improved, total sleep time tended to increase but remained somewhat unpredictable, REM latency and percentage stage 4 increased somewhat, and the number of sleep stage changes decreased. The return of REM latency toward normal values suggests that REM pressure was reduced as he recovered.

Hartmann and his colleagues (1966) studied a 39-year-old manic-depressive patient (depressed type) who was studied for 30 weeks. As his depression gradually improved, percentage REM sleep fell from about 35% to 25% and REM latency increased from about 25 minutes to 60–80 minutes. These data suggest that he was in a state of REM compensation initially, which decreased as he improved.

Since these initial longitudinal studies, several investigators have undertaken the laborious task of making consecutive nightly sleep recordings of severely ill hospitalized depressed patients. Snyder (1972) studied a 58-year-old man with an agitated involutional depression. When first studied, the patient slept less than three hours per night; percentage REM sleep was high, about 30%, while REM sleep first appeared almost immediately after sleep onset. Over the next three weeks, as he became increasingly psychotic, his total sleep time remained about the same, but his percentage REM sleep increased dramatically, reaching 59% on one night. In addition, REM sleep periods tended to appear unusually rapidly after sleep onset and were characterized by the marked intensity of eye movements (REM storms).

In a second patient, a 49-year-old male who was studied shortly after the onset of an acute brief psychotic depressive illness, Snyder reported that nearly complete lack of REM sleep accompanied the severe loss of sleep at the onset of the study. As the psychosis subsided and sleep began to reappear, the patient exhibited extremely short REM latencies and unusually high levels of REM sleep.

In yet a third patient, a 65-year-old manic-depressive woman who was studied over a 45-day period of subsiding depression prior to a hypomanic episode, REM sleep increased to unusually high levels as depressive ratings gradually fell.

Based on observations such as these, Snyder suggested that many of the sleep disturbances of psychotically depressed patients might be expressions of REM deprivation and REM compensation. As is well known, when REM sleep is prevented from taking place, the propensity for its occurrence becomes stronger and stronger (see chap. 1). REM sleep deprivation has been shown to increase the frequency of REM sleep, reduce the REM latency, increase REM sleep in absolute terms and as proportion of total sleep time, and, in animals, increase the intensity of eye movements during REM sleep.

Snyder proposed that with sleep disturbance in depression some degree of REM deprivation would be inevitable. Thus, during the waxing phases of a depressive illness, REM deprivation would occur. Later, with the beginning of clinical remission, REM compensation would occur during the waning phases.

This attractive hypothesis accounts for many of the observed abnormalities of sleep in psychotic depression, particularly the great variability of total REM sleep, percentage REM sleep, and REM latency, and perhaps, the fragmentation of sleep. Unfortunately, the evidence from other longitudinal studies does not provide clear confirmation or refutation of the hypothesis (see Table 7-2). In part, this is because no patient has ever been studied longitudinally with sleep studies from the time before the inception of the depressive episode until recovery.

For example, Lowy *et al.* (1971) collected 83 all-night EEG sleep recordings from six previously unmedicated female patients with severe unipolar depression (all six were initially considered psychotic, although the diagnosis of psychosis proved to be unequivocal in only four cases). Following baseline recordings without medication, they first received 0.75-mg of dexamethasone (a long-acting adrenal cortical glucocorticoid steroid) and then imipramine (150 mg/day), an antidepressant agent. All-night sleep recordings were obtained several times each week. During the initial drug-free period, sleep findings varied considerably from patient to patient. As shown in Table 7-2, mean total sleep, delta sleep, and REM percentage were generally low. REM latency was high. With clinical improvement following treatment with imipramine, total sleep, delta sleep, and REM sleep all increased. REM latency was essentially unchanged. The individual variability of sleep change over time was highlighted by one patient whose sleep improved significantly long before any clinical improvement was observed. In three of the other four patients who had initial reduction of total sleep, lengthening of sleep coincided with clinical improvement. Two of the six patients, both of whom were admitted to the hospital following suicide attempts, however, had no initial reduction of total sleep (mean total sleep was 370 min.). Five patients initially had low levels of stage 3

TABLE 7-2. Longitudinal Sleep Studies in Depression: Comparison of Selected Sleep Variables Early and Late in Clinical Course

Authors	Patients	No.	Treatment	Time	Total sleep	REM%	Delta%	REM latency
Lowy *et al.*, 1971	Psychotic or severely depressed	6	None	Early	238 min	14	18	117 min
			Imipramine	Late	458 min	23	20	109 min
Mendels and Hawkins, 1971a[a]	Depressed	5[b]	None	Early	270 min	22	13	89 min
			ECT or Drugs	Late	325 min	23	19	45 min
Kupfer and Foster, 1973	Psychotic depression	1	None	Early	345 min	20	9.5[c]	16 min
			None	Late	471 min	27	33.7	6 min

[a] Data averaged from tables: Early—all nights before treatment; late—last three nights on study, except for Patient 4, for whom Nights 16–18 were averaged since drug treatment and/or awakenings interfered with later nights.
[b] Patient 6 presented graphically in a separate publication (Hawkins *et al.*, 1967).
[c] All stage 3 both early and late.

and 4; in four, the absolute amounts of stage 3 and 4 increased after improvement; in the fifth, this change took place several days prior to improvement. In three patients, REM sleep was initially low and returned to normal levels with improvement. In three other patients, REM sleep values were normal throughout the study.

.Interpretation of the sleep changes in the Lowy *et al.* (1971) study was complicated by the administration of dexamethasone and, later, imipramine, both of which suppress REM sleep in normals. The authors concluded that their data showed no consistent pattern of REM sleep in psychotic depression and neither supported nor contradicted Snyder's hypothesis on the relationship of REM sleep deprivation to psychotic depression.

In an even more intensive longitudinal study, Mendels and Hawkins (1971a) studied six hospitalized depressed patients for a total of 153 nights. All subjects were treated with ECT or tricyclic antidepressants. Considerable variability in sleep parameters was again noted between subjects and from night to night. Before treatment, sleep was fragmented and light with increased awake and drowsy times (see Table 7-2). There were marked fluctuations in REM sleep, suggesting a long-standing deficiency of this sleep stage, although the expression of the heightened pressure for REM sleep appeared to be blocked in some cases. In addition, successful treatment leads to increased amounts of REM sleep, at times greater than normal amounts in several patients. Individual differences must again be stressed, however. In two patients (numbers 2 and 4), REM sleep times were initially higher than normal, while REM latency was low; over time, REM (both as absolute minutes and percentage of total sleep) actually decreased, although in one patient (number 2), this was attributed to the patient's increasing antagonism to the sleep laboratory and clinical deterioration. As shown in Table 7-2, the overall results suggested increased total sleep and delta sleep improvement. While REM percentage was stable, REM latency fell with treatment.

In a longitudinal study of a psychotically depressed patient, Kupfer and Foster (1973) measured nightly EEG sleep changes and 24-hour telemetric activity measurements in a 54-year-old unmedicated woman. During the first half of the study (days 1–20), she was floridly delusional and severely depressed. She believed she was being "held" in the hospital while awaiting transfer to a prison for execution, she "confessed" to having murdered her entire family, to being a drug addict and to being "injected with gonorrhea and syphilis." During the second half of the hospitalization (nights 21–43) her psychosis abated and her mood improved spontaneously without drugs. As she improved, she slept longer and more efficiently, nonREM sleep increased significantly, especially stage 3 (both in terms of absolute minutes and as a percentage of total sleep) (Table 7-2). Total REM sleep tended to increase but did not reach statistical significance. A particularly striking change was in REM activity, a measure of total eye movement activity during REM sleep, which increased coincident with her sudden spontaneous improvement. REM latency was sh   both early and late in the study. Psychomotor activity decreasec as she improved, especially during the nighttime hours. It was interesting that the shift from the first to the second phase of her clinical course was marked by one or two nights of atypical sleep associated with either increased or decreased REM activity.

To summarize these longitudinal studies, tremendous variability exists from patient to patient and from night to night in the same patient. With improvement most patients show increased total sleep, delta sleep, and REM sleep. Whether or not a REM sleep rebound occurs during the waning phases of a depressive episode cannot definitely be decided. Markedly increased REM sleep or REM phasic events have been observed in a few patients who suddenly improved clinically either spontaneously or after ECT, but have not been observed when improvement was more slowly induced by treatment with imipramine. The REM-sleep suppressive effects of imipramine, seen in normal patients, may have, however, prevented the excessive elevation of REM sleep.

In view of the reported relationship between the phasic events of REM sleep and clinical improvement of depressed patients (Snyder, 1972; Kupfer and Foster, 1973) it is particularly interesting that Hauri and Mendels (1971) found a significant correlation between nightly patterning of eye movements in REM and clinical ratings of depression. As a measure of eye movement activity during REM episodes, they used percentage of phasic REM, the percentage of 30-second epochs during REM containing at least one eye movement. In a study of nine depressed patients, who slept from 10 to 32 nights each in the laboratory, the greater the percentage of phasic REM a patient showed, the less waking depression he indicated on the Beck Inventory both before sleep and on the following evening. No other sleep measure correlated with day-to-day fluctuations in Beck depression scores. These results suggested that depression might be correlated with malfunctioning of the phasic event system.

Sleep of Depressed Patients in Remission

Since unipolar depression is often a recurrent illness, the study of depressed patients in remission may reveal important information about predisposing personality or physiological factors. Previous studies had demonstrated that the sleep of depressed patients reverted toward normal as they improved during hospitalization or shortly following discharge. Hauri et al. (1974) studied a group of 14 remitted patients, hospitalized more than six months previously with unipolar depression. All patients were carefully screened to determine that they were living in the community, working, and socializing at least as well as they had before hospitalization. The patients were drug free. They were matched with normal subjects by sex, age, and education. As compared with controls, the former patients showed delayed sleep onset, shallower sleep (more stage 1, less delta sleep), a slower sleep cycle, more wakefulness, and increased variability from night to night for almost all sleep parameters. It is impossible to conclude, however, that these sleep abnormalities are a biological trait in depression-prone individuals, independent of clinical state. Psychological testing revealed that the former patients remained, at best, mildly depressed; compared with controls, they scored significantly higher on depression rating scales (the Beck, Zung, and MMPI D scales).

Chemical Correlates of Sleep in Depression

There has been considerable interest in the relationship between the biogenic amines, affective disorders, and sleep. According to the catecholamine hypothesis of affective disorders, depression is associated with a functional deficit of norepinephrine, while mania is associated with an excess (Schildkraut, 1965; Bunney and Davis, 1965).

In a study of 12 hospitalized, unmedicated depressed patients, Schildkraut et al. (1973) correlated EEG sleep measures and 24-hour urinary excretion of 3-methoxy-4-hydroxyphenylglycol (MHPG), a principal metabolite of norepinephrine in the brain (see Fig. 2-8). MHPG excretion was significantly lower in bipolar patients than in patients with chronic dysphoric characterologic depressions. Moreover, excretion of MHPG was inversely related to time spent in REM sleep, particularly in patients with bipolar illness. MHPG excretion did not correlate with total sleep time or delta sleep time. These results are compatable with data indicating an inverse relationship between REM sleep and central catecholamine activity (see chap. 2). In addition, the same authors noted an inverse relationship between MHPG excretion and REM sleep in a small number of amphetamine addicts during withdrawal, although statistical significance was not reached (Watson et al., 1972).

Other studies have also shown a negative relationship between

REM sleep and urinary catecholamine excretion. An inverse relationship has been noted between urinary norepinephrine excretion and REM sleep in three patients with periodic catatonia (Takahashi and Gjessing, 1972) and in a small number of bipolar patients "switching" from depression to mania (Bunney et al., 1972).

Using a different approach, Weiss et al. (1974) correlated metabolites of serotonin (5-hydroxy-indoleacetic acid, 5HIAA; see Fig. 2-1) and dopamine (homovanillic acid, HVA; see Fig. 2-8) in cerebrospinal fluid (CSF) with EEG sleep records in 11 unmedicated, hospitalized depressed patients. Neither the CSF metabolite concentrations nor the ratio (HVA/5HIAA) correlated significantly with any sleep parameter. While these data do not support the hypothesized relationship between sleep and biogenic amines, it is well to remember that CSF concentrations of 5HIAA or HVA in lumbar space may not reflect activity of the parent compounds in relevant areas of the central nervous system.

Further Sleep Studies in Bipolar Illness

Very little information exists about the sleep of manic patients. This is unfortunate because manic patients, with their remarkable energy levels, may go for weeks or months with little sleep and little subjective fatigue. Any theory about need for sleep and the functions of sleep must be able to account for the remarkable changes in energy levels, feelings of fatigue, and subjective need for sleep observed in these patients.

One reason there have been few studies is that manic patients are often uncooperative, particularly as the severity of the mania increases. In a useful clinical longitudinal analysis of the manic episode, Carlson and Goodwin (1973) described three major stages in the evolution of a manic episode: stage 1, characterized predominately by euphoria; stage 2, by anger and irritability; and stage 3 by severe panic. Polygraphic sleep studies, needless to say, are extremely difficult in stages 2 and 3.

Platman and Fieve (1970) investigated the sleep patterns of 31 bipolar depressed patients and 21 hypomanic or manic patients by nurses' ratings of sleep and by subjective ratings by patients. The authors concluded that the depressed patient perceived his sleep to be poorer than did the staff, while the manic patient saw his sleep as better than did the staff. Although the manic patient appeared to sleep less (201 minutes of "sound sleep" as compared with 258 minutes for depressed patients), he woke up feeling rested whereas the depressed patients woke up feeling fatigued. The staff noted fewer interruptions of sleep in mania than depression.

In two studies in which polygraphic recordings were possible, the authors concluded that the sleep of the hypomanic or manic patient resembled that of psychotically depressed patients in some respects (Table 7-3). Muratorio *et al.* (1968c) studied five patients for two nights each, whereas Mendels and Hawkins (1971b) studied an unmedicated 45-year-old hypomanic man for 17 of 25 consecutive nights. Like psychotically depressed patients studied in the same laboratories, the manic patients showed a marked reduction of total sleep time and stage 4 and in increase in awake and drowsy. While Muratorio *et al.* (1968c) reported REM percentage to be low both in their manic patients and in their psychotically depressed patients, Mendels and Hawkins (1971b) found that mean REM percentage in their hypomanic patient was between normal controls and psychotically depressed patients. These two investigators, like Hartman (1968a), found REM latency to be normal, although Mendels and Hawkins observed that it was frequently abbreviated early in the study. In their longitudinal study, Mendels and Hawkins (1971b) did not, apparently, observe any REM sleep rebound at the end, although their patient suffered considerable loss of REM sleep early in the study.

In a longitudinal sleep study of six manic-depressive patients, Hartmann (1968a) collected 162 all-night recordings that were made about once a week over periods of 10 to 26 months. Four patients were

TABLE 7-3. Polygraphic Sleep Studies of Manic or Hypomanic Patients with Comparison Groups

Author	Subjects	Number	Total sleep (min)	REM%	Stage 4%	REM latency
Muratorio, Maginni, and Pappagallo, 1968c	Manic Psychotic	5	253	16	5	82
	depressives	—	224	16	3	—
	Normals	—	408	28	18	—
Hartmann, 1968a[a]	Manic		300	19	12	103
	Normal	4	350	21	8	95
	Depressed	same patients	379	23	10	65
Mendels and Hawkins, 1971b	Hypomania	1	282	15	1.3	103
	Psychotic depressives	4	216	9	0.2	—
	Normals	14	414	25	19.7	—

[a] Data based on four patients studied in normal, depressed, and manic periods, calculated from Table 7-2 (Hartmann, 1968a).

studied while manic, normal, and depressed. As shown in Table 7-3, manic periods were characterized by low total sleep, slightly low REM sleep and REM percentage, and normal or elevated REM latency, as compared with normal periods in the same patients. Depressed periods showed normal total sleep, relatively high REM sleep and REM percentage, and low REM latency. Interpretation of his results is complicated by treatment with chlorpromazine or ECT in five patients, by the infrequent sampling of sleep, and by uncertainty as to severity of illness. Although rated as manic, one patient was studied as an outpatient. Furthermore, Hartmann's findings of increased REM sleep and REM percentage in depression, particularly severe depression, is at variance with the results of most other studies.

Somewhat different results, however, were reported by Jovanovic et al. (1973) who studied 10 female manic-depressive patients. In a brief report, they suggested that patients slept longer, better, and more deeply while manic than while depressed.

Sleep during the Switch Process in Manic-Depressive Illness

The *switch process* in bipolar illness is one of the most dramatic events in psychiatry. It refers to the change from a depressed state to a manic state or vice versa. A bipolar depressed woman, withdrawn, taciturn, appearing like a wizened old lady, may suddenly blossom into an energetic, joking, seductive young woman after switching into mania. Though less common, the switch from mania to depression may be equally sudden and dramatic.

Sitaram, Gillin, and Bunney (unpublished data) have observed that a rapid switch, either into mania or out of mania, is more likely to occur during the hours of 7:00 A.M. to 3:00 P.M. than at any other time of day (Fig. 7-2). Whether this clustering is due to biological factors or to psychosocial ones is not known. When examining sleep changes before and after the switch, total sleep, as estimated by nurses' ratings, fell slightly for several nights before the switch into mania and was especially low during the first few days of mania (see Fig. 7-3). Many patients experience total insomnia for a day or two at the onset of mania. Patients who switched into mania at night (11:00 P.M. to 7:00 A.M.) showed higher ratings for mania and greater loss of sleep than patients who switched at other times of the day (7:00 A.M. to 3:00 P.M. or 3:00 P.M. to 11:00 P.M. [see Table 7-4]). The sleep changes accompanying the switch from mania to depression were less dramatic.

Little data is published about EEG sleep changes during the switch process. Snyder (1972) reported a dramatic fall in REM time with little

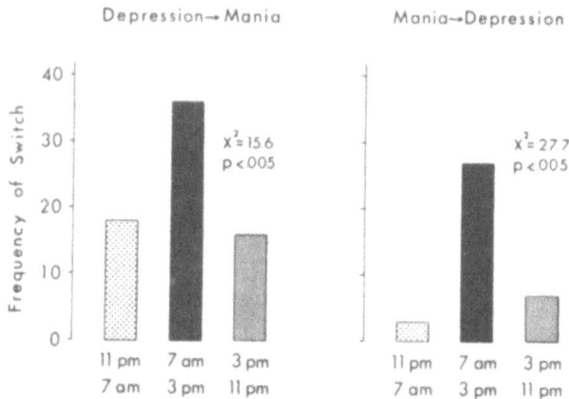

FIGURE 7-2.   Clustering of switch into and out of mania in daytime (7:00 A.M.–3:00 P.M.) as compared with evening (3:00 P.M.–11:00 P.M.) or nighttime (11:00 P.M.–7:00 A.M.) (Sitaram, Gillin, Bunney, unpublished data).

change in nonREM sleep during a "slow" switch (over 10 days) from depression to hypomania in a 65-year-old unmedicated woman. Bunney *et al.* (1972) reported a more dramatic fall in REM sleep at the onset of mania in a single patient who switched rapidly. In addition, in a second patient they showed an increase in REM sleep to normal levels and a lesser increase in nonREM coinciding with the switch out of

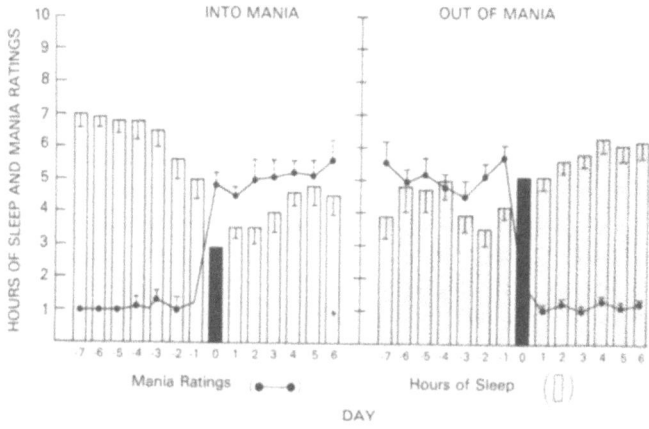

FIGURE 7-3.   Decreased total sleep before, during, and after switch into mania and increased sleep during and following switch out of mania in bipolar patients. Hours of sleep based on nurses' estimates (Sitaram, Gillin, and Bunney, unpublished data).

TABLE 7-4. The Rapid Switch into Mania: Manic Ratings and Nurses'
Estimate of Total Sleep as a Function of Time of Switch

	Time of switch		
	11:00 P.M.– 7:00 A.M.	7:00 A.M.– 3:00 P.M.	3:00 P.M.– 11:00 P.M.
Manic ratings[a]	6.8 ± 0.4	4.6 ± 0.2	5.4 ± 0.4
Total sleep (hr)[b]	2.6 ± 0.4	4.7 ± 0.3	3.7 ± 0.6

Mean ± sem for first four days of mania
[a] $p < .001$, $F = 11.03$, df 2,69 ANOVA
[b] $p < .005$, $F = 6.9$, df 2,53 ANOVA
From Sitaram, Gillin, Bunney (unpublished data).

mania. Gillin and Wyatt (1975) demonstrated marked reduction in REM
sleep and nonREM sleep in a 19-year-old bipolar girl who was studied
on consecutive nights through two manic episodes. During the periods
of depression without mania, REM and nonREM returned to relatively
normal values. Although she suffered considerable loss of REM sleep
during periods of insomnia, no REM rebound was observed. Since she
remained clinically depressed, however, a marked elevation of REM
sleep may not have occurred until a later time of relative clinical
remission.

As shown in Fig. 7-4, a sudden switch from depression into severe
mania may be associated with severe insomnia. The patient, a 51-year-
old woman with a long history of severe bipolar illness, unresponsive
to conventional pharmacologic treatments, had depressions characterized by mutism, anorexia, withdrawal, low mood, self-deprecatory
remarks, and negativism. During the switch process she passed quickly
into "Stage 3" mania. During the first seven days of mania, she had
total insomnia for five days. On the two nights on which she did sleep,
she had virtually no REM sleep despite elevated amounts of nonREM
sleep (344 and 448 minutes, respectfully). As the patient's mania
abated, her sleep returned toward normal.

Studies such as these indicate that it is particularly difficult to
generalize about the sleep of the manic. There is clearly an evolution of
sleep during the manic episode. As the patient gets farther away from
the switch period, sleep tends to return to normal, in part because of
improvement in clinical condition.

The switch process may actually occur during sleep. As shown in
Fig. 7-5, a 36-year-old bipolar patient was studied with polygraphic
recordings on five nights when she went to bed with a severe, retarded
depression and woke up in a wildly manic state. On four of the five

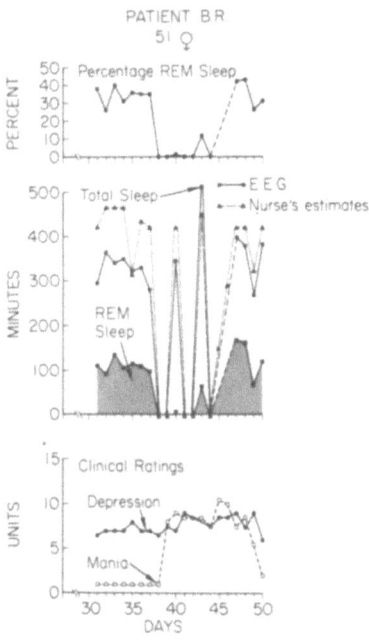

FIGURE 7-4. All-night polygraphic sleep records during switch into mania in a 51-year-old woman with severe bipolar illness (Gillin and Snyder, unpublished data).

occasions, the last recorded sleep state was REM sleep while on the fifth night, she lay in bed in a drowsy condition (a mixture of alpha EEG, wakefulness, and stage 1) before appearing at the nursing station with clear signs of mania. We cannot be certain that the switch occurred during EEG arousal (either REM or awake-stage 1 as compared with nonREM sleep); she may have switched earlier in the night and continued sleeping, although this seems unlikely in this patient whose daytime switches were always rapid and dramatic.

Hartmann (1968a) studied two bipolar patients who went to bed in a mixed hypomanic-depressed state and arose with a much greater degree of clinical mania. Both patients awoke out of nonREM sleep (Hartmann, written communication, 27 October 1975). Interestingly, one patient (Mrs. V.) reported a nightmare that involved her killing her mother, but prior to waking up in a manic state she had had about 50 minutes of stage 2, 3, and 4 since the only REM period of the night. Thus, the evidence to date does not clarify whether or not the switch during sleep occurs during a unique stage of sleep or whether it would be related, in a psychodynamic way, to REM sleep or nonREM mentation. These data do suggest, however, that the switch into mania may occur during sleep in the absence of concurrent environmental influences.

Besides the "fast" and the "slow" switches, there are recorded cases of patients with regular, 48-hour cycles. Table 7-5 summarizes the available data on the time of switch in 48-hour cycling patients. With one exception (the case reported by Folin and Shaffer), all of the patients typically switched during the evening or bedtime hours. In many cases, the switch occurred during sleep. Nevertheless, the switch does not appear to depend upon sleep *per se* since Jenner *et al.* (1967) reported that their patient continued to switch even when he was prevented from sleeping. Moreover, Jenner *et al.* (1968) demonstrated that the 48-hour mood cycle was not the product of an immutable "clock" within the patient that was impervious to environmental influence. When the patient was studied in an isolation chamber on a 22-hour day rather than a 24-hour day, his 48-hour mood cycle became a 44-hour mood cycle. This result did suggest that environmental events do influence the underlying biological process.

In the case of one 48-hour cycling bipolar patient (originally reported for 40 days by Bunney and Hartmann, 1965), behavioral data and "time of switch" was analyzed for two years. The switch from depression to mania occurred predominately between 2:00 A.M. and 4:00 A.M. and was preceded by an average of four hours sleep (as estimated by nurses). The switch from mania to depression usually

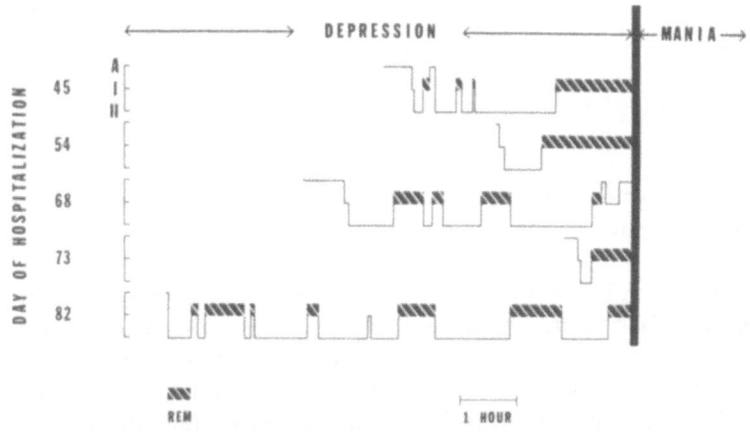

FIGURE 7-5. Switch into mania occurring during sleep in a bipolar patient (Gillin, Post, Jimerson, Mazure, and Bunney, unpublished data).

TABLE 7-5. Time of Day at Which Switch Occurs in Patients with 48-Hour Mood Cycles.

Author	Patient	Time of Switch
MacLulich, 1899	45-yr.-old woman	Midnight.
Scheiber, 1901	63-yr.-old man with 48-hr cycles since 2nd stroke	Bad day begins and ends at midnight.
Folin and Shaffer, 1902		"Nervous behavior" began suddenly between 10:00 and 11:00 A.M.
Starobinski, 1921	67-yr.-old man with 48-hr cycles	Bad day begins at 2:00–4:00 A.M.
Wiesel, 1927	40-yr.-old man	Transition from depression to mania always took place at night, usually 1:00 A.M. after 3–4 hr sleep.
Richter, 1938	Case W (59-yr.-old woman with 48-hr cycles)	Switch apparently occured during bedtime hours. Sleepless nights preceded bad days.
	Case B (60-yr.-old woman)	Switch apparently occurred during bedtime hours, such as 6:00 A.M. Bad days preceded by sleepless night.
Delay et al., 1961	58-yr.-old manic, 48-hr cycles for 3 yr.	Switch into mania: 3:00 A.M. When high, goes to sleep with difficulty but wakes up depressed at 8:00 A.M.
Jenner et al., 1967, 1968	56-yr.-old man with 12-yr. history of 48-hr cycle	Switch tended to occur during sleep, took place even if he were prevented from sleeping. On active day, he woke up early and elated; on inactive day, he woke late and lethargic. When he lived in an artificial environment on a 22-hr day rather than a 48-hr day, his cycle length changed from 48 to 44 hr.
Kupfer and Heninger, 1972	70-yr.-old man with 4-yr. history of 48-hr cycle	Largest changes in mood occurred between 7:00 P.M. and 7:00 A.M.
Sitaram et al., 1976 (unpublished)	43-yr.-old woman with 2-yr. history of 48-hr cycles	Switch into mania occurred between 2:00 A.M. and 4:00 A.M. Switch out of mania occurred between 4:00 A.M. and 6:00 A.M.

occurred between 4:00 A.M. and 6:00 A.M. and was preceded by an average 4.6 hours of sleep (Sitaram, Gillin, and Bunney, unpublished data).

Kupfer and Heninger (1972) obtained all-night sleep records from a 70-year-old man with a four-year history of 48-hour cyclic change in mood. On nights preceding depressed days, early morning awakening was increased while REM activity (a measure of total REM eye movements per night) and REM index (a measure of average number of eye movements per minute of REM sleep) were significantly decreased. The more depressed the patient was in the morning, the less REM activity and the more early morning awakening he had the night before. Despite the relationship of REM activity to depression, REM deprivation did not alter the mood cycles. This result appears to be consistent with the report of Jenner et al. that deprivation of sleep did not prevent the continuation of the 48-hour mood cycle in their patient.

In summary, the sleep of manic and hypomanic patients is variable from day to day and from patient to patient. In general, total sleep tends to be short, with insomnia varying with the intensity of mania. REM sleep is particularly prone to reduction. Insomnia is likely during the switch process from depression to mania. The degree of insomnia at that time appears to vary with the time of day at which the switch occurred, with the intensity of mania, and with the speed with which the manic episode evolves. The switch process can occur during sleep. In the case of regular 48-hour cycling patients, the switch is particularly likely during the nighttime hours.

Experimental Deprivation of Sleep in Depression

Total sleep deprivation or selective REM sleep deprivation appears to have antidepressant effects. If this finding appears contrary to common sense and to the ideas that originally motivated sleep investigations of depressed patients, the evidence for this unanticipated conclusion, nevertheless, is becoming stronger.

In perhaps the first careful study of therapeutic sleep deprivation, Pflug and Tölle (1971a,b) studied 23 hospitalized patients with endogenous depression, 11 with neurotic depression, and 23 normal controls (Table 7-6). The subjects were deprived of sleep for one night (approximately 36 hours). All of the endogenously depressed patients improved clinically. The clinical amelioration was long-lasting in some patients, transient in others, and followed by brief but substantial deterioration on the second day after sleep deprivation in still other patients. Neither the neurotically depressed patients nor the normals showed significant changes in mood, although five neurotically depressed patients improved and one worsened. In addition, sleep deprivation produced a significant rise in blood pressure in the opthalmic artery as compared with the brachial artery in endogenously depressed patients, but not in neurotically depressed patients or normals (Bojanovsky et al., 1973). In a later study, Pflug (1972) reported good results in ambulatory patients.

Several other investigators have also reported generally good results (Voss and Kind, 1974; Bhanji and Roy, 1975; Matussek et al., 1974; van den Burg and van den Hoofdakker, 1975; Post et al., 1976).

TABLE 7-6. Effects of Deliberate Sleep Deprivation on Depressed Patients[a]

Authors	Subjects	Total no.	No. improved
Pflug and Tölle, 1971a,b	Endogenously depressed	23	23
	Neurotically depressed	11	5
	Normal controls	23	0
Pflug, 1972	Ambulatory, endogenously depressed	12	10
Voss and Kind, 1974	Endogenously depressed	9	7
	Mixed endogenously–reactively depressed	4	1
Matussek et al , 1974	Chronic and involutional	14	7
Zimanova and Vojtechovsky, 1974	Endogenous or secondary to alcoholism	20	3
Bhanji and Roy, 1975	Mixed depression	28	17
Van den Burg and van den Hoofdakker, 1975	Endogenously depressed	10	10
Post et al., 1976	Primary depression	19	10

[a] Sleep deprivation was for approximately 36 hours Van den Burg and van den Hoofdakker (1975) performed sleep deprivation twice in each patient, separated by one night of sleep

Matussek et al. (1974) observed clinical improvement in 7 of 14 endogenously depressed patients who were sleep deprived. In a 12-hour urine collection before sleep deprivation, the group that improved had a significantly higher ratio of norepinephrine to epinephrine than the group that did not improve. Moreover, following sleep deprivation, responders had increased urinary excretion of epinephrine and norepinephrine, while nonresponders did not.

Van den Burg and van den Hoofdakker (1975) deprived 10 endogenous patients on each of two nights, with one night of sleep in between. The overall results were of mild but consistent improvement, except in two patients who showed clear-cut, sustained improvement. They also suggested that sleep deprivation might be most beneficial in patients with clear diurnal mood swings.

Post, Kotin, and Goodwin (1976) reported clear improvement of depressive symptomotology in 10 of 19 patients who were sleep deprived for one night. Those who improved had higher depressive ratings and tended to be older than nonresponders. CSF concentrations of 5-hydroxyindoleacetic acid (5-HIAA) and homovanillic acid (HVA) were not affected by sleep deprivation. There was, however, a significant interaction between change in 3-methoxy-4-hydroxyphenylglycol (MHPG) and clinical response, with good responders showing a decrease in MHPG concentration and poor responders an increase. While total sleep (estimated by nurses) was not different in responders as compared with nonresponders before sleep deprivation, nonresponders slept significantly longer on the night after sleep deprivation than did responders.

Not all investigators have reported good clinical effects with sleep deprivation. In a study of 20 inpatients suffering from endogenous depression or depression in chronic alcoholics, Zimanova and Vojtechovsky (1974) found clinical deterioration in nine and marked improvement in only three.

In some studies, sleep deprivation has been reported to precipitate hypomania or mania in depressed bipolar patients (van den Burg and van den Hoofdakker, 1975; Pflug, 1973; Zimanova and Vojtechovsky, 1974), although the switch into mania did not always occur immediately coincident with the sleep deprivation. Fig. 7-6 shows total EEG sleep time in a bipolar woman studied through several cycles of depression and mania. As shown, she switched from depression to mania when deprived of sleep for one night. This figure also illustrated the gradually increasing length of total sleep as the patient progresses through the manic episode. Whether or not sleep deprivation per se has been responsible for these reports of switch cannot be determined. Nonspecific factors may be important or endogenous, uncontrolled mechanisms may play a role.

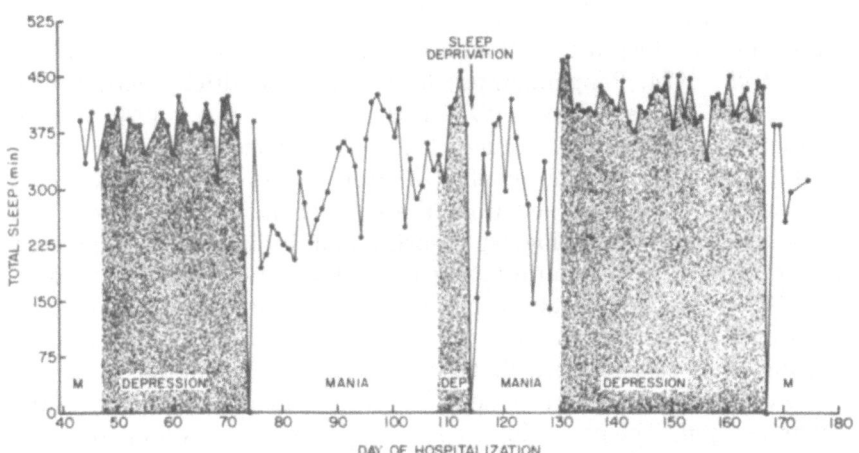

FIGURE 7-6.   All-night polygraphic sleep studies showing total sleep time in a bipolar patient studied nightly during manic and depressed phases. Onset of manic phase was marked by spontaneous total insomnia and was apparently precipitated by experimental sleep deprivation. (Gillin, Post, Stoddard, Bunney, unpublished data.)

The mechanisms by which sleep deprivation alleviates depression are not clear. Several hypotheses have been considered.

1. Sleep deprivation produces psychological effects such as the sense of accomplishment in completing a difficult task, or, through paradoxical intention, in doing the very thing that is most frightening to an insomniac depressed patient, going without sleep.

2. Biochemical effects of sleep deprivation are possible but remain hypothetical and unproven. While urinary catecholamine metabolites were increased before and after sleep deprivation in responders, these changes probably reflect peripheral sympathetic activity. It is of interest that a significant interaction was found between CSF MHPG concentration and clinical response, suggesting that clinical response to sleep deprivation might be related to central norepinephrine metabolism. CSF metabolites of dopamine and serotonin did not change. The effects of sleep deprivation on biogenic amines in brains of animals are slight and controversial, probably reflective of stress or severe exhaustion (Bliss, 1967; Radulovacki, 1973). In addition, using other biochemical indices, Bojanovsky, Koch, and Tölle (1974) reported that sleep deprivation increased serum calcium concentration and decreased hematocrit (a measure of the number of red blood cells), that these changes were more pronounced than those produced by amitriptyline, and that these and other electrolytes correlated with good clinical response.

Animal studies also suggest that sleep deprivation leads to the elaboration of sleep factors (Monnier and Schoenenberger, 1972; Monnier et al., 1974; Pappenheimer, Miller, and Goodrich, 1967; Fence, Koski, and Pappenheimer, 1971; Drucker-Colin et al., 1970; Matsumoto, Sogabe, and Hori-Santiago, 1972). These factors might be related to the short-term clinical benefits. If sleep factors are involved and if they act by producing sedation, these biochemical speculations are consistent with psychological theories that indicate that depressed patients are excessively aroused (van den Burg and van den Hoofdakker, 1975). Sleep deprivation may tend to decrease arousal levels and return the patients to an arousal level more conducive to normal functioning. It is also relevant that Zung et al. (1964) suggested that the sleep disturbance of depression resulted from increased activity of the arousal system. The physiological affects of sleep deprivation, however, remain controversial. This confusing state of affairs is reflected in the question of whether sleep deprivation does or does not increase physiological indices of arousal, such as a rise in palm or skin conductance, respiration, and a fall in alpha EEG amplitude (see Malmo and Bilanger, 1967).

3. Sleep deprivation may interrupt certain biorhythms that have been implicated in affective illness (Kripke, 1975; Curtis, 1972). As suggested earlier, sleep deprivation was reported to affect patients with diurnal mood swings more than patients without.

Effects of REM Sleep Deprivation on Depression

That REM sleep deprivation might have antidepressant effects was suggested by several lines of evidence (summarized by Vogel, Traub, and Ben-Horin, 1968): (a) major antidepressants in normals and ECT in animals were reported to suppress REM sleep; (b) reserpine, which can cause depression in some patients who receive it for treatment of hypertension, elevated REM sleep; and (c) REM deprivation in animals increased drive-related behavior, such as motor activity, feeding, and sex.

In a pilot, uncontrolled study, Vogel and his collegues (1968) REM deprived five severely depressed patients by the awakening method for seven to fourteen days. Two patients improved substantially, and three showed little or no clinical change.

In a later, carefully designed study, Vogel et al. (1975b) showed that REM sleep deprivation significantly alleviated depression in endogenous patients, but not in reactively depressed patients. Patients were essentially unmedicated and were assigned to either an experimental group who were REM sleep deprived by arousals or to a control group who were awakened from nonREM sleep. Following three weeks of experimental REM deprivation or nonREM awakenings, the endogenously depressed patients who were REM deprived had improved significantly on the Global and Hamilton scores and rated significantly better than controls (Table 7-7). Three weeks after being crossed over to the REM sleep deprivation procedure, the controls were significantly less depressed than before. By the end of the project, 17 of 34 endogenously depressed patients were discharged after receiving REM sleep deprivation as the only specific treatment (an average of seven weeks of REM sleep awakenings). Among the endogenously depressed patients who failed to respond to REM sleep deprivation, most of those who later received imipramine also failed to respond. ECT was effective in most of the nonresponders to either imipramine or REM sleep deprivation.

Among the reactively depressed patients, REM sleep deprivation produced no significant clinical changes over time or in comparison with nonREM awakenings. After reviewing the effects of imipramine in

TABLE 7-7. Effects of Experimental REM
Deprivation on Endogenously Depressed Patients
(Vogel *et al.*, 1975b)

	Controls	Experimental
Number	17	17
Age	56	59
REM %		
Baseline	23.4%	22%
Deprivation	26.7%	8.1%[a]
Recovery	25.8%	31.9%[b]
Global Scale		
Baseline	4.4	4.6
3 weeks	4.1	3.4[c]
Hamilton Scale		
Baseline	47.8	49.9
3 weeks	42.3	35.5[d]

[a] $p < .001$ } paired comparison with baseline
[b] $p = .005$
[c] $p = .018$ (comparison between controls and experimental)
[d] $p = .029$ (comparison between controls and experimental)

depression, Vogel and his colleagues also concluded that the efficacy of imipramine in treating depression was about the same as that of REM sleep deprivation.

Effects of Antidepressant Medication and Lithium Salts on Human Sleep

As shown in Table 7-8 and discussed chapter 2, there is general agreement that tricyclic antidepressant medications and monoamine oxidase inhibitors, in high doses, profoundly suppress REM sleep in normal subjects. This has been demonstrated with the monoamine oxidase inhibitors isocarboxide and pargyline (Wyatt *et al.*, 1969), and nialamide (Toyoda, 1964), and with the tricyclic antidepressants chlori-mipramine (clomipramine) (Passouant *et al.*, 1975; Dunleavy *et al.*, 1972), imipramine (Dunleavy *et al.*, 1972; Toyoda, 1964), amitriptyline (Hartmann, 1968b; Hartmann and Cravens, 1973a; Nakazawa *et al.*, 1975b; Toyoda, 1964), desipramine (Dunleavy *et al.*, 1972; Zung, 1966; Toyoda, 1964), and doxepin (Dunleavy *et al.*, 1972). Imipramine has also been shown to suppress REM sleep in eneuretic boys (Ritvo *et al.*, 1967). Furthermore, with extended administration for two weeks, pargyline and

TABLE 7-8. Effects of Monoamine Oxidase Inhibitors and Tricyclic Antidepressants on Sleep in Man

Authors	Patients	No.	Drug/dose	Major findings
Toyoda, 1964	Normals (3) Psychiatric patients (3)	6	Imipramine 50 mg once	↓REM%. ↑Body movements.
	Depressed patient	1	Desmethylimipramine 50 mg	↓REM%, to lesser degree than imipramine.
LeGassiche et al., 1965	Normal / Normal / Tranylcypromine addict	1 / 1 / 1	Nialamide 50 mg / Amitriptyline 25–50 mg / Tranylcypromine (> 120–320 mg)	On high dose, REM near zero. During withdrawal, ↑REM% (up to 75.7% or 215 min one night; 67.5% or 403 min on another). REM onset sleep, nightmares.
Zung, 1966	Normals	7	Desipramine 25 mg three times a day	↓REM% but ↑no. of REM periods. ↑Stage E (Stage 4). ↓Sleep stage changes.
Cramer and Kuhlo, 1967	Depressed	2	Nialamide (100–500 mg) for 36–56 days	↓REM, especially in first cycles of night, coincided with improvement of depression and, in one case, switch into mania. ↑Delta.
Ritvo et al., 1967	Eneuretic boys	7	Imipramine 25 mg at bedtime	↓REM%, ↑REM Latency.↑Stage 2.
Cramer and Ohlmeier, 1967	28-year-old addict	1	Addiction to Jatrosom (tranylcypromine up to 205 mg/day and trifluoperazine, up to 17 mg/day)	While on drug, REM sleep was zero. On 7th day off drug, total sleep was 417 min, REM sleep 106 min and REM latency zero. Urinary 5-HIAA was reduced during withdrawal.
Muratorio, Maggini, and Murri, 1968b	Depressives (4-endogenous, 6-neurotic)	10	P-3693A (Pfizer) 75–300 mg/day	At 7 and 14 days of treatment, patients were improved (Hamilton Scale) and showed significantly REM%,↑stage 4.
Hartmann, 1968b	Normals	8	Amitriptyline 75 mg at bedtime for 2 days	↓REM and REM%. ↑REM Latency.

continued

TABLE 7-8 (continued)

Authors	Patients	No.	Drug/dose	Major findings
Zung, 1969	Depressed males	6	Desipramine 25 mg 4 times a day for 4 weeks	REM% decreased during first week of treatment but increased during 4th week. ↑ Stage E (Stage 4). ↓ Wakefulness.
Wyatt et al., 1969	Normal Depressed	2 2	Isocarboxide 30–60 mg for 14 days, Pargyline 50–100 mg for 14 days Mebanazine 15 mg for 24 days Phenelzine 15–45 mg for 14 days	Extended REM reduction or suppression with extended treatment, REM rebound noted after mebanazine but not after other drugs (8–11 days).
Akindale et al., 1970	Normal volunteers	2	Nialamide 75 mg po for 17 days and 500 mg IM for 1 day	No effect.
Wyatt et al., 1971	Depressed patients	3	Phenelzine 60–90 mg/day for 5–22 days	Total REM suppression after 5–22 days. Mood improvement coincided with REM suppression in depressed patients. REM rebound on withdrawal.
	Anxious-depressed	9	Phenelzine, up to 75 mg	Total REM suppression for 14–40 nights beginning 6–47 days after drug started and coinciding with clinical improvement. Large REM rebound on discontinuation.
Kupfer and Bowers, 1972	Psychiatric patients	9	Phenelzine 45–60 mg for 5 weeks	↑ NREM, ↑ stage 2. ↓ REM and REM% (both near zero). ↑ NREM, ↑ stage 2. ↓ CSF HVA, no change in 5-HIAA. During withdrawal, REM rebound correlated with ↑ CSF HVA.
Dürrigl et al., 1973b	Endogenous depression	10	Imipramine 150 mg for 5 days	↑ Wakefulness. ↓ REM and REM%, ↓ no. of REM periods.

Reference	Group	N	Drug/dose	Findings
Hartmann and Cravens, 1973a	Normals	10	Amitriptyline 50 mg at bedtime for 28 days	↑Total sleep, ↓REM, ↓REM% throughout drug administration. REM rebound on withdrawal. ↑Delta sleep, ↓sleep latency early.
Dunleavy and Oswald, 1973	Endogenous depression	22	Phenelzine 60–90 mg	Total REM suppression within days to weeks. Date of onset of sustained mood improvement coincided with REM suppression.
Shirakura, 1973	Manic-depressive, depressed	3	Isocarboxide (0.5 mg/day) for 10 days	↓REM% initially. ↑Delta %.
Passouant et al., 1975	Normals	7	Clorimipramine 25–175 mg for 4 days	Total or near total prolonged suppression of REM. ↑Stage 2, ↓stage 4. No REM rebound in first 3 days.
	Narcoleptic	1	25–100 mg for 4 days	Total or near total suppression of REM.
	Depressed	3	25–200 mg/day for 16–27 days	Total suppression of REM without much or any rebound in the first 3–7 nights.
Nakazawa et al., 1975b	Normals	5	(1) Amitriptyline 25 mg hs for one night	↓REM% and REM. ↑Total sleep, ↑stage 2, ↑stage 3. No REM rebound on 2 recovery nights.
			(2) Partial differential REM deprivation for one night	REM rebound on first recovery night but not second.
			(3) Amitriptyline 25 mg po at bedtime on night after partial differential REM deprivation	↓REM% on night of drug administration and REM rebound next night.
Gillin and Wyatt, 1975	Anxious-depressed	6	Phenelzine 60–90 mg per day for 4–8 weeks	Total REM suppression on drug. Marked REM rebound lasting at least 17 days; one patient had zero REM for 12 days after drug was stopped and then had a REM rebound.

isocarboxide were reported to completely suppress REM sleep. In the case of imipramine, desipramine, chlorimipramine, and doxepin, the REM suppressive effects lessened somewhat over the course of a month, but complete tolerance did not develop. Although pargyline and isocarboxide were administered for only two weeks in the normal volunteer study, tolerance did not appear since, if anything, the REM suppressive effects were still increasing.

During withdrawal, normal volunteers showed significant REM sleep rebounds following omission of imipramine, desipramine, chlorimipramine, and doxepin (Dunleavy et al., 1972), and amitriptyline (Hartmann and Cravens, 1973a). The rebound lasted as long as a month. No REM sleep rebound developed during the first eight or nine nights following discontinuation of pargyline and isocarboxide (Wyatt et al., 1969).

Nakazawa et al. (1975b) performed an interesting experiment on the effect of amitriptyline on the REM sleep rebound in normal subjects. The drug itself, administered for one night, suppressed REM sleep but did not produce a REM sleep rebound on two following recovery nights. In contrast, following one night of partial differential REM deprivation by restricting the length of the sleep period, a REM rebound was observed on the first but not the second recovery night. In the third part of the experiment, the subjects again underwent partial differential REM deprivation; on the first recovery night amitriptyline was administered, producing a significant reduction in REM sleep as compared with baseline. On the second recovery night, however, an excess of REM sleep in comparison to baseline was noted. These results suggest that a single dose of amitriptyline may delay the REM sleep rebound of REM sleep-deprived persons but does not eliminate it. Perhaps the same phenomena occur in depressed patients, REM sleep deprived in the waxing phases of the illness who are given amitriptyline later.

Monoamine oxidase inhibitors produce profound REM sleep suppression and a REM sleep rebound after administration in therapeutic doses to depressed patients (see Fig. 2-13). These phenomena have been observed with ixocarboxide (Shirakura, 1973), mebanazine (Wyatt et al., 1969), nialamide (Cramer and Kuhlo, 1967), and phenelzine (Wyatt et al., 1969, 1971; Kupfer and Bowers, 1972; Akindale et al., 1970; Dunleavy and Oswald, 1973; Gillin and Wyatt, 1975). Indeed, the mood-elevating clinical response appears to coincide with abolition of REM sleep. Although patients have been followed for months with neither recollection of dreams in the morning nor evidence of REM sleep during polygraphic recordings at night, no adverse effects have been reported that are attributable directly to REM suppression by monoamine oxidase inhibitors. During withdrawal, some depressed patients have experienced frightening dreams and nightmares in association with markedly elevated amounts of REM sleep, but these have subsided with time (Wyatt et al., 1971; Gillin and Wyatt, 1975).

In addition, following omission of phenelzine in depressed patients, REM sleep may continue to be suppressed for periods as long as two weeks, or no REM rebound may be observed at all in occasional patients (Kupfer and Bowers, 1972; Gillin and Wyatt, 1975). These deviations from the expected REM rebound may be related to genetically determined differences in the rate at which phenelzine is metabolized (Vesell, 1972) and to biochemical factors, particularly involving dopamine (Kupfer and Bowers, 1972).

The evidence from these studies of monoamine oxidase inhibitors in depressed patients is consistent, therefore, with the hypothesis that deprivation of REM sleep and increased REM pressure have antidepressant effects (Vogel, 1975; Vogel et al., 1975b).

In two separate studies of addicts to tranylcypromine or to Jatrosom (a tranylcypromine-containing compound), LeGassiche et al. (1965) and Cramer and Ohlmeier (1967) reported complete REM sleep suppression while the patients were maintained on high doses. LeGassiche and his colleagues also reported extremely high amounts of REM sleep during withdrawal, although Cramer and Ohlmeier did not on a single night seven days after omission of the drug.

In contrast to their effects in normals, the tricyclic antidepressants do not clearly suppress REM sleep in depressed patients. The only tricyclic drug that has been shown to produce a profound REM suppressive effect in these patients is chlorimipramine (Passouant et al., 1975), which also appears to be the most powerful REM-sleep suppressor in normals (Dunleavy et al., 1972). Passouant and his colleagues found total REM-sleep suppression during 16 to 27 days of treatment but no REM rebound during the first three to seven nights of withdrawal. In one of the few other studies in which tricyclic antidepressants have been studied in depressed patients, Zung (1969b) reported that REM percentage was decreased the first week of treatment with desipramine but was elevated by the fourth week of treatment. During initial administration, both imipramine (Dürrigl et al., 1973b) and desmethylimipramine (Toyoda, 1964) were observed to reduce REM sleep but the effects of long-term administration were not reported.

In one other long-term study of the effects of an antidepressant drug on the sleep of depressed patients, Muratorio *et al.* (1968) reported that P-3693A produced significant clinical improvement and increased REM percentage and stage 4 at 7 and 14 days of treatment.

As discussed earlier in this chapter, both Lowy *et al.* (1971) and Mendels and Hawkins (1971a) observed normal or high levels of REM sleep in patients receiving tricyclic antidepressant medication during longitudinal studies.

Lewis and Oswald (1969) studied the sleep changes in three women who had taken overdoses of tricyclic antidepressants (amitriptyline 3925 mg, nortriptyline 5000 mg, and imipramine 1000 mg, respectfully). REM sleep was markedly suppressed during the first five days or so following ingestion. A REM sleep rebound then occurred, peaking at about 9 to 12 nights, and was accompanied by vivid, unpleasant sexual dreams. Accentuated sleep spindles were also noted for the first 6 to 12 days. The REM sleep rebound lasted about one month. While this prolonged elevation of REM percentage could be related to protein synthesis, as the authors suggest, it may also reflect, in part, the sleep changes ascribed by Snyder to the waning phases of depression.

The effects of antidepressant medication upon nonREM parameters have been variable. Delta sleep has been increased by short- and long-term administration of amitriptyline in normals (Nakazawa *et al.*, 1975b; Hartmann and Cravens, 1973a); by short- and long-term administration of desipramine in normals (Zung, 1966) and depressed patients (Zung, 1969b), respectfully; by long-term administration of P-3693A in depressed patients (Muratorio *et al.*, 1968b); by the monoamine oxidase inhibitors isocarboxide and nialamide in depressed patients (Shirakura, 1973; Cramer and Kuhlo, 1967). By way of contrast, delta sleep was reduced both by chlorimipramine in normals (Passouant, 1975) and by imipramine in depressed patients (Dürrigl *et al.*, 1973b). In this respect, it is interesting that both imipramine and chlorimipramine have been reported to increase wakefulness and body movements during sleep in normals (Dunleavy *et al.*, 1972; Toyoda, 1964), thus reminding us that these drugs have stimulant properties. Phenelzine has generally increased nonREM sleep, by elevating stage 2 rather than delta sleep (Wyatt *et al.*, 1971; Kupfer and Bowers, 1972).

With regard to the other major somatic treatment of depression, electroshock therapy (ECT) does not appear to reduce REM sleep predictably in depressed patients (Green and Stajduher, 1966; Mendels and Hawkins, 1971a; Vogel *et al.*, 1975). Some patients actually show markedly increased REM sleep during and following ECT treatment.

In one other report on treatment, Hauri and Hawkins (1972) studied the effects of leucotomy in the sleep of a 59-year-old woman suffering from a severe refractory depression with obsessive thoughts and ruminations. Prior to surgery, she had little delta sleep or REM sleep. Although her clinical condition improved dramatically immediately after surgery, stages 3 and 4 increased only gradually beginning about 10 days after surgery and required about six months to reach normal levels. This slow return of stage 4 to normal was in agreement with earlier reports from this group of investigators that clinical improvement precedes normalization of delta sleep in depressed patients (Mendels and Hawkins, 1967b). These data suggest that the suppression of delta sleep in depression is not caused directly by depressed mood but perhaps by a third, slow to change variable, and that some bodily functions remain abnormal for periods up to six months after recovery from depression.

The effects of lithium carbonate on human sleep are shown in Table 7-9. Except for the first study (Brebbia et al., 1969) in which serum lithium concentrations were below the accepted therapeutic range of 0.6 to 1.2 mEq/1, all subsequent reports agree that lithium in therapeutic doses suppresses REM sleep and REM percentage, increases REM latency and delta sleep, and is not followed by a REM sleep rebound once it is discontinued. REM sleep reduction is achieved by shorter REM sleep periods. The effects of lithium on sleep parameters are intimately related to either serum levels or red blood cell concentrations of lithium. [The latter measure is thought to be a better indication of intracellular lithium than serum lithium concentrations (Chernik et al., 1974).] The REM suppressive effects of lithium appear to be independent of the patients' initial sleep characteristics. For example, in the study of Chernik and Mendels (1974) REM percentage was "normalized" (reduced from a high value of 25.6% before lithium to 19.8% with treatment), while in the study of Kupfer et al. (1974) it was reduced to subnormal levels (from 19.5% to 12.5%). Although lithium increases delta sleep in patients who initially exhibit some delta sleep, it apparently cannot induce delta sleep in patients who lack it before treatment.

Concluding Comments on Affective Disorders

The exact relationship of sleep disturbance to affective disorders remains elusive. Altered sleep is a major symptom of most patients with affective illness, but not all. Even when it is present, the direction of change is variable, with some patients exhibiting insomnia and others hypersomnia. (Exact definitions of these terms are still required.) More specific sleep indices of depression also seem to be missing. While a shortened REM latency remains one of the most predictable

TABLE 7-9. Effects of Lithium Salts on the Sleep of Man

Authors	Subjects	No.	Drug/dose	Plasma levels	Major findings
Brebbia et al., 1969	Normals	3	Lithium carbonate 750 mg/day for 8 days	0.33 to 0.49	No significant effects.
	Remitted manic-depressives	3	"Comparable" doses for 10 days to 18 months	0.34 to 0.46	
Kupfer et al., 1970a	Manic-depressive or depressed	7	Lithium carbonate 900–1800 mg/day	0.7 to 1.3	↓REM and REM%, ↑REM latency. ↑Delta sleep. ↓REM activity. No REM rebound.
Mendels and Chernik, 1973	Depressed patients	5	Lithium carbonate dose not stated	Not stated	↑REM Latency (34 to 53 min). ↑Delta (from 5.1 to 10.4%). ↓REM% (27.5 to 20.4%).
Chernik and Mendels, 1974	Endogenous depression (8 bipolar, 2 unipolar)		Lithium carbonate 900–2400 mg/day		↓REM and REM% (25.6 to 19.8%). ↑REM latency (38 to 52 min). ↑Sleep efficiency. ↓Wakefulness. ↓Stage I. ↑Delta sleep. ↓Phasic REM%. No REM rebound.
	Insomniac	1	Lithium carbonate 900 mg/day for 7 nights	0.27 to 0.53	↑Subjective ratings of sleep as good.
Chernik et al., 1974	Affective illness Psychiatric	15 2	Lithium carbonate 900–3700 mg/day	Low < 0.7 Medium 0.7 to 1.1 High > 1.1	↓REM and REM%. ↑Delta. ↑REM latency. No REM rebound. Sleep changes correlated better with lithium concentration in red blood cells than in plasma.
Kupfer et al., 1974	Affective disorders	6	Lithium carbonate 1250–2400 mg/day	Serum lithium negatively correlated with REM% and REM latency	↓REM and REM% (19.5 to 12.5%). ↑REM Latency (70 to 104 min). ↓Duration of REM periods. No REM rebound.

findings, even this measure is not present in all patients with depression and it is found, at times, in many schizophrenic patients (see below), manic patients, normal short sleepers (Jones and Oswald, 1968), and even in normal volunteers sleeping on altered rest–activity schedules (Weitzman *et al.*, 1970; 1974; Carskadon and Dement, 1975). When the REM latency is short and/or REM sleep elevated in depressed patients, it is not clear whether this heightened REM pressure results from past deprivation of REM sleep, increased propensity toward REM as an inherent part of depression, biochemical changes, a reflection of the waning phase of a depressive episode, a desynchronization of rest–activity rhythms from light-dark cues, or what. With regard to a biochemical mechanism for a shortened REM latency, enhanced cholinergic activity has been shown to shorten the REM latency (Sitaram *et al.*, 1976) and has been implicated in the pathophysiology of depression (Davis, 1975; Janowsky *et al.*, 1972). This interpretation might also be consistent with the beneficial effects of REM sleep deprivation in depression. A significant fall in acetylcholine in telencephalon has been reported following 96 hours of REM deprivation in two studies in rats (Bowers *et al.*, 1966; Tsuchiya *et al.*, 1969) but not in total brain in the mouse (Sagales and Domino, 1973). Either regional differences or species differences may be responsible for these discrepant results. To confuse matters, however, Tsuchiya *et al.* reported that 24 hours of total sleep deprivation slightly increased acetylcholine in the telencephalon.

It is proper to remember at this point that affective disorders are a heterogeneous collection of illnesses and syndromes and that our failure to pinpoint specific sleep disorders to specific subclassifications of affective illness may reflect our poor understanding of the underlying illnesses. While this may be true, it remains to be proven. Moreover, it appears that all or some of the sleep disorders (such as decreased delta) result not from depression *per se* but from accessory symptoms, such as anxiety or nonspecific change in the brain. This also remains to be clarified.

As confusing as the current evidence is, loss of sleep does not appear to be a general cause of depression. Natural short sleepers are not depressed (Jones and Oswald, 1968; Hartmann *et al.*, 1972; Webb and Friel, 1971; Meddis *et al.*, 1973), and sleep deprivation of normals is more likely to produce delerium than depression. Ironically, therapeutic benefits may result from further disturbing the already disturbed sleep of depressed patients, such as by deliberate sleep deprivation, REM sleep deprivation, or drugs that reduce REM sleep levels. These results, as well as those that indicate sleep deprivation exacerbates epilepsy, at least demonstrate that sleep deprivation "does something," a conclusion that seems obvious but that has been amazingly difficult to establish in normal subjects.

An important clinical implication is that treatment should be directed toward the depression rather than the sleep disturbance. For example, i̇ ̣ ṵ̇ents with insomnia or excessive daytime sleepiness, the diagnosis of depression must be carefully considered before beginning treatment for the presenting symptom.

Extrapolating fr˙ ʋ̇ sleep deprivation studies to date, it does not seem likely that sleep deprivation will ˙ come part of the clinical armamentarium. It does produce salutory effects in one-third to one-half of endogenously depressed patients, but only a minority of patients enjoy significant, prolonged benefits.

The evidence does support the hypothesis that prolonged REM deprivation, whether by drugs or by awakenings, may have antidepressant effects. As Vogel (1975) has suggested, there are probably no known drugs that produce profound, prolonged REM suppression with a REM rebound upon discontinuation that are not antidepressant. On the other hand, successful treatment of depression does not appear to depend upon deprivation of REM sleep in depressed patients. Vogel *et al.* (1975b) showed that about 10 to 20 days of REM-sleep deprivation by arousals were required before salubrious effects were observed in depressed patients. Although a night of sleep deprivation or administration of tricyclic antidepressants reduce REM sleep initially, total loss of REM sleep appears to be small. Moreover, the clinical efficacy of antidepressant therapies does not correlate well with the degree of REM sleep deprivation. Electric shock therapy does not reduce REM sleep appreciably. Tricyclic antidepressants are better clinically in most patients than monoamine oxidase inhibitors, but do not suppress REM sleep as well. The hypothesis that REM sleep deprivation has antidepressant properties is of heuristic value, however, and further research will be required to establish its validity and generalizability.

SLEEP STUDIES IN SCHIZOPHRENIA

The early polygraphic sleep studies of schizophrenia focused on REM sleep. This orientation reflected the hope and expectation that an abnormality of REM sleep might be involved with or even responsible for much of the behavior of schizophrenic patients that is dreamlike, such as hallucinations. The hypotheses took two forms: first, that schizophrenics might have too much REM sleep, perhaps as a manifestation of an "overactive" dream center or from failure of inhibition of dreams; and, secondly, that schizophrenics might have too little REM sleep with the psychosis developing when the normal "safety valve function" of dreams failed.

These hopes have yet to be realized, although, as in the case with affective disorders, some intriguing findings have entered and await further evaluation. In particular, evidence suggests that some schizophrenics fail to have a normal REM rebound after deprivation of REM sleep.

Cross-Sectional Studies of Schizophrenia

In the first all-night polygraphic study of schizophrenic patients since the discovery of REM sleep, Dement (1955) compared 17 chronic schizophrenics with 13 medical students. Although this study was conducted before the formulation of the current definition of sleep stages, the data suggested that periods of rapid eye movements were the same during sleep in patients and controls, although some schizophrenic patients appeared to show REMs earlier than controls. Upon awakenings during REM sleep, schizophrenics reported dreams as frequently as controls, but their dreams more often were of isolated, inanimate objects, apparently hanging in space, with no overt action whatsoever.

Subsequent studies have failed to establish any unique or even consistent abnormalities in the sleep of schizophrenic patients. No physiological manifestation of REM sleep has been found in waking schizophrenic patients (Rechtschaffen et al., 1964b), and, as shown in Table 7-10, no consistent difference in REM percentage during sleep has been found in most studies between chronic schizophrenic patients and normals (Feinberg et al., 1964; 1965a; Hartmann et al., 1966; Caldwell and Domino, 1967; Caldwell, 1969; Jus et al., 1968; 1973; Vincent et al., 1968; Traub, 1972; Dürrigl et al., 1973a) or between schizophrenic or psychotic children and normal controls (Onheiber et al., 1965; Ornitz et al., 1965a and b). When hallucinating and nonhallucinating schizophrenic patients have been compared, no difference in REM percentage was reported in two studies (Koresko et al., 1963; Feinberg et al., 1964, 1965a) but in a third, hallucinating subjects had low normal values whereas nonhallucinating subjects had very low values (Penati et al., 1968).

Contrasting amounts of REM sleep have been reported in some other studies. Gulevich et al. (1967) reported an increased amount of REM sleep, short REM latencies, and REM storms in a group of 13

TABLE 7-10. Polygraphic Sleep Studies in Schizophrenia

Authors	Type of subjects	Total sleep		REM%	Δ%	REM latency (min)	Comments
		No.	(min)				
Koresko et al., 1963	Schizophrenics:						
	hallucinating	7	372	22.2			
	nonhallucinating	4	389	22.5			
Feinberg et al.	Actively ill schizophrenics	18	383	22.0	15.4%	76	Short-term = <1 year.
1964	short-term	9	368	19.6[b]		79	Actively ill patients have less rapid eye movement activity than nonschizophrenics. REM and REM% significantly shorter in short-term than long-term. Sleep latency significantly longer in actively ill than controls. Variance of REM latency significantly greater in actively ill schizophrenics than controls. Eye movement density low in nonhallucinating patients. ↓ Stage 4 in schizophrenics (especially first nonREM period), normal stage 3.
1965a	long-term	9	398	24.4[b]		74	
1969b	hallucinating	10	366	22.2		73	
	nonhallucinating	8	403	21.7		84	
	Schizophrenics in remission	4	379	26.5			
	Nonschizophrenics	10	403	24.7		66	
	Normal controls	17			22.2		
Onheiber et al., 1965	Schizophrenic children	6		19.7	21.3	154	No differences compared with published age norms. Children sedated with promazine.
Ornitz et al., 1965a	Psychotic children	7	498	22.2		151	
	Nonpsychotic children	6	490	20.2		201	
Feinberg et al., 1965b	Elderly, deluded, hallucinated man	1	339	41		16	
Lairy et al., 1965	"Acute delirium"	10	132	16	16		Diagnosis is not certain.

Reference	Group	n					Findings
Caldwell and Domino, 1967	Chronic schizophrenics	25	322[c]	19.3	18.0[c]	93–101	40% of schizophrenics had no stage 4. Patients showed more awakenings, stage changes, and longer latency to sleep and to delta sleep.
Caldwell, 1969	Normal controls	10	376[c]	19.7	25.2[c]	88	
Gulevich et al., 1967	Chronic schizophrenics in remission	13	420	27.4[c]		81[a]	Schizophrenics showed ↑REM & REM%, no "first night effect." ↓REM latency. 6 of 13 had REM storms and 10 showed partial EMG tonus during REM.
	Nonpsychotic controls	7	411	20.8[c]		112[a]	
Jus et al., 1968	Chronic schizophrenics	42	356	18.3	30.4		Compared with published norms, ↓stage 3 and 4,↑stage 1 and 2.
Vincent et al., 1968	Acute schizophrenics	15		17.4	29.9	67	Schizophrenics show significantly ↑sleep latency, ↓REM latency, ↓length of first REM period.
	Chronic hallucinatory psychosis	4		25.6	21.4	94	
	Normal controls	11		18.2	32.8	125	
Penati et al., 1968	Schizophrenics hallucinating	10	406	17.9	40.3		↓Stage 4, ↑stage 3.
	nonhallucinating	10		7.9	28.1		
Stern et al., 1969	Acute, unmedicated schizophrenics	8	352[a]	19.5	7	53	Patients had significantly ↓total sleep, ↓REM latency, ↑sleep latency, ↓awakening. No first night effect.
	Normal controls	6	408[a]	21.9	9.5	94	
Kupfer et al., 1970b	Acute, unmedicated schizophrenics*	6	235[c]	9[a]	5[c]	177[c]	Patients' data is from waxing psychotic phase.
	Normal controls	15	416[c]	19[c]	10[c]	77[c]	
Traub, 1972	Chronic schizophrenics	9	378	21.5	1	99	Low doses of chlorpromazine.
Jus et al., 1973	Aged, unmedicated schizophrenics	11	323	18.9	27.6	53[b]	Patients show significantly ↓sleep latency,↓REM latency, ↑number REM periods,↓duration REM period.
	Normal controls	10	336	17.8	26.5	93[b]	

continued

TABLE 7-10 (continued)

Authors	Type of subjects	Total sleep No.	Total sleep (min)	REM%	Δ%	REM latency (min)	Comments
Dürrigl et al., 1973a	Acute, unmedicated schizophrenics	10	373	20.5		95.7	Patients showed ↑sleep latency, and ↓REM latency and ↑variability of REM latency, ↓duration of REM periods.
	Normal controls	10	419	19.7		150	
Reich et al., 1975	Schizophrenias (all)	29	335	19.4	31	79	The greater the REM activity, the greater dose of phenothiazines required. Baseline REM latency was lower in pts. later given antidepressants. Schizoaffective pts. differed significantly in REM latency and REM intensity. Latent pts. fell asleep faster, slept longer and more efficiently.
	acute	14	305	17.4	29	98	
	latent	9	375	20.0	43	81	
	schizoaffective	6	346	23.2	18	32^c	

^{a} $p < .05$
^{b} $p < .025$
^{c} $p < .01$

chronic, unmedicated schizophrenics in remission as compared with nonpsychotic controls. Feinberg (1964) also reported high levels of REM sleep in four schizophrenics in remission. On the other hand, Azumi (1966) found less REM sleep in a group of 35 chronic schizophrenics than in 33 normals. This discrepancy between the reports seems, however, to be compatible with the finding of Feinberg *et al.* (1964) that *short-term* (less than one year) schizophrenics have significantly lower REM sleep than *long-term* (greater than one year) schizophrenics. Azumi's patients appear to be more acute and more disturbed than the patients of Gulevich *et al.* (1967). Insomnia and loss of REM sleep have been reported during acute phases or at times of psychic turmoil. While Fisher and Dement (1963) reported a REM percentage of 50 in a patient at the beginning of an acute paranoid psychosis, Dement later reexamined the sleep records and concluded that the patient had very little REM sleep at that time (Dement, 1966). Feinberg (1965a) also found high amounts of REM sleep in a single, elderly psychotic patient, but the diagnosis was unclear. Nevertheless, the presence of low amounts of REM in disturbed patients was subsequently confirmed by Lairy *et al.* (1965) in 10 patients at the onset of an acute psychosis or "delirium"; by Vincent *et al.* (1968) in four disturbed patients; by Rogina *et al.* (1968) in three schizophrenics during an acute period; by Kupfer *et al.* (1970c) in six acute unmedicated schizophrenic patients; and in 19 chronic male schizophrenics at the time of a clinical exacerbation (Kunugi, 1970). Not all so-called acute schizophrenics, however, have had low amounts of REM sleep [the less disturbed patients of Vincent *et al.* (1968); the previously untreated patients of Jus *et al.* (1968); and seven of the eight acute patients of Stern *et al.* (1969)]. It is not clear at this time whether these discrepant results reflect differences in symptomatology, severity, length of illness, phase of illness, past use of drugs, previous loss of REM sleep, or other factors.

Some of the remitted schizophrenic patients studied by Gulevich *et al.* (1967) failed to demonstrate muscle atonia at times during periods of REM sleep (defined on the basis of typical EEG patterns and bursts of rapid eye movements). This anomaly has not been reported by other investigators, and brings into question their report of elevated amounts of REM sleep.

The REM latency in schizophrenia is also highly variable. The data from Dement's original study (1955) suggested it might be short in some schizophrenics, but Feinberg (1964, 1965a) was the first to systematically investigate this parameter, which he found to be significantly more variable in actively ill schizophrenics than in controls. Subsequent studies appear to confirm his conclusion. Some patients show sleep onset REM periods, some normal REM latencies, while still others must sleep unusually long before the first REM period. Reich *et al.* (1975) have suggested that the REM latency might be abbreviated in schizophrenic patients with affective features. This would be consistent with their hypothesis of an inverse relationship between depression and the REM latency. For example, they found that schizoaffective patients showed short REM latencies in comparison with acute and latent schizophrenics. Moreover, baseline REM latency was shorter in patients who later required antidepressant medications than in those who did not. Further data will be required to evaluate these interpretations. Aside from Feinberg's original reports, short REM latencies have also been reported by Gulevich *et al.* (1967) in 13 remitted schizophrenics as compared with seven nonpsychotic controls and by Dürrigl *et al.* (1973a) in 10 acute schizophrenic patients as compared with 10 normal controls (interpretation in these two studies is complicated by the fact that the absolute values for REM latency were about normal for schizophrenics and high for controls); by Stern *et al.* (1969) in eight unmedicated acute schizophrenics as compared with normal controls; and by Jus *et al.* (1973) in 11 chronic aged, never medicated schizophrenics as compared with age-matched normal controls. Azumi (1966) also reported the early appearance of REM in some chronic schizophrenics. In contrast, Kupfer *et al.* (1970c) reported significantly elevated REM latency in six severely ill, acute, unmedicated schizophrenic patients during the waxing phase of psychosis.

A number of investigators have reported reduced amounts of delta sleep in schizophrenics (Caldwell and Domino, 1967; Caldwell, 1969; Lairy *et al.*, 1965; Jus *et al*, 1968; Feinberg *et al.*, 1969b; Stern *et al.*, 1969; Itil *et al.*, 1970; Kupfer *et al.*, 1970c; Kunugi, 1970), but the meaning of this finding is unclear since reduced delta sleep has also been reported in mental retardates (Feinberg *et al.*, 1969c), in patients with chronic brain syndrome (Feinberg, 1967), in the normal elderly (Feinberg *et al.*, 1967), in students under stress (Lester *et al.*, 1967), and in depressed patients (see earlier discussion of sleep in affective disorders). The low levels of delta sleep in schizophrenic patients, as well as aged normal subjects, results from loss of delta sleep during the first nonREM period (Feinberg, 1969b, 1975). Caldwell (1969) suggested that stage 4 sleep in chronic schizophrenics correlated negatively with a biochemical abnormality reported in the blood of schizophrenics, i.e., the effect of schizophrenic plasma upon the uptake of tryptophan and 5-hydroxy-tryptophan by chicken erythrocytes. This correlation has apparently not been pursued or confirmed.

Other abnormalities of sleep in schizophrenia have also been reported: Spontaneous skin potentials show marked fluctuations during REM sleep in acute schizophrenics although in normals these are usually inhibited during REM (Wyatt et al., 1970c); evoked potentials show increased amplitude during REM sleep in autistic children although they are normally reduced (Ornitz et al., 1968); and the *intermediate stage* of sleep (a mixture of stage 2 and REM) is elevated in schizophrenics as compared with normals (Lairy et al., 1965; de Barros-Ferreira et al., 1973).

Both Itil et al. (1970) and Jus et al. (1975) have observed a significant increase in deep sleep stages (stage 4) in the lobotomized schizophrenic patients as compared with the nonlobotomized schizophrenic patients. This observation appears to be consistent with the increase in stage 4 observed in a depressed patient treated with lobotomy (Hauri and Hawkins, 1972).

Longitudinal Studies of Sleep in Schizophrenia

The cross-sectional studies suggest that REM sleep is reduced in many schizophrenic patients at times of psychic turmoil. The longitudinal studies indicate no REM compensation during recovery in those schizophrenic patients who lost REM sleep during the acute psychosis phases. Kupfer et al. (1970b) studied six acute schizophrenic patients with nightly polygraphic sleep recordings during the psychotic episodes. Three of the patients did not receive medication at any time. During the "waxing" phase of the psychotic episode, patients suffered considerable insomnia and a disproportionate loss of REM sleep. As the psychotic episode waned, both REM and nonREM gradually returned to normal values. In the postpsychotic and remission periods, the schizophrenics slept relatively well. Although the patients had little REM sleep during the early phases of psychosis, they did not show evidence of a REM rebound during the recovery phases. Similar findings were present in two acutely ill schizophrenic patients studied longitudinally by Gillin and Wyatt (1975).

No other longitudinal sleep studies of schizophrenics during a psychotic episode have been reported. There are studies that suggest that REM sleep is reduced during acute phases of psychosis but normal during recovery and remission (Lairy et al., 1965; Kunugi, 1970; and one patient studied longitudinally by Stern et al., 1969).

The failure to observe elevated amounts of REM during recovery in schizophrenic patients appears to contrast with such findings in depressed patients (see earlier discussion of sleep in affective disorders). These data suggest that schizophrenic patients fail to compensate

for lost REM sleep. Many difficulties, however, preclude definite conclusions at this time. First, as mentioned earlier, interpretation of the
sleep data from depression is difficult. Secondly, the study of Gulevich
et al. (1967) suggests that a REM rebound might occur late in the
recovery process of schizophrenia rather than early; they reported
elevated REM, REM storms, and short REM latencies in remitted
schizophrenics.

If abnormalities in the level of REM sleep or REM latency do exist in
schizophrenia, these abnormalities may not be associated with psychosis per se but with nonspecific clinical features such as acute psychotic turmoil, panic, depressive symptoms, or a past history of REM
sleep deprivation, yet even here it is impossible to resolve the discrepancies. In terms of the hypothesis that schizophrenics fail to compensate for lost REM sleep, the evidence is clearer and more readily
interpretable in experimental studies of REM deprivation.

Experimental REM Deprivation in Schizophrenia

The longitudinal studies of schizophrenic patients and depressed
patients suggested that schizophrenic patients did not show a REM
rebound following loss of REM whereas depressed patients did. This
interpetation is open to many criticisms because of the uncertainties of
the longitudinal method. Since the REM rebound is defined as an
increase of REM above the individual's normal levels, it is necessary to
know the normal level of REM in order to determine whether an
individual has had a REM rebound or not. Determination of this normal
level is difficult if not impossible, however, during a longitudinal sleep
study. Sleep records obtained during nonpsychotic or remitted periods
provide inadequate information about the patients' natural level of
REM sleep. Although the psychosis is remitted, the patient may continue to be depressed, anxious, or otherwise disturbed. Furthermore,
adequate control data with which to compare these results does not
currently exist. Few longitudinal studies of sleep in depressed patients
have been published, and no sleep studies have been done on normal
individuals who have attempted to simulate the insomnia of an acute
psychotic episode or of depression.

Experimental REM deprivation is one method of overcoming the
limitations of the longitudinal study. Sleep in the recovery period can
be compared with that of the baseline period in order to determine
whether or not REM compensation has occurred. As shown in Table 7-
11, there have been five experimental studies of REM deprivation in
schizophrenic patients. In two of the studies, schizophrenics appeared

TABLE 7-11. Experimental REM Deprivation in Schizophrenia

Authors	Subjects	Duration of REM deprivation	Parameter	Time period	Schizophrenic	Controls	P
Azumi et al., 1967	Schizophrenics-3 Normals-3	5 nights	REM%	Baseline Recovery night 1	24.9% 29.2%	22.1% 27.8%	NS NS
Vogel and Traub, 1968	Schizophrenics-5	7 nights	REM%	Baseline Recovery night 1[a] Recovery night 1–5	23.1% 35.5% 29.3%		
			REM (min)	Baseline Recovery night 1[a] Recovery night 1–5	100 180 141		
Zarcone et al., 1968, 1975	Actively ill Schizophrenics-9 Nonpsychotic control patients-7	2 nights	REM (min)	Baseline	108	85	NS
			ΔREM (min)	Recovery nights 1 and 2	−3	22	.01
			REM%	Baseline	25.2%	19.1%	NS
			ΔREM%	Recovery night 1 and 2	−0.9%	3.6%	.01
De Barros-Ferreira et al., 1973	Schizophrenics-11 Normals-5	3 nights	REM%[b]	Recovery night 1 3 Recovery nights	7% ~5%	8% ~5%	NS
Gillin et al., 1974c	Actively ill Schizophrenics-8 Nonpsychotic psych. pts.-8	2 nights	REM (min)	Baseline 1st night 2nd night	93 91 83	99 137 116	NS .0025 .05
			REM%	Baseline Recovery night 1	25% 24.5%	25.5% 30.8%	NS .01
			ΔREM (min)	Recovery night 1 Recovery night 2 Recovery nights 1–5	−2 −10 1	38 17 14.5	.01 .05 .05
			ΔREM%	Recovery night 1	−0.8%	5.8%	.05

[a] Data calculated from table. [b] Data estimated from Figure 3. ΔREM = change of REM sleep time (recovery REM minus baseline REM). ΔREM% = change of REM% (recovery REM% minus baseline REM%).

to have normal REM rebounds. Vogel and Traub (1968) REM deprived five chronic schizophrenic patients for seven nights by awakenings and by administration of nighttime phenobarbital and amphetamine, drugs that partially suppress REM sleep. Four of the five patients were treated with phenothiazines at the time of the study. All patients had an increase in REM sleep and REM percentage during the recovery period as compared with baseline. De Barros Ferreira *et al.* (1973) REM deprived 11 chronic schizophrenic patients and five normals for three nights and reported that all had a REM sleep rebound. Eight of the eleven patients were on phenothiazine medications at the time of the study.

In the three other studies, the schizophrenic patients showed an abnormal response to REM deprivation. Azumi *et al.* (1967) REM deprived three chronic unmedicated schizophrenic patients for five nights. Only one of the patients had a "rebound" of REM sleep, and it was more marked than that of normal controls. Zarcone *et al.* (1968, 1975) REM sleep deprived nine actively ill schizophrenics and seven nonschizophrenic psychiatric controls for two nights. Most patients received phenothiazines. The actively ill schizophrenic patients did not show a significant change in REM sleep or REM percentage during recovery as compared with baseline. In contrast, the nonschizophrenic controls did have a REM rebound and differed significantly from the actively ill schizophrenic patients. Finally, in a replication and confirmation of the Zarcone *et al.* study, Gillin *et al.* (1974c) REM deprived eight actively ill schizophrenic patients and 8 age, sex matched nonpsychotic psychiatric controls for 2 nights. Except for one control patient who received a low dose of chlorpromazine, the patients were drug free. No significant differences in sleep were observed during baseline between schizophrenics and controls. On the first night of REM sleep deprivation, both groups required the same number of awakenings to achieve REM deprivation, but on the second deprivation night the controls had to be awakened significantly more frequently than the schizophrenic patients, thus indicating that the controls had the normally expected increase in the number of entries into REM sleep while the schizophrenics did not.

During the postdeprivation recovery period, the control patients showed the normal REM sleep rebound patterns: a large increase in REM sleep and percentage of REM on the first night following REM sleep deprivation with a gradual decline in REM sleep and percentage of REM to the normal baseline levels after 3–5 nights (Fig. 7-7). In striking contrast, the actively ill schizophrenic patients showed almost exactly the same amount of REM sleep and percentage of REM on the first night after deprivation as during the baseline period and remained at or near

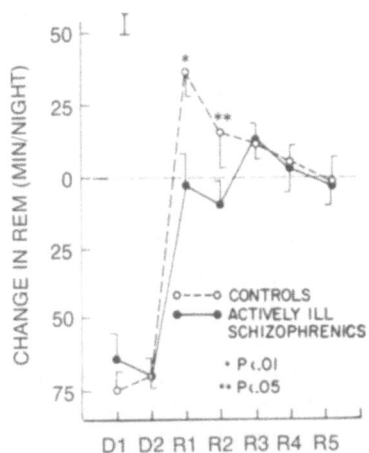

FIGURE 7-7. REM sleep rebound during Recovery Night (R_1-5) in control patients but not in actively ill schizophrenics for two nights (D_1-2). Each value represents change in REM sleep as compared with baseline. (Described in Gillin *et al.*, 1974.)

baseline levels for the five recovery nights. Though the control patients had a significantly greater increase in REM sleep than the actively ill schizophrenics, there was considerable overlap between the two groups. Three actively ill schizophrenic patients had moderate-to-average increases in REM sleep following REM sleep deprivation. One of the control patients averaged less REM sleep during the recovery period than during the baseline period.

REM deprivation did, however, affect one aspect of REM sleep in the actively ill schizophrenics during recovery. It led to a three-night reduction of the REM latency in the actively ill schizophrenics, although REM sleep did not increase significantly. In contrast, the REM latency was reduced only on the first recovery night in the control patients. Short REM latencies have been reported in some previous studies of the sleep of schizophrenics and have been interpreted as evidence of uncompensated REM sleep deprivation (Gulevich *et al.*, 1967; Stern *et al.*, 1969). These data support this interpretation. Among the acutely ill schizophrenics, the REM latency returned to normal following the modest elevation of REM sleep on the third recovery night. This finding suggests that the mechanisms determining the onset of REM sleep may be partially independent of mechanisms determining the amount of REM sleep. As discussed in chapter 2, cholinergic activity could underlie such phenomena. Infusion of physostigmine during nonREM sleep in normal volunteers induces REM sleep without affecting the length of REM sleep (Sitaram et al., 1976).

How are these discrepant results from these five studies to be resolved? There are several factors to be considered. First, the clinical status of the patients at the time of the study was not specified in three of the reports (Vogel and Traub, 1968; de Barros Ferreira et al., 1973; Azumi et al., 1967). (In the Vogel and Traub study, however, unpublished psychological tests indicate that the patients were actively ill.) As Zarcone et al. (1968) showed, only actively ill schizophrenics fail to show a REM rebound. Second, the effects of psychoactive medication and amphetamines on REM compensation are not fully understood. In cats, phenothiazines enhance the magnitude of REM compensation (Cohen et al., 1968). Small doses of chlorpromazine, however, do not affect the REM rebound in normal volunteers (Naiman et al., 1972). In humans, amphetamine administration does suppress REM sleep, but has not been followed by a REM rebound in some studies (Feinberg et al., 1974a; Small et al., 1971; Gillin et al., 1975b) while it has been in other studies (Rechtschaffen and Maron, 1964; Oswald and Thacore, 1963; Watson et al., 1972). These factors, therefore, complicate interpretation of the four studies in which either phenothiazines or amphetamines were administered to schizophrenic patients. Third, in the de Barros-Ferreira et al. (1973) study the sleep records were not scored or analyzed according to standard criteria. Their laboratory has been particularly interested in a stage of sleep that they call the *intermediate stage*, which appears to be transitional between nonREM and REM. Their method of scoring REM appears to differ from the other studies. Fourth, in studies reporting normal REM compensation, total sleep time increased from baseline to recovery periods. Verdone (1968) has shown in normal subjects that the proportion of total sleep spent in REM rises as total sleep time increases. Therefore, the REM rebound in schizophrenics reported by Vogel and Traub and de Barros-Ferreira et al. may merely reflect an increase in total sleep following REM deprivation with its accompanying loss of total sleep. In the case of subjects who had a REM rebound, both Zarcone et al. (1975) and Gillin et al. (1974c) also observed an initial increase in total sleep during recovery that correlated significantly with the increase of REM sleep and REM percentage. Gillin et al. were able to show, however, that the controls had a significant REM rebound as compared with actively ill schizophrenics after the changes in total sleep time had been controlled for by a variety of statistical techniques. Fifth, statistical comparisons between schizophrenics and controls were performed only in the studies of Zarcone et al. (1975) and Gillin et al. (1974c).

In summary, in two studies in which a statistical comparison was made between a carefully defined group of actively ill schizophrenics and controls, no REM rebound was observed in the schizophrenic patients whereas a REM rebound was observed in the controls. Before attaching greater importance to this finding we have just described, several issues await clarification. Even in normals, individual differences appear to play an important role in determining whether or not a subject has a REM rebound. Cartwright *et al.* (1967) reported, in a study of normal volunteers, that "good REM compensators" tended to be field independent; that is, they tended to see foreground relatively independent of background, in comparison to "poor REM compensators." In eight of the patients in their REM deprivation study, Gillin *et al.* (1974c) found a significant correlation between a measure of field independence (the portable rod and frame test) and the magnitude of the REM sleep rebound. Although this finding was tentative, it suggested that some third factor other than active schizophrenic symptoms might be responsible for the failure of REM rebound in most schizophrenic patients and its presence in most control subjects. In addition to the study by Cartwright *et al.* (1967) other investigations indicate considerable individual differences in REM compensation among normal subjects (Dement, 1960; Kales *et al.*, 1965; Sampson, 1965; Rechtschaffen and Maron, 1964). In a careful study of the relationship between personality characteristics and REM compensation, Nakazawa *et al.* (1975a) subjected 14 normal university students to one night of partial REM sleep deprivation by limiting the time allowed for sleep. On the night following partial REM sleep deprivation, the group as a whole showed a substantial increase in REM percentage as compared with baseline. Fairly marked individual differences were evident, however, and these persisted from one experimental trial of REM sleep deprivation to the next, thus suggesting that the degree of REM sleep rebound is a stable characteristic of an individual. Psychological assessment (the Maudsley Personality Inventory) indicated that good REM compensators were extraverted, active, optimistic, and showy, without neurotic tendencies. In contrast, the subjects who had less or no REM sleep rebound were found to be introverted, inactive, nervous, modest, and restrained, with neurotic tendencies. These findings appeared to be in agreement with those of Cartwright *et al.* (1967). Since schizophrenics often share many of the personality characteristics observed in the poor REM rebounders (Nakazawa *et al.*, 1975a), the failure of REM rebound in schizophrenics could be related to a third variable, such as personality.

If failure to have a REM rebound is a characteristic of most actively ill schizophrenics, then it is important to determine whether it is a trait or state characteristic. So far, no one has made a systematic attempt to REM deprive schizophrenic patients while ill and recovered. Zarcone *et al.* (1968) did REM deprive six remitted schizophrenics and found exaggerated REM rebounds in them as compared with nonschizophrenic controls. In three remitted schizophrenics studied by Gillin *et al.* (1974c), however, a normal REM rebound was observed, not an exaggerated one.

The physiological mechanisms underlying the REM rebound are not well understood. Serotonin has been implicated in the REM rebound, and if this is true, the failure of a REM rebound in schizophrenia would be consistent with the hypothesis that schizophrenics suffer from an abnormality of serotonin metabolism. The serotonin theory of schizophrenia was first proposed by Woolley and Shaw (1954) and was given new impetus by Dement and his collaborators (Dement *et al.*, 1969, 1970). After inhibiting serotonin synthesis with p-chlorophenyl-alanine (PCPA), Dement and his collaborators demonstrated behavioral abnormalities in cats, including apparent "hallucinations," which could be reversed by administration of chlorpromazine or by 5-hydroxy-tryptophan (5-HTP), the precursor of serotonin that bypassed the PCPA block (Fig. 2-1). More pertinent to the present discussion, the PCPA-treated animals failed to have a REM rebound after experimental deprivation of REM sleep. This failure of REM compensation was in contrast to the normal REM rebounds observed in these animals prior to PCPA administration. Furthermore, PCPA administration in man (in low doses compared with those given cats) suppresses REM sleep but is not followed by a REM rebound after termination of administration (Wyatt *et al.*, 1969a), a change in sleep which appears to be similar to the deficiency of REM compensation observed in longitudinal studies of sleep during acute schizophrenic psychosis. Psychological disturbances, including depression, anxiety, confusion, and hallucinations, have been described in patients with carcinoid syndrome who were treated with PCPA (Engelman *et al.*, 1967). Moreover, hallucinogenic agents, such as lysergic acid diethylamide, mescaline, and dimethyl-tryptamine, slow the spontaneous firing of serotonin containing neurons within the raphe nuclei of the brain stem (Aghajanian *et al.*, 1970).

The serotonin theory of schizophrenia does not currently enjoy much popular support. The concentration of 5-HIAA in CSF of schizophrenic patients appears to be normal (Goodwin and Post, 1975). Although administration of 5-hydroxytryptophan (5-HTP) had modest beneficial effects in some unmedicated schizophrenic patients (Wyatt *et al.*, 1972b), some patients became worse and no significant clinical effects were observed when 5-HTP was given to chronic schizophrenic patients who were being treated with haloperidol (Walls et al., 1976). In addition, treatment with tryptophan (the normal precursor to serotonin via 5-HTP) had no significant clinical effects in unmedicated schizophrenic patients (Gillin, Kaplan, and Wyatt, 1976). These findings do not disprove a role for serotonin in schizophrenia or the REM rebound, but do indicate that no straightforward therapeutic or research approach has so far emerged from the REM deprivation studies in schizophrenia.

REM deprivation in man has not been shown to produce significant changes in eye movement patterns in REM sleep (REM density) during recovery from REM deprivation. REM density is a measure of the phasic events of REM sleep, an important aspect of Dement's hypothesis relating serotonin to schizophrenia and REM compensation. Since PGO spikes appear outside of REM in waking behavior following PCPA administration, Dement postulated that hallucinations were associated with waking PGO spikes and that REM deprivation–compensation is actually PGO spike deprivation–compensation. No widely accepted measure of phasic events of REM sleep now exists in man, since it is impossible to measure PGO spikes directly without depth electrodes. Whether REM density measures crucial phasic events in man is unknown. The development of new measures of phasic events in man (Rechtschaffen et al., 1970; Pessah and Roffwarg, 1972), however, suggests that it may be possible to test the hypothesis relating phasic events to hallucinations and REM compensations.

Little is known about the role of dopamine and norepinephrine in the REM rebound. Kupfer and Bowers (1972) have suggested a role for dopamine. Several other studies indicate that norepinephrine turnover is increased during recovery from REM deprivation in the rat (Pujol et al., 1968; Schildkraut and Hartmann, 1972), although the effect may be due less to REM deprivation than to the stress of the REM deprivation procedure (Stern et al., 1971). Marantz et al. (1968) were unable to alter the REM rebound by administration of α-methylparatyrosine, an inhibitor of tyrosine hydroxylase, the rate-limiting enzymic step in the synthesis of dopamine and norepinephrine from tyrosine; the dose, however, was small. It is also of interest that Nakazawa et al. (1973) found that L-DOPA prevented the REM rebound in normal subjects after partial REM sleep deprivation although an identical dose had no effect on normal sleep. In the present context, more information on the roles of dopamine and norepinephrine in the REM rebound would be useful since both neurotransmitters have been implicated in schizophrenia. Snyder (1976) has suggested that some types of psychosis may be mediated by dopamine, and Stein and Wise (1971; Wise and Stein, 1973) have suggested that a functional deficit of norepinephrine exists in schizophrenic patients. Response to REM deprivation may therefore be a physiological indicator of serotonin, dopamine, or norepinephrine metabolism.

Finally, even if failure of REM rebound is characteristic of actively ill schizophrenia, it is important whether this characteristic occurs in other psychiatric categories. Although experimental REM deprivation has not been tried in hypomanic patients—perhaps for obvious reasons—the evidence from longitudinal studies suggests that no REM rebound occurs with recovery. Since REM rebounds have been reported during longitudinal sleep studies of psychotically depressed patients (Snyder, 1968, 1969a and b, 1972; Mendels and Hawkins, 1971a) and following experimental REM deprivation in actively ill childhood schizophrenic patients (Zarcone et al., 1973b), psychosis per se does not explain the absence of a REM rebound.

In summary, the experimental REM deprivation studies suggest that the actively ill schizophrenics are less likely to exhibit a REM rebound than control subjects. This abnormality is not pathognomonic of schizophrenia, however, since some actively ill patients do have a REM rebound while some normals apparently do not. The mechanisms underlying the REM rebound remain to be elucidated.

Experimental Sleep Deprivation in Schizophrenia

Although many depressed patients have been sleep deprived for therapeutic and experimental purposes, few schizophrenic patients have been deliberately deprived of sleep. Nevertheless, schizophrenic patients appear to respond with modest initial improvement, just as many depressed patients do. Koranyi and Lehmann (1960) as well as Luby and Caldwell (1967) reported clinical improvement with continuous sleep deprivation up to about 72 hours (in the first study) and up to 85 hours (in the second). Koranyi and Lehmann (1960), however, noted progressive deterioration and remanifestation of acute psychotic symptoms between 72 and 100 hours of deprivation, when the study was scheduled to end.

Luby and Caldwell (1967) obtained all-night sleep studies before and after sleep deprivation. None of the schizophrenic subjects responded with the anticipated increase in stage 4, seen following sleep deprivation in normals (Berger and Oswald, 1962). Sleep deprivation in normal subjects has generally not produced psychosis. It has, however, been reported to lower the threshold to psychotomimetic agents such as LSD (Bliss et al., 1959).

Effects of Neuroleptics on Sleep

The neuroleptics do not affect sleep in a characteristic manner (Table 7-12). Although some neuroleptics change a particular sleep stage in a consistent direction, other neuroleptics may not or may even have variable effects.

Reserpine, for example, has increased REM sleep in most studies, but chlorpromazine has not. The increase of REM sleep did not always occur on the first night of reserpine administration, but was consistently observed therafter whether or not administration of reserpine was continued beyond one night (Tissot, 1965; Hartmann, 1966; Hoffman and Domino, 1969; Williams et al., 1969; Coulter et al., 1971; Hartmann and Cravens, 1973c). The significant increase in REM sleep remained even if change in total sleep was controlled (Williams et al., 1969). In the only study of reserpine in schizophrenic patients, Jus et al. (1975a) found that it increased REM percentage and decreased REM latency in nonlobotomized patients but not in lobotomized patients, who showed no changes in REM sleep. Chlorpromazine has also been reported to increase REM percentage in some studies (Toyoda, 1964; Lewis and Evans, 1969), but in other studies it has had either no effect (Lester and Guerrero-Figuerroa, 1966; Sagales et al., 1969; Kupfer et al., 1971; Lester et al., 1971; Naiman et al., 1972; Hartmann and Cravens, 1973b; Kaplan et al., 1974) or has even decreased REM sleep (Feinberg et al., 1969a; Lewis and Evans, 1969). This variability is apparently not determined by the type of subjects since chlorpromazine decreased REM sleep in one study with schizophrenics (Feinberg et al., 1969a) but not in other studies (Kupfer et al., 1971; Kaplan et al., 1974). In a brief report, Blum and Girke (1973) found that clozapine markedly increased REM percentage (beyond 85% of total sleep) in association with an expected small rise in body temperature. Clozapine is a neuroleptic that rarely produces extrapyramidal side effects, often seen with other neuroleptics. Since thioridazine likewise rarely produces extrapyramidal side effects, it is of interest that it has also been reported to increase REM sleep initially in schizophrenics (Brannan and Jewitt, 1969) and insomniacs (Kales et al., 1974b) and that its metabolite, mesoridazine, also increased REM sleep during a three-week trial (Oswald et al., 1974). Against this line of reasoning, however, is the report that perphenazine, a phenothiazine neuroleptic with a high incidence of extrapyramidal side effects, also increased REM sleep in two normal subjects (Toyoda, 1964). Other neuroleptics have produced no change in REM sleep: pimozide (Sagales and Erill, 1975), sulpiride (Schneider et al., 1974b), promethazine, and trifluoperazine (Brannan and Jewett, 1969).

In the case of delta sleep, reserpine has been reported to decrease it

TABLE 7-12. Effects of Reserpine, Chlorpromazine, and Other Neuroleptics on Human Sleep

Authors	Subjects	No.	Drug/dose	Results
			Reserpine	
Tissot, 1965	Patients (type unspecified)	?	Reserpine 3–4 mg for 5 nights	↑ REM%.
Hartmann et al., 1966	Normals	6	Reserpine 1–2 mg at bedtime	↓ Stage 3 and 4. ↑ REM and REM%.
Hoffman and Domino, 1969	Prisoners	20	Reserpine .01–.14 mg/kg given once at bedtime	Dose related, prolonged ↓ nonREM sleep, ↓ stage 2, and ↓ stage 4, and ↑ stage 1. Dose related ↓ REM on night of drug administration, ↑ REM on recovery nights.
Williams et al., 1969	Normals	16	Reserpine 1 mg	↑ REM on second night.
Coulter et al., 1971	Normals	10	Reserpine 1 mg at bedtime for 1 night	Little acute effect, but ↑ REM%, ↓ REM latency and ↓ delta% on night after drug.
	Normals	10	Resperpine 1 mg at bedtime for 3 nights	Progressive ↑ REM%, ↓ delta%, ↓ REM latency, ↓ cycle length, ↑ arousals.
Hartmann and Craven 1973a	Normals	14	Reserpine 0.5 mg at bedtime for 28 days	↓ Sleep latency, ↑ REM, ↑ number of REM periods, ↑ stage shifts, body movements ↓ cycle length.
Jus et al., 1975a	Lobotomized schizophrenics	9	Reserpine 1 mg at bedtime for 3 nights	Reserpine caused ↑ REM%, ↓ REM latency, and ↓ sleep latency in nonlobotomized patients and ↓ stage 4 and ↓ sleep latency in lobotomized patients.
	Nonlobotomized schizophrenics	9		

Chlorpromazine

Reference	Subjects	N	Dose	Findings
Toyoda, 1964	Normals	5	Chlorpromazine 12.5–50 mg once	↑REM%, ↑ duration of REM periods (no statistics).
	Neurotic	2		
	Schizophrenic	1		
Lester and Guerrero-Figueroa, 1966	Normals	6	Chlorpromazine 100 mg once	↓REM latency, ↑ duration first REM period, ↑stage 4%.
Lewis and Evans, 1969	Normals	4	Chlorpromazine 25 mg for 6–7 nights	↑REM% (effect greater in females than males) ↑ total sleep, no changes on withdrawal.
	Normals	3	Chlorpromazine 100 mg for 3 nights	↓REM%, no changes on withdrawal.
Sagales et al., 1969	Normals	6	Chlorpromazine 0.4 mg/kg by injection once	↑Stage 3 (from 9.8% to 17.6%), ↓ stage 2 (from 39.4% to 33.6%).
Feinberg et al., 1969a	Schizophrenics	3	Chlorpromazine 200 mg 40 min before bed for 4–5 nights	↓Stage 1%, ↓ REM%, ↑ stage 4%.
	Character disorders	3		
Lester et al., 1971	Normals	12	Chlorpromazine 150 mg once	↑Delta sleep, ↓ REM latency, ↓ body movements.
Kupfer et al., 1971	Schizophrenics	2	Chlorpromazine 100 mg at bedtime for 6–12 nights	↑Total sleep, ↑nonREM sleep, ↓wakefulness, ↓early morning awakening. Over six nights, tolerance developed to sleep-promoting effect. Daytime administration of chlorpromazine had no effect.
	Insomniac neurotics	2		
Naiman et al., 1972	Normals	5	Chlorpromazine 1 mg/kg at bedtime plus 25–150 mg during day for 10 days	No change in total sleep, REM sleep, REM latency, or REM%.
Hartmann and Craven, 1973c	Normals	14	Chlorpromazine 50 mg for 28 nights	↑Stage 3, ↑ cycle length, ↓ body movements, initial ↑ total sleep for 5 nights.
Kaplan et al., 1974	Chronic schizophrenics	11	Chlorpromazine 100 mg 4 times a day for 1 month	↓Sleep latency, ↓ wakefulness, ↑ total sleep, ↑nonREM, ↑ stage 2, ↑ delta, ↑ REM latency, ↑REM density and activity.

continued

TABLE 7-12 (*continued*)

Authors	Subjects	No.	Drug/dose	Results
			Other Neuroleptics	
Toyoda, 1965	Normals	2	Perphenazine 8 mg once	↑ REM%, ↓ nonREM between REM periods.
	Normals	2	Levomepromazine 25–50 mg once	↓ REM%.
Brannan and Jewett, 1969	Young, chronic schizophrenics	4	Promethazine 50 mg at bedtime once	↑ Total sleep, ↑ cycle length.
		4	Trifluoperazine 5 mg at bedtime once	No significant effects, tended to increase REM and REM%.
		2	Thioridazine 25–50 mg four times daily	↑REM and REM% on first night but not on 6th night.
Blum and Girke, 1973	Neurotics	4	Clozapine up to 500 mg per day for 10 nights	Markedly ↑ REM% (85%) coincident with drug induced rise in body temperature.
Schneider *et al.*, 1974b	Psychotic	1		
	Schizophrenics	3	Sulpiride 200–400 mg intravascular (acute) or oral 300–600 mg (chronic)	Acute effect: ↓ Wakefulness, ↓ sleep latency. After 3 weeks, ↓ wakefulness, ↑stage 4.
	Endogenous depression	6		
	Neurotics	2		
Sagales and Erill, 1975	Normals	6	Pimozide 1 mg or 4 mg at bedtime once	No significant changes in stages 1–4 or REM.
Jus *et al.*, 1975b	Chronic schizophrenics	10	Various neuroleptics (chlorpromazine equivalent, mean = 495 mg)	Study compared single nighttime dose versus divided doses 3–4 times per day. With single dose, ↓ stage 2%, ↑ stage 4%, ↑ REM%.
Jus *et al.*, 1975c	Schizophrenics	15	Penfluridol 40–120 mg once weekly	No significant changes between first night and seventh night after treatment.

in two studies in normals (Hoffman and Domino, 1969; Coulter *et al.*, 1971) but not in two other studies (Hartmann, 1966; Hartmann and Cravens, 1973c). Jus *et al.* (1975a) reported that reserpine decreased stage 4 in lobotomized schizophrenic patients but not in nonlobotomized schizophrenic patients, who had significantly low amounts of stage 4 before treatment as compared with lobotomized patients. Tissot (1965) reported that it decreased delta sleep, but did not provide information about the patients or their baseline delta levels. In contrast to reserpine, chlorpromazine has generally been reported to increase delta sleep (Feinberg *et al.*, 1969a; Sagales *et al.*, 1969; Lester and Guerrero-Figueroa, 1966; Hartmann and Cravens, 1973b; Kaplan *et al.*, 1974), as has sulpiride (Schneider *et al.*, 1974b).

Chlorpromazine, in particular, has been reported to increase total sleep time, both in normals (Lewis and Evans, 1969 for low dose, not high dose; Hartmann and Cravens, 1973b) and in patients (Kupfer *et al.*, 1971; Kaplan *et al.*, 1974). Tolerance appears to develop to this chlorpromazine-induced increase in total sleep time (Kupfer *et al.*, 1971; Hartmann and Cravens, 1973b). In the study by Kaplan *et al.* (1974), increased total sleep was still observed a month after initiating chlorpromazine treatment in chronic schizophrenics, but higher doses (400 mg) were used than in the other two studies (50–100 mg) and, furthermore, sleep time may have increased because the clinical condition of the patients improved markedly.

Kaplan *et al.* (1974) also observed a significant increase in REM density and REM activity, two measures of eye movement activity during REM sleep. This finding is consistent with the hypothesis that chlorpromazine forces phasic events, such as PGO spikes, into REM sleep (Cohen *et al.*, 1973).

Many clinicians routinely administer neuroleptics in one dose at bedtime rather than in divided doses throughout the day. In part, the hope is that the single dose will increase sleep time and decrease extrapyramidal side effects. Kupfer *et al.* (1971) compared the effect of a low dose of chlorpromazine (100 mg) given at bedtime and in the morning. As expected, bedtime administration significantly increased total sleep and nonREM sleep and decreased wakefulness during the night and early morning awakening. Administration of chlorpromazine in the morning had no effect on sleep at night. These time-dependent effects appeared to correlate with blood chlorpromazine levels. Jus *et al.* (1975b) compared the effects of various neuroleptics (the mean dose was equivalent to 495 mg of chlorpromazine) given at night in a single dose with the same doses divided into three–four doses throughout the day. With the single nighttime dose, the percentage of stage 2 was significantly reduced and those of stage 4 and REM were significantly increased. Clinical benefits and the role of tolerance have not yet been rigorously compared in these two different methods of drug administration.

Penfluridol is a new, largely experimental neuroleptic that appears to be clinically active with once-a-week oral adminstration. In a brief report, Jus *et al.* (1975c) found no changes in sleep on the seventh day following oral administration as compared with the first day. Baseline sleep characteristics prior to treatment were not studied adequately.

In summary, the neuroleptic medications, as well as antidepressants, have been reported to produce diverse effects on sleep. It is not clear if the discrepant findings are apparent or real. Major methodological problems confound meaningful interpretations of many results from different laboratories (Freeman, 1972, pp. 96–116). The number of subjects has often been small in some studies, dose response relationships have rarely been reported, the time of day at which the drug was administered has varied, carry-over effects from one night to another have not always been controlled, double-blind administration and scoring has not always been observed, the relative effects of acute versus chronic administration have not been compared frequently enough to make statements about tolerance in some cases and the slow development of sleep changes in other cases, the differing response of normals and patients to the same drug and dose has not always been taken into account, the interraction between one sleep variable (for example, total sleep) and another (for example, REM time) has not been considered in some studies, and pharmacokinetic correlations have rarely been made.

With these limitations in mind, it does not appear that neuroleptics, as a class of drugs, produce common changes in human sleep. All neuroleptics, however, do apparently share the biochemical property of interfering with dopaminergic transmission, whether this is by blockade of postsynaptic receptors, inhibition of dopamine release, or disruption of dopamine storage in the presynaptic neuron. These results suggest that dopamine plays little role in the regulation of sleep states (see chapter 2).

Concluding Remarks about Sleep in Schizophrenia

As with affectively ill patients, schizophrenic patients often sleep poorly, particularly at times of acute psychotic decompensation or psychic turmoil. In general, no specific abnormalities of sleep have emerged from the cross-sectional studies of schizophrenic patients, although there have been occasional reports suggesting such deviations as high muscle potential and REM storms in remitted schizophrenics (Gulevich et al., 1967).

The longitudinal studies have documented the remarkable turmoil experienced by acutely disturbed patients suffering through a florid, psychotic episode. We do not know whether the sleep disturbance of these patients is similar to that of acutely manic patients.

The longitudinal studies also suggest the absence of a REM rebound in schizophrenic patients and this has been confirmed, to some extent, in experimental REM deprivation studies of actively ill schizophrenic patients. The significance of this finding remains to be demonstrated.

Although there have been few sleep deprivation studies in schizophrenia as compared with depression, the results suggest that it produces clinical improvement in schizophrenics, at least initially. As with the effects of sleep deprivation in depression, this procedure may be of greater theoretical interest than potential long-term, clinical benefit.

Neither the phenomenological descriptions of sleep in schizophrenia nor the effects of drugs upon the sleep of schizophrenics has resulted in any major new hypotheses about the cause or pathophysiology of schizophrenia. Dement's serotonin-phasic event hypothesis, born mostly from laboratory studies of animals, has had important heuristic benefits, however, for both clinical studies and basic science.

SUMMARY

In this chapter, we have reviewed EEG sleep studies in patients suffering from affective illnesses and schizophrenia. We examined cross-sectional studies that have compared patients with normals or with other patients, longitudinal studies that have followed patients over time, total sleep deprivation studies, REM deprivation studies, and observations on the effects of medications used in treating these disorders.

Tolstoy began Anna Karenina by writing "Happy families are all alike; every unhappy family is unhappy in its own way." Perhaps we will not be amiss to end this review by saying, "Happy people sleep alike; every unhappy person sleeps unhappily in his own way." Few generalizations can be made about the sleep of psychiatric patients that apply to all patients or that distinguish clinically defined subgroups of patients from controls. Compared with other depressed and schizophrenic patients, psychotically depressed patients probably have the most distinctively disturbed sleep patterns with their extreme fragmentation and shallowness of sleep and variability of REM sleep parameters. Still, some nonpsychotic depressed patients show no change in sleep or even increased sleep. More attention has been given to hypersomnia among depressed patients than among schizophrenic patients. Since loss of energy and apparent sleepiness is a common clinical feature of many chronic schizophrenics, the issue of hypersomnia in schizophrenia should be studied. Loss of delta sleep is a common finding in depressed and schizophrenic patients, but is hardly distinctive since it also occurs in a variety of other disorders. A short REM latency is also common in both, particularly in depression.

Formidable difficulties would exist in proving that a distinctive sleep disorder characterizes a particular clinical syndrome. Comparison groups would have to include both normal subjects and patients with other syndromes, and would have to control for variables such as age, sex, medications, and in the case of patients, factors such as clinical stage (waxing, stable, or waning phases of the illness), psychotic versus nonpsychotic features, or acute versus chronic history. Much of the confusion about current results may have resulted from the failure to study carefully defined groups of patients in comparison to carefully defined controls. Very few studies have attempted to compare depressed patients with, say, schizophrenic patients, a contrast that might shed light on sleep features that distinguish clinically defined diagnostic groups. Furthermore, it would be useful to compare the sleep of psychiatric patients with nonpsychiatric controls, such as natural long or short sleepers or primary insomniacs. In addition, while most investigators have compared groups according to one variable at a time (univariate techniques), few have attempted to compare groups according to combinations of variables (multivariate techniques). For example, it might be the combination of low delta sleep, short REM latency, short sleep time, and poor sleep efficiency that characterizes the sleep of most depressed patients rather than any one single feature taken alone.

The hypothesis that affective disorders and schizophrenia might result from a disorder of sleep is attractive. At the present time, however, the data is inconclusive. Nor does it seem likely that either prophylaxis of affective disorders and schizophrenia or clinical recovery depends upon normalization of sleep. Sleep deprivation may actually improve some depressed and schizophrenic patients, at least briefly. This observation only highlights our general ignorance about the functions of sleep and the effects of sleep deprivation.

Bibliography

Abramson, E. A., Arky, R. A., and Woeber, K. A. Effects of propanolol on the humoral and metabolic responses to insulin-induced hypoglycemia. *Lancet 2:* 1386–1388, 1966.

Adamson, J., and Burdick, J. A. Sleep of dry alcoholics. *Arch. Gen. Psychiatry 28:* 146–149, 1973.

Aghajanian, G. K., Rosecrans, J. A., and Sheard, M. H. Serotonin: Release in the forebrain by stimulation of midbrain raphe. *Science 156:* 402–403, 1967.

Aghajanian, G. K., Foote, W. E., and Sheard, J. H. Action of psychotogenic drugs on single midbrain raphe neurons. *J. Pharmacol. Exp. Ther. 171:* 178–187, 1970.

Aghajanian, G. K., Kuhar, M. J., and Roth, R. H. Serotonin-containing neuronal perikarya and terminals: Differential effects of p-chlorophenylalanine. *Brain Res. 54:* 85–101, 1973.

Agnew, H. W., Webb, W. B., and Williams, R. L. The effects of stage four sleep deprivation. *Electroencephalogr. Clin. Neurophysiol. 27:* 68–70, 1964.

Agnew, H. W., and Webb, W. B. Sleep latencies in human subjects: Age, prior wakefulness, and reliability. *Psychonomic Science 24:* 253–254, 1971.

Ahlenius, S., Carlsson, A., Engle, J., Svensson T., and Sobersten, P. Antagonism by alpha methyltyrosine of the ethanol-induced stimulation and euphoria in man. *Clin. Pharmacol. Ther. 14:* 586–591, 1973.

Ahtee, L., and Erikkson, K. Regional distribution of brain 5-hydroxytryptamine in rat brains selected for their alcohol intake. *Ann. N.Y. Acad. Sci. 215:* 126–134, 1973.

Akimoto, H., Honda, Y., and Takahashi, Y. Pharmacotherapy in narcolepsy. *Dis. Nerv. Syst. 21:* 704–706, 1960.

Akindale, M. O., Evans, J. I., and Oswald, I. Mono-amine oxidase inhibitors, sleep and mood. *Electroencephalogr. Clin. Neurophysiol. 29:* 47–56, 1970.

Alford, F. P., Baker, H. W., Burger, H. G., de Kretser, D. M., Hudson, B., Johns, M. W., Masterton, J. P., Patel, Y. C., and Rennie, G. C. Temporal patterns of integrated plasma hormone levels during sleep and wakefulness. II. Follicle-stimulating hormone, luteinizing hormone, testosterone and estradiol. *J. Clin. Endocrinol. Metab. 37:* 848–854, 1973a.

Alford, F. P., Baker, H. W., Burger, H. G., de Kretser, D. M., Hudson, B., Johns, M. W., Masterton, J. P., Patel, Y. C., and Rennie, G. C. Temporal patterns of integrated plasma hormone levels during sleep and wakefulness. I. Thyroid stimulating hormone, growth hormone and cortisol. *J. Clin. Endocrinol. Metabl. 37:* 841–847, 1973b.

Allen, C., and Scharf, M. B., and Kales, A. The effect of flurazepam (Dalmane) administration and withdrawal on REM density. Paper presented at the Annual Meeting of Assoc. For Psychophysiological Study of Sleep. Bruges, Belgium, 1971a.

Allen, R. P., Wagman, A., Faillace, L. A., and McIntosh, M. Electroencephalographic (EEG) sleep recovery following prolonged alcohol intoxication in alcoholics. *J. Nerv. Ment. Dis. 153:* 424–433, 1971b.

Anden, N-E., Butcher, S. G., Corrode, H., Fuxe, K., Ungerstedt, R. Receptor activity and turnover of dopamine and noradrenaline after neuroleptics. *Europ. J. Pharmacol. 11:* 303–314, 1970.

Anton-Tay, F., Chou, C., Anton, S., and Wurtman, R. J. Brain serotonin concentration: Elevation following intraperitoneal administration of melatonin. *Science 162:* 277–178, 1968.

Anton-Tay, F., Diaz, J. L., and Fernandez-Guardiola, A. On the effect of melatonin upon human brain. Its possible therapeutic implications. *Life Sci. 10:* 841–850, 1971.

Armstrong, R. H., Burnap, D., Jacobson, A., Kales, A., Ward, S., and Golden, J. Dreams and gastric secretions in duodenal ulcer patients. *New Physician 14:* 241–243, 1965.

Aserinsky, E., and Kleitman, N. Regularly occurring periods of eye motility, and concomitant phenomena during sleep. *Science 118:* 273–274, 1953.

Axelrod, J. The pineal gland: A neurochemical transducer. *Science 184:* 1341–1348, 1974.

Ayd, F. J., Jr. A clinical evaluation of the hypnotic efficacy and safety of mebutamate. *Dis. Nerv. Syst. 33:* 684–693, 1972.

Azumi, K. A polygraphic study of sleep in schizophrenics (English abstract). *Seishin Shinkeigaku Zasshi 68:* 69–75, 1966.

Azumi, K., Takahashi, S., Takahashi, K., Maruyama, N., and Kikuti, S. The effects of dream deprivation on chronic schizophrenics and normal adults: A comparative study. *Folia Psychiat. Neurol. Jap. 21:* 205–225, 1967.

Azumi, K., Jinnai, S., and Takahashi, S. The effects of L-DOPA on sleep patterns and SPR in normal adults. *Sleep Res. 1:* 40, 1972.

Baekeland, F. Pentobarbital and dextroamphetamine sulfate: Effects on the sleep cycle in man. *Psychopharmacologia 11:* 388–396, 1967.

Baekeland, F., and Lundwall, L. Effects of methyldopa on sleep patterns in man. *Electroencephalogr. Clin. Neurophysiol. 31:* 269–273, 1971.

Bailey, E., Jenner, F. A., and Wheeler, M. J. Renal function during the stages of sleep. *J. Physiol. (Lond.) 218:* 40–42, 1971.

Ball, Thomas. *An Inaugural Dissertation on the Causes and Effects of Sleep.* Budd and Bartram, Philadelphia, 1796, p. 8.

Bardin, C. W. Hormonal control of gonadal function, in *Best and Taylor's Physiological Basis of Medical Practice,* Brobick, J. R. (ed.), Williams and Wilkins, Baltimore, 1973, pp. 776–787.

Barnes, C. D., and Meyers, F. H. Eserine and amphetamine: Interactive effects on sleeping time in mice. *Science 144:* 1221–1222, 1964.

Bates, R. C. Delirium tremens and sleep deprivation. *Mich. Med. 71:* 941–944, 1972.

Batini, C., Moruzzi, G., Palestini, M., Rossi, G. F., and Zanchetti, A. Persistent patterns of wakefulness in the pretrigeminal midpontine preparation. *Science 128:* 30–32, 1958.

Batini, C., Magni, F., Palestini, M., Rossi, G. F., and Zanchetti, A. Neural mechanisms underlying the enduring EEG and behavioral activation in the midpontine pretrigeminal cat. *Arch. Ital. Biol. 97:* 13–25, 1959.

Bazelon, M., Barnet, A., Lodge, A., and Shelburne, S. A. The effect of high doses of 5-hydroxytryptophan on a patient with trisomy 21. *Brain Res. 11:* 397–411, 1968.

Berger, H. Über das Elektroencephalogramm des Menschen. *Arch. Psychiatr. Nervenkr. 87:* 527–570, 1929.

Berger, H. Das Elektroencephalogramm des Menschen. *Nova Acta Leopoldina 6:* 173–309, 1938.

Berger, R. J. Tonus of extrinsic laryngeal muscles during sleep and dreaming. *Science 134:* 840, 1961.

Berger, R. J. Physiological characteristics of sleep, in *Sleep: Physiology and Pathology,* Kales, A. (ed.), J. B. Lippincott Co., Philadelphia, 1969, pp. 66–79.

Berger, R. J., and Oswald, I. Effects of sleep deprivation on behavior, subsequent sleep, and dreaming. *J. Ment. Sci. 108:* 457–465, 1962.

Bergonzi, P., Chiurulla, C., Cianchett, C., and Tempesta, E. Clinical pharmacology as an approach to the study of biochemical sleep mechanisms: The action of L-DOPA. *Confin. Neurol. 36:* 5–22, 1974.

Berson, S. A., and Yalow, R. S. Radioimmunoassay of ACTH in plasma. *J. Clin. Invest. 47:* 2725–2751, 1968.

Bert, J. Action de la p-chlorophenylalanine sur le sommeil du babouin papio. *Electroencephalogr. Clin. Neurophysiol. 33:* 99–103, 1972.

Bhanji, S., and Roy, G. A. The treatment of psychotic depression by sleep deprivation: A replication study. *Br. J. Psychiatry 127:* 222–226, 1975.

Bignotti, N., Bocci, U., and Luzi, T. Il flurazepam da mg 30 nil frattamento dill insomnia. *Riv. Sper. Freniat. 96:* 1543–1577, 1972.

Binns, Edward. *The Anatomy of Sleep; or the Art of Procuring Sound and Refreshing Slumber at Will.* John Churchill, London, 1852, p. 146.

Bivens, C. H., Lebovitz, H. E., and Feldman, J. M. Inhibition of hypoglycemia-induced growth hormone secretion by the serotonin antagonists cyproheptadine and methysergide. *N. Eng. J. Med. 289:* 236–239, 1973.

Bixler, E., Scharf, M. B., and Kales, A. The effect of prolonged use of flurazepam (Dalmane) on eye movement density. *Sleep Res. 2:* 48, 1973.

Blackard, W. G., and Heidingsfelder, S. A. Adrenergic receptor control mechanisms for growth hormone secretion. *J. Clin. Invest. 47:* 1407–1414, 1968.

Bliss, E. L. Sleep in schizophrenia and depression—studies of sleep loss in man and animals, in *Sleep and Altered States of Consciousness,* Kety, S. S., Evarts, E. V., Williams, H. C. (eds.), Research Publication of Assoc. Res. *Nerv. Ment. Dis. 45:* 195–210, 1967.

Bliss, E. L., Clark, L. D., and West, C. D. Studies of sleep deprivation—relation to schizophrenia. *Arch. Neurol. Psychiatry 81:* 348–356, 1959.

Blum, A., and Girke, W. Marked increase in REM sleep produced by a new antipsychotic compound. *Clin. Electroencephalogr. 4:* 80–84, 1973.

Blum, K., Merritt, J. H., Wallace, J. E., Owen, R., Hahn, J. W., and Geller, I. Effects of catecholamine synthesis inhibition on ethanol narcosis in mice. *Curr. Ther. Res. 14:* 324–329, 1972.

Bloom, F. E., Hoffer, B. J., Nelson, C. N., Sheu, Y., and Siggins, G. R. The physiology and pharmacology of serotonin mediated synapses, in *Serotonin and Behavior,* Barchas, J., and Usdin, E. (eds.), Academic Press, New York, 1973, pp. 249–261.

Bodenheimer, W. S., Winter, J. S. D., and Faiman, C. Diurnal rhythms of serum gonadotropins, testosterone, estradiol and cortisol in blind men. *J. Clin. Endocrinol. Metab. 37:* 472–475, 1973.

Bojanovsky, J., Pflug, B., Toelle, R., and Uber, T. Autonomic effects of therapeutic sleep deprivation in depression patients. Ophthalmodynamography and pupillometry. *Nervenarzt 44:* 161–163, 1973.

Bojanovsky, J., Koch, W., and Tölle, R. Electrolyte changes with antidepressive therapy. Sleep deprivation and thymoleptic medication. *Arch. Psychiatr. Nervenkr. 218:* 379–386, 1974.

Bonasegla, F., and Menegati, E. Effect of administration of L-DOPA on the phases of sleep. *Rass. Stud. Psichiat. 57:* 797–804, 1968.

Bordeleau, J. M., Charland, P., and Tetreault, L. Hypnotic properties of nitrazepam (Mogadon). (A comparative study of chlordiazepoxide, diazepam, nitrazepam, secobarbital and placebo in psychiatric patients.) *Dis. Nerv. Syst. 31:* 318–323, 1970.

Bowers, M. B., Jr., Hartmann, E. L., and Freedman, D. X. Sleep deprivation and brain acetylcholine. *Science 153:* 1416–1417, 1966.

Bowling, G., and Richards, N. G. Diagnosis and treatment of the narcolepsy syndrome: Analysis of seventy-five case records. *Cleve. Clin. Quart. 28:* 38–45, 1961.

Boyar, R., Finkelstein, J., Roffwarg, H., Kapen, S., Weitzman, E., and Hellman, L. Synchronization of augmented luteinizing hormone secretion with sleep during puberty. *N. Eng. J. Med. 287:* 582–586, 1972a.

Boyar, R., Perlow, M., Hellman, L., Kapen, S., and Weitzman, E. Twenty-four hour pattern of luteinizing hormone secretion in normal men with sleep stage recording. *J. Clin. Endocrinol. Metab. 35:* 73–81, 1972b.

Boyar, R. M., Finkelstein, J. W., David, R., Roffwarg, H., Kapen, S., Weitzman, E. D., and Hellman, L. Twenty-four hour patterns of plasma luteinizing hormone and follicle-stimulating hormone in sexual precocity. *N. Eng. J. Med. 289:* 282–286, 1973.

Boyar, R. M., Rosenfeld, R. S., Kapan, S., Finkelstein, J. W., Roffwarg, H. P., Weitzman, E. D., and Hellman, L. Human puberty: Simultaneous augmented secretion of luteinizing hormone and testosterone during sleep. *J. Clin. Invest. 54:* 609–618, 1974.

Boyar, R. M., Finkelstein, J. W., Kapen, S., and Hellman, L. Twenty-four hour prolactin (PRL) secretory patterns during pregnancy. *J. Clin. Endocrinol. Metab. 40:* 1117–1120, 1975.

Branchey, M. H., Begleiter, H., and Kissin, B. The effects of various doses of alcohol on sleep in the rat. *Comm. Behav. Biol. 5:* 75–79, 1970.

Branchey, M., and Kissin, B. The effects of alpha-methyl-paratyrosine on sleep and arousal in the rat. *Psychonomic Science 19:* 281–282, 1970.

Branchey, L., Branchey, M., and Nadler, R. D. The influence of sex hormones on brain activity in male and female rats, in *Influence of Hormones on the Nervous System.* Proc. Int. Soc. Psychoneuroendocrinol, Ford, D. H. (ed.), Karger, Basel, 1971a, pp. 334–340.

Branchey, M., Branchey, L., and Nadler, R. D. Effects of estrogen and progesterone on sleep patterns of female rats. *Physiol. Behav. 6:* 743–746, 1971b.

Branchey, L., Branchey, M., and Nadler, R. D. Effects of sex hormones on sleep patterns of male rats gonadectomized in adulthood and in the neonatal period. *Physiol. Behav. 11:* 609–611, 1973.

Brannan, J. O., and Jewett, R. E. Effects of selected phenothiazines on REM sleep in schizophrenics. *Arch. Gen. Psychiatry 21:* 284–290, 1969.

Brazeau, P., Vale, W., Burgus, R., Ling, N., Butcher, M., Rivier, J., and Guillemm, R. Hypothalamic polypeptide that inhibits the secretion of immunoreactive pituitary growth hormone. *Science 179:* 77–79, 1973.

Brazier, M. A. B. *The Electrical Activity of the Nervous System.* Pittman Publishing Corp., New York, 1973, pp. 240–292.

Brebbia, D. R., and Altshuler, K. Z. Oxygen consumption rate and electroencephalographic stage of sleep. *Science 150:* 1621–1623, 1965.

Brebbia, D. R., Altshuler, K. Z., and Kline, N. S. Lithium and the electroencephalogram during sleep. *Dis. Nerv. Syst. 30:* 541–546, 1969.

Breese, G. R., Colt, J. M., Cooper, B. R., Prange, A. J., and Lipton, M. A. Antagonism of ethanol narcosis by thyrotropin-releasing hormone. *Life Sci. 14:* 1053–1063, 1974.

Bremer, F. Historical development in ideas on sleep, in *Basic Sleep Mechanisms*, Petre-Quadens, O. and Schlag, J. D. (eds.), Academic Press, New York, 1974, pp. 3–11.

Brewer, V., and Hartmann, E. Variable sleepers: When is more or less sleep required. Paper presented to Assoc. for Psychophysiological Study of Sleep. San Diego, California, 1973.

Brezinova, V., Loudon, J., and Oswald, I. Tryptophan and sleep. *Lancet 2:* 1086–1087, 1972.

Bricolo, A., Turella, G., Mazza, C. A., Buffatti, P., and Grosslercher, J. C. Modification del sonno noturno in parkinsoniani trattati con L-DOPA. *Sist. Nerv. 2–3:* 181–190, 1970.

Bridges, P. K., and Jones, M. T. The diurnal rhythm of plasma cortisol concentration in depression. *Br. J. Psychiatry. 112:* 1257–1261, 1966.

Brod, J. *The Kidney*, Butterworth and Co., London, 1973, pp. 125–149.

Brodie, B. B., Comer, M. S., Costa, E., and Dlabac, A. The role of brain serotonin in the mechanism of the central action of reserpine. *J. Pharmacol. Exp. Ther. 152:* 340–349, 1966.

Brodie, H. K. H., Murphy, D. L., Goodwin, F. K., and Bunney, W. E. Catecholamines and mania: The effect of alpha-methyl-para-tyrosine on manic behavior and catecholamine metabolism. *Clin. Pharmacol. Exp. Ther. 12:* 218–224, 1971.

Broughton, R. J. Sleep disorders: Disorders of arousal? *Science 159:* 1070–1078, 1968.

Broughton, R., and Mamelak, M. Gamma-hydroxy-butyrate in the treatment of compound narcolepsy. *Sleep Res. 4:* 211, 1975.

Brown, G. M., and Reichlin, S. Psychologic and neural regulation of growth hormone secretion. *Psychosom. Med. 34:* 45–61, 1972.

Bruhova, S., and Roth, B. Heredo-familial aspects of narcolepsy and hypersomnia. *Arch. Suiesse. Neurol. Neurochir. Psychiat. 110:* 45–54, 1972.

Bunney, W. E., and Davis, J. M. Norepinephrine in depressive reactions. *Arch. Gen. Psychiatry 13:* 483–494, 1965.

Bunney, W. E., and Hartmann, E. L. Study of a patient with 48-hour manic-depressive cycles. *Arch. Gen. Psychiatry 12:* 611–618, 1965.

Bunney, W. E., Goodwin, F. K., Murphy, D. L., House, K. M., and Gordon, E. K. The "switch process" in manic depressive illness. II Relationship to catecholamines, REM sleep, and drugs. *Arch. Gen. Psychiatry 27:* 304–309, 1972.

Byck, R. Drugs and the treatment of psychiatric disorders, in *The Pharmacological Basis of Therapeutics*, Fifth Edition, Goodman, L. S., and Gilman, A. (eds.), Macmillan Publishing Co., New York, 1975, pp. 152–200.

Caldwell, D. F. Differential levels of stage IV sleep in a group of clinically similar chronic schizophrenic patients. *Biol. Psychiatry 1:* 131–141, 1969.

Caldwell, D., and Domino, E. Electroencephalographic and eye movement patterns during sleep in chronic schizophrenic patients. *Electroencephalogr. Clin. Neurophysiol. 22:* 414–420, 1967.

Caldwell, J., and Sever, P. S. The biochemical pharmacology of abused drugs II. Alcohol and barbiturates. *Clin. Pharmacol. Ther. 16:* 737–749, 1974.

Camjanovich, R. P., and MacInnes, J. W. Factors involved in ethanol narcosis: Analysis of mice of three inbred strains. *Life. Sci. 13:* 55–65, 1973.

Carlson, G. A., and Goodwin, F. K. The stages of mania. *Arch. Gen. Psychiatry* 28: 221–228, 1973.

Carlson, H. E., Gillin, J. C., Gorden, P., and Snyder, F. Absence of sleep-related growth hormone peaks in aged normal subjects and in acromegaly. *J. Clin. Endocrinol. Metab.* 34: 1102–1105, 1972.

Carlsson, A., Jonason, J., Lindquist, M., and Fuxe, K. Demonstration of extra-neuronal 5-hydroxytryptamine accumulation in brain following membrane pump blockage by chlorimipramine. *Brain Res.* 12: 456–460, 1969a.

Carlsson, A., Corrodi, H., Fuxe, K., Hokfelt, T. Effects of some antidepressant drugs on the depletion of intraneuronal brain catecholamine stores. *Europ. J. Pharmacol.* 5: 367–373, 1969b.

Carskadon, M. A., and Dement, W. C. Sleep studies on a 90-minute day. *Electroencephalogr. Clin. Neurophysiol.* 39: 145–155, 1975.

Cartwright, R. D., Monroe, L. J., and Palmer, C. Individual differences in response to REM deprivation. *Arch. Gen. Psychiatry* 16: 297–303, 1967.

Castaldo, V., Krynicki, V. E., and Crade, M. L-DOPA and REM sleep in normal subjects and mentally retarded subjects. *Biol. Psychiatry* 6: 295–299, 1973.

Castellotti, V., and Pittaluga, E. Studio EEG del sonno spontaneo notturno negli state depressivi. *Riv. Neurol.* 36: 417–436, 1966.

Cazzullo, C. L., Penati, G., Bozzi, A., and Mangoni. A. Sleep patterns in depressed patients treated with a MAO inhibitor: Correlation between EEG and metabolites of tryptophan, in *The Present Status of Psychotrophic Drugs*, Cerletti, A., and Bove, F. J. (eds.), *Excerpta Med. Int. Congr. Ser.* 180: 199–203, 1969.

Ceresa, F., Angeli, A., Boccuzzi, G., and Molino, G. Once-a-day neurally stimulated and basal ACTH secretion phases in man and their response to corticoid inhibition. *J. Clin. Endocrinol.* 29: 1074–1082, 1969.

Cerone, G., Murri, L., Rossi, B., and Fraioli, F. Gonadotropin secretion during sleep in chronic schizophrenic patients. Presented at Second. Int. Sleep Res. Congress, Edinburgh, June 30–July 4, 1975.

Cervello, V. Über die physiologische Wirkung des Parceldehyds und Beiträge zu den Studien über das Chloralhydrat. *Arch. Exp. Path. Pharmacol.* 16: 265–290, 1883.

Chen, C. N., Kalucy, R. S., Hartman, M. K., Lacey, J. H., Crisp, A. H., Bailey, J. E., Eccleston, E. G., and Coppen, A. Plasma tryptophan and sleep. *Br. J. Med.* 4: 564–566, 1974.

Chernik, D. A., Ramsey, T. A., and Mendels, J. Effect of parachlorophenylalanine on the sleep of a methadone addict. *Br. J. Psychiatry* 122: 191–199, 1973.

Chernik, D. A., Cockrane, C., and Mendels, J. Effects of lithium carbonate on sleep. *J. Psychiatr. Res.* 10: 133–146, 1974.

Chernik, D. A., and Mendels, J. Longitudinal study of the effects of lithium carbonate on the sleep of hospitalized depressed patients. *Biol. Psychiatry* 9: 117–123, 1974.

Chu, N. S., and Bloom, F. Activity patterns of catecholamine-containing pontine neurons in the dorso-lateral tegmentum of unrestrained rats. *J. Neurobiol.* 5: 527–544, 1974.

Clemens, J. A., Shaar, C. J., Smalstig, E. D., Tandy, W. A., and Roush, M. E. Preoptic area multiple unit activity and LH release during the sleep cycle of the rat. *Endocrinology* 91: 621–625, 1972.

Clemes, S., and Dement, W. The effect of REM sleep deprivation on psychological functioning. *J. Nerv. Ment. Dis.* 144: 485–491, 1967.

Coccagna, G., Mantovani, M., Berti-Ceroni, G., Pazzaglea, P., Petrella, A., and Lugaresi, E. Sindrome ipersonniche-ipoventilatore. *Men. Med.* 61: 1073–1084, 1970.

Cohen, H., Mitchell, G., and Dement, W. C. Chlorpromazine and sleep in the cat. *Psychophysiology* 5: 207, 1968.

Cohen, H., Thomas, J., and Dement, W. C. Sleep styles, REM deprivation, and electroconvulsive threshold in the cat. *Brain Res.* 19: 317–321, 1970.

Cohen, H. B., Dement, W. C., and Barchas, J. D. Effects of chlorpromazine on sleep in cats pretreated with para-chlorophenylalanine. *Brain Res.* 53: 363–371, 1973.

Colvin, G. B., Whitmoyer, D. I., and Sawyer, C. H. Circadian sleep-wakefulness patterns in rats after ovariectomy and treatment with estrogen. *Exp. Neurol.* 25: 616–625, 1969.

Coppola, J. A. Brain catecholamines and gonadotropin secretion, in *Frontiers in Neuroendocrinology*, Martini, L., and Ganong, W. F. (eds.), Oxford University Press, New York, 1971, pp. 129–143.

Costello, C. G., and Smith, C. M. The relationships between personality, sleep and the effects of sedatives, *Br. J. Psychiatry* 109: 568–571, 1963.

Coulter, J. D., Lester, B. K., and Williams, H. L. Reserpine and sleep. *Psychopharmacologia* 19: 134–147, 1971.

Coursey, R., Buchsbaum, M., and Frankel, B. L. Personality measures and evoked responses in chronic insomniacs. *J. Abnorm. Psychol.* 84: 239–249, 1975.

Cramer, H., and Kuhlo, W. Effets des inhibiteurs de la mono-aminoxydase sur le sommeil et l'électroencephalogramme chez l'homme. *Acta Neurol. Belg.* 67: 658–669, 1967.

Cramer, H., and Ohlmeier, D. Ein Fall von Tranylcypromin- und Trifluoperazin (Jatrosom^R)-Sucht: Psychopathologische, schlafphysiologische, und biochemische Untersuchungen. *Arch. Psychiat. Nervenkr.* 210: 182–197, 1967.

Cramer, H., Rudolph, J., Consbruch, U., and Kendel, K. On the effects of melatonin on sleep and behavior in man. *Adv. Biochem. Psychopharmacol.* 11: 187–191, 1974.

Crisp, A. H., and Stonehill, E. Aspects of the relationship between psychiatric status, sleep, nocturnal motility, and nutrition. *J. Psychosom. Res.* 15: 501–509, 1971.

Crowley, T. J., Pegram, G. V., and Smith, D. E. The biogenic amines and sleep in the monkey. Preliminary report, in *Primate Electrophysiology Particularly Related to Sleep*. Holloman Air Force Base, New Mexico, 5761 Aeromedical Research Laboratory, Dept. ARL TR-69-3, Rept. 163, 1969.

Cryer, P. E., and Daughaday, W. H. Regulation of growth hormone secretion in acromegaly. *J. Clin. Endocrinol. Metab.* 29: 386–393, 1969.

Curtis, G. C. Psychosomatics and chronobiology: Possible implications of neuroendocrine rhythms. *Psychosom. Med.* 34: 235–256, 1972.

Daly, D. D., and Yoss, R. E. The treatment of narcolepsy with methyl phenylpiperidylacetate: A preliminary report. *Proc. Staff Meetings of the Mayo Clinic* 31: 620–625, 1956.

Daughaday, W. H. The Adenohypophysis, in *Textbook of Endocrinology*, Williams, R. H. (ed.), W. B. Saunders Co., Philadelphia, 1974, pp. 31–79.

Daughaday, W. H. Regulation of growth by endocrines. *Ann. Rev. Physiol.* 37: 211–244, 1975.

Daughaday, W. H., Othmer, E., and Kipnis, D. M. Hypersecretion of growth hormone during REM deprivation. *Abst. 51st Mtg. Endocrine Soc.*, New York, 1969, p. 126.

Davis, V. E. Neuroamine-derived alkaloids: A possible common denominator in alcoholism and related drug dependencies. *Ann. N.Y. Acad. Sci.* 215: 111–115, 1973.

Davis, V. E., Brown, H., Huff, J. A., and Cashaw, J. L. The alteration of serotonin metabolism to 5-hydroxytryptophol by ethanol ingestion in man. *J. Lab. Clin. Med.* 69: 132–140, 1967a.

Davis, V. E., Brown, H., Huff, J. A., and Cashaw, J. L. Ethanol-induced alterations of norepinephrine metabolism in man. *J. Lab. Clin. Med.* 69: 787–789, 1967b.

BIBLIOGRAPHY

Davis, V. E., and Walsh, M. J. Alcohol, amines, and alkaloids: A possible biochemical basis for alcohol addiction. *Science 167:* 1005–1007, 1970.

Dawson, S., Kaplan, J., Semel, C., Green, R., Woodrow, K., Gillin, J. C., and Wyatt, R. Sleep changes in chronic schizophrenics. Effects of 5-hydroxytryptophan (5-HTP). *Sleep Res. 3:* 37, 1974.

De Barros-Ferreira, M., Goldsteinas, L., and Lairy, G. C. Rem sleep deprivation in chronic schizophrenics: Effects on the dynamics of fast sleep. *Electroencephalogr. Clin. Neurophysiol. 34:* 561–569, 1973.

Deguchi, T., and Axelrod, J. Induction and superinduction of serotonin N-acetyltransferase by adrenergic drugs and denervation in rat pineal organ. *Proc. Natl. Acad. Sci., USA 69:* 2208–2211, 1972.

Deguchi, T., Sinha, A. K., and Barchas, J. Biosynthesis of serotonin in raphe nuclei of rat brain: Effect of p-chlorophenylalanine. *J. Neurochem. 20:* 1329–1336, 1973.

De Lacerda, L., Kowarski, A., Johanson, A. J., Athanasiou, R., and Miceon, C. J. Integrated concentration and circadian variation of plasma testosterone in normal men. *J. Clin. Endocrinol. Metab. 37:* 366–371, 1973.

Delay, J., Pichot, P., Deniker, P., and Jousseln, D. Psychoses cycliques avec inversions quotidiennes de l'humez. *Ann. Med. Psychol. 119:* 125–129, 1961.

Delorme, F. Monoamines et sommeils. *Etude Polygraphique Neuropharmacologique et Histochimique des Etats de Sommeil Chez le Chat.* Thèse Université de Lyon, Imprimerie LMD, 1966.

Dement, W. Dream recall and eye movements during sleep in schizophrenics and normals. *J. Nerv. Ment. Dis. 122:* 263–269, 1955.

Dement, W. The effect of dream deprivation. *Science 131:* 1705–1707, 1960.

Dement, W. C. Experimental dream studies, in *Academy of Psychoanalysis: Science and Psychoanalysis.* Grune & Stratton, Inc., New York, 1964, vol. 7, pp. 129–184.

Dement, W. Recent studies on the biological role of REM sleep. *Amer. J. Psychiatry 122:* 404–408, 1965.

Dement, W., and Kleitman, N. Cyclic variations in EEG during sleep and their relation to eye movements, body motility and dreaming. *Electroencephalogr. Clin. Neurophysiol. 9:* 673–690, 1957.

Dement, W. C., and Fisher, C. Experimental interference with the sleep cycle. *Can. Psychiat. Assoc. J. 8:* 400–405, 1963.

Dement, W., Greenberg, S., and Klein, R. The effect of partial REM sleep deprivation and delayed recovery. *J. Psychiat. Res. 4:* 141–152, 1966a.

Dement, W., Rechtschaffen, A., and Gulevich, G. The nature of the narcoleptic sleep attack. *Neurology (Minneap) 16:* 18–33, 1966b.

Dement, W., Zarcone, V., Ferguson, J., Cohen, H., Pivik, T., and Barchas, J. Some parallel findings in schizophrenic patients and serotonin-depleted cats, in *Schizophrenia—Current Concepts and Research,* Siva, D. V. (ed.), PJD Publications, Ltd., New York, 1969, pp. 775–811.

Dement, W. C., Ferguson, J., Cohen, H., and Barchas, J. Non-chemical methods and data using a biochemical model: The REM quanta, in *Some Current Issues in Psychochemical Research Strategies in Man,* Mandell, A. (ed), Academic Press, New York, 1970, pp. 275–325.

Dement, W. C., Carskadon, M., and Ley, R. The prevalence of narcolepsy II. *Sleep Res. 2:* 147, 1973a.

Dement, W., Guilleminault, C., and Mitler, M. Cataplectic attack: Polygraphic recording in man and experimental induction in cat. *Neurology (Minneap) 23:* 403–404, 1973b.

Dement, W., Zarcone, V. P., Hoddes, E., Smithe, H., and Carskadon, M. Sleep laboratory and clinical studies with flurazepam, in *The Benzodiazepines*, Garattini, S., Mussini, E., and Randall, L. O. (eds.), Raven Press, New York, pp. 599–611, 1973c.

Dement, W. C., and Mitler, M. M. An introduction to sleep, in *Basic Sleep Mechanisms* Petre-Quadens, O., and Schlag, J. D. (eds.), Academic Press, New York, 1974, pp. 271–296.

Detre, T., Himmelhock, J., Swartzburg, M., Anderson, D. M., Byck, R., and Kupfer, D. J. Hypersomnia and manic-depressive disease. *Amer. J. Psychiat.* 128: 1303–1305, 1972.

Diaz-Guerrero, R., Gottlieb, J. S., and Knott, J. R., The sleep of patients with manic depression. *Br. J. Psychiatry* 112: 1263–1267, 1966.

Doig, R. J., Mummery, R. V., Willis, M. R., and Elkes, A. Plasma cortisol levels in depression. *Br. J. Psychiatry* 112: 1263–1267, 1966.

Douglas, W. W. Histamine and antihistamines; 5-hydroxytryptamine and antagonists, in *The Pharmacological Basis of Therapeutics*, Goodman, L. S., and Gilman, A. (eds.), Macmillan, London, 1970, pp. 621–662.

Dragstedt, L. L. Causes of peptic ulcer. *JAMA* 169: 203–209, 1959.

Drucker-Colin, R. R., Rojas-Ramairez, J. A., Vera-Trueba, J., Monroy-Ayala, G. and Hernandez-Peon, R. Effects of crossed perfusion of the midbrain reticular formation upon sleep. *Brain Res.* 23: 269–273, 1970.

Drucker-Colin, R. R., Spanis, C. W., Shkurovich, M., and Ugartechea, J. C. Central neuro-protein regulation of REM sleep. Presented at the Second International Sleep Research Congress, Edinburgh, June 30–July 4, 1975.

Dundee, J. W. The influence of body weight, sex and age on the dosage of thiopentone. *Br. J. Anesth.* 26: 164–173, 1954.

Dunleavy, D. L. F., Maclean, A. W., and Oswald, I. Debrisoquine, quanethidine, propanolol and human sleep. *Psychoharmacologia* 21: 101–110, 1971.

Dunleavy, D. L., Březinová, V., Oswald, I., Maclean, A. W., and Tinker, M. Changes during weeks in effects of tricyclic drugs on the human sleeping brain. *Br. J. Psychiatry* 120: 663–672, 1972.

Dunleavy, D. L., and Oswald, I. Phenelzine, mood response, and sleep. *Arch. Gen. Psychiatry* 28: 353–356, 1973.

Dunleavy, D. L., Oswald, I., Brown, P., and Strong, J. A. Hyperthyroidism, sleep and growth hormone. *Electroencephalogr. Clin. Neurophysiol.* 36: 259–263, 1974.

Duron, B. La fonction respiratoire pendant le sommeil physiologique. *Bull. Physiolpathol. Resp.* 8: 1277–1288, 1972.

Dürrigl, V., Buranji, I., and Stojanovic, V. Characteristics of paradoxical sleep in schizophrenic patients, in *Sleep: Physiology, Biochemistry, Psychology, Pharmacology, Clinical Implications*, Koella, W. P., and Levin, P., (eds.), Karger, Basel, 1973a, pp. 587–591.

Dürrigl. V., Rogina, V., Stojanovic, V., Hajnšek, F., Gubarev, N., Jovanovic, U. J. Drugs—A study of two substances, in *The Nature of Sleep*, Jovanovic, U. J. (ed.), Stuttgart, 1973b, 203–208.

Dusan-Peyrethon, D., and Jouvet, M. Etude quantitative des phénomènes phasiques du sommeil paradoxal pendant et après sa déprivation instrumentale. *C.R. Soc. Biol. (Paris)* 16: 2530–2533, 1967.

Eastman, C. J., and Lazarus, L. Growth hormone release during sleep in growth retarded children. *Arch. Dis. Child.* 48: 502–507, 1973.

Eccleston, D., Reading, W. H., and Ritchie, I. M. 5-Hydroxytryptamine metabolism in brain and liver slices and the effects of ethanol. *J. Neurochem.* 16: 274–276, 1969.

Efron, D. H., and Gerson, G. L. Failure of ethanol and barbiturates to alter brain monoamine content. *Arch. Int. Pharmacodyn.* 142: 111–116, 1963.

Eitinger, L. *Concentration Camp Survivors in Norway and Israel*. Allen and Unwin, London, 1964.

Ekbom, K. A. Restless legs syndrome. *Neurology 10:* 868–873, 1960.

Erickson, C. K., and Burnam, W. L. Cholinergic alteration of ethanol-induced sleep and death in mice. *Agents and Actions 2:* 8–13, 1971.

Erickson, C. K., and Matchett, J. A. Correlation of brain amine changes with ethanol-induced sleep-time in mice. *Adv. Exp. Med. Biol. 59:* 419–430, 1974.

Ersmark, B., and Lidvall, H. Trial with amantime in narcolepsy. *Psychopharmacologia 28:* 308, 1973.

Evans, J. I., and Oswald, I. Some experiments in the chemistry of narcoleptic sleep. *Br. J. Psychiatry. 112:* 401–404, 1966.

Evans, J. I., MacLean, A. M., Ismail, A. A. A., and Love, D. Circulating levels of plasma testosterone during sleep. *Proc. Royal Soc. Med. 64:* 841–842, 1971a.

Evans, J. I., MacLean, A. W., Isamil, A. A. A., and Love, D. Concentrations of plasma testosterone in normal men during sleep. *Nature 229:* 261–262, 1971b.

Everett, G. M., and Borcherding, J. W. L-DOPA: Effect on concentrations of dopamine, norepinephrine, and serotonin in brains of mice. *Science 168:* 849–850, 1970.

Falck, B., Hillarp, N. A., Thieme, G., and Torp. A. Fluorescence of catecholamines and related compounds condensed with formaldehyde. *J. Histochem. Cytochem. 10:* 348–354, 1962.

Falk, J. L., Samson, H. H., and Winger, G. Behavioral maintenance of high concentrations of blood ethanol and physical dependence in the rat. *Science 177:* 811–813, 1972.

Faure, J. La phase "paradoxale" du sommeil chez le lapin (ses relations neuro-hormonales). *Rev. Neurol. 106:* 190–197, 1962.

Faust, V., and Hole, G. Meteorologisch bedingte Schlaf-störungen bei psychiatrischen Patienten. *Psychiatr. Clin. 5:* 265–288, 1972.

Feinberg, I. Sleep electroencephalographic and eye movement patterns in patients with schizophrenia and with chronic brain syndrome. *Res. Publ. Assoc. Nerv. Ment. Dis. 45:* 211–240, 1967.

Feinberg, I. The ontogenesis of human sleep and the relationship of sleep variables to intellectual function. *Compr. Psychiatry 9:* 138–147, 1968.

Feinberg, I. Sleep in organic brain conditions, in *Sleep: Physiology and Pathology*, Kales, A. (ed.), Lippincott Co., Philadelphia, 1969a, pp. 131–147.

Feinberg, I. Recent sleep research: Findings in schizophrenia and some possible implications for the mechanism of action of chlorpromazine and for the neurophysiology of delirium. Reprinted from *Schizophrenia: Current Concepts and Research*, Siva-Sanker, D. V. (ed.), PJD Pub. LTD., Box 581, Hicksville, N.Y. 11802, 1969b.

Feinberg, I. Changes in sleep cycle patterns with age. *J. Psychiat. Res. 10:* 283–306, 1974.

Feinberg, I. Across-night changes in the sleep EEG in man. Presented at the Second International Sleep Research Congress, Edinburgh, Scotland, June 30–July 4, 1975.

Feinberg, I. Functional implications of changes in sleep-physiology with age, in *The Neurobiology of Aging*, Gershon, S., and Terry, R. (eds.), Raven Press, New York, 1976.

Feinberg, I., Koresko, R., Gottlieb, F., and Wender, P. Sleep electroencephalographic and eye-movement patterns in schizophrenic patients. *Compr. Psychiatry 5:* 44–53, 1964.

Feinberg, I., Koresko, R., and Gottlieb, F. Further observations on electrophysiological sleep patterns in schizophrenia. *Compr. Psychiatry 6:* 21–24, 1965a.

Feinberg, I., Koresko, R. L., Heller, N., and Steinberg, H. R. Unusually high dream time in a hallucinating patient. *Am. J. Psychiatry 121:* 1018–1020, 1965b.

Feinberg, I., Koresko, R. L., and Heller, N. EEG sleep patterns as a function of normal and pathological aging in man. *J. Psychiat. Res. 5:* 107–144, 1967.

Feinberg, I., and Carlson, V. R. Sleep variables as a function of age in man. *Arch. Gen. Psychiatry 18:* 239–250, 1968.

Feinberg, I., Wender, P. H., Koresko, R. L., Gottlieb, F., and Piehuta, J. A. Differential effects of chlorpromazine and phenobarbital on EEG sleep patterns. *J. Psychiat. Res. 7:* 101–109, 1969a.

Feinberg, I., Braun, M., Koresko, R. L., and Gottlieb, F. Stage 4 sleep in schizophrenia. *Arch. Gen. Psychiatry 21:* 262, 1969b.

Feinberg, I., Braun, M., and Shulman, E. EEG sleep patterns in mental retardation. *Electroencephalogr. Clin. Neurophysiol. 27:* 128–141, 1969c.

Feinberg, I., Hibi, S., Cavness, C., and March, J. Absence of REM rebound after barbiturate withdrawal. *Science 185:* 534–535, 1974a.

Feinberg, I., Hibi, S., Braun, M., Cavness, C., Westerman, G., and Small, A. Sleep amphetamine effects in MBDS and normal subjects. *Arch. Gen. Psychiatry 31:* 723–731, 1974b.

Feldman, J. M., and Lebovitz, H. E. Antagonism of catecholamine inhibition of insulin secretion by methysergide. *Experientia 28:* 433–434, 1972.

Feldstein, A. Ethanol-induced sleep in relation to serotonin turnover and conversion to 5-hydroxyindoleacetaldehyde, 5-hydroxytryptophol, and 5-hydroxyindoleacetic acid. *Ann. NY. Acad. Sci. 215:* 71–76, 1973.

Feldstein, A., Chang, F. H., and Kucharski, J. M. Tryptophol, 5-hydroxytryptophol and 5-methoxytryptophol induced sleep in mice. *Life Sci. 9:* 323–329, 1970.

Felger, H. L. Chlorprothixene-enforced sleep for newly admitted patients with acute mental decompensation. *Dis. Nerv. Syst. 32:* 46–51, 1971.

Fencl, V., Koski, G., and Pappenheimer, J. R. Factors in cerebrospinal fluid from goats that affect sleep and activity in rats. *J. Physiol. 216:* 565–589, 1971.

Figurelli, F. A. Delirium tremens: Reduction of mortality and morbidity with promacine. *JAMA 166:* 747–750, 1958.

Finkelstein, J. W., Roffwarg, H. P., Boyar, R. M., Kream, J., and Hellman, L. Age-related change in the twenty-four hour spontaneous secretion of growth hormone. *J. Clin. Endocrinol. Metab. 35:* 665–670, 1972.

Fischer-Perroudon, C., Mouret, J., and Jouvet, M. Four months without sleep (Agrypnia) in a case of "chorée fibrillaire de Morvan"—Improvement after 5-HTP, in *Sleep Research,* Chase, M. H., Stern, W. C., and Walter, P. L. (eds.). Brain Information Service, UCLA, Los Angeles, 1973, p. 148.

Fischer-Perroudon, C., Mouret, J., and Jouvet, M. Sur un cas d'agrypnie (4 mois sans sommeil) au cours d'une maladie de Morvan. Effet favorable du 5-hydroxytryptophane. *Electroencephalogr. Clin. Neurophysiol. 36:* 1–18, 1974.

Fisher, C., and Dement, W. C. Studies in the psychopathology of sleep and dreams. *Am. J. Psychiatry 119:* 1160–1168, 1963.

Fisher, C., Byrne, J., Edwards, A., and Kahn, E. A psychological study of nightmares. *J. Am. Psychoanal. Assoc. 18:* 747–782, 1970.

Fisher, C., Kahn, E., Edwards, A., and Davis, D. A psychological study of nightmares and night terrors. *Arch. Gen. Psychiatry 28:* 252–259, 1973.

Fisher, E., and von Mering, S. Über eine neue Klasse von Schlafmitteln. *Ther. Ggw. 44:* 97, 1903.

Fiszer, S., and DeRobertis, E. Subcellular distribution and chemical nature of the receptor for 5-hydroxytryptamine in the central nervous system. *J. Neurochem. 16:* 1201–1209, 1969.

Florio, V., Scotti, A., Carolis, A., and Longo, V. G. Observations on the effect of D,L-Parachlorophenylalanine on the electroencephalogram. *Physiol. Behav. 3:* 861–863, 1968.

Fodor, N. Motives of insomnia. *J. Clin. Psychopath.* 7: 395–406, 1945.

Folin, O., and Shaffer, P. A. On phosphate metabolism. *Am. J. Physiol.* 7: 135–151, 1902.

Foster, F. G., and Kupfer, D. J. Psychomotor activity and serum creatine phosphokinase activity. *Arch. Gen. Psychiatry* 29: 752–758, 1973.

Foulkes, D., Pivik, T., Aherns, J. G., and Swanson, E. M. Effects of dream deprivation on dream content: An attempted cross night replication. *Psychophysiology* 4: 386–387, 1968.

Fram, D. H., Murphy, D. L., Goodwin, F. K., Brodie, H. K., Bunney, W. E., and Snyder, F. L-DOPA and sleep in depressed patients. *Psychophysiology* 7: 316–317, 1970.

Fram, D., Gillin, J. C., Wyatt, R. J., and Snyder, F. The waking action of histidine: Evidence to the contrary. *Psychophysiology* 9: 85, 1972.

Franchimont, P. The regulators of follicle stimulating hormone and luteinizing hormone secretions in humans, in *Frontiers in Neuroendocrinology*, Martini, L., and Ganong, W. F. (eds.), Oxford University Press, New York, 1971, pp. 331–358.

Frankel, B. L., Buchbinder, R., and Snyder, F. Ineffectiveness of electrosleep in chronic primary insomnia. *Arch. Gen. Psychiatry* 29: 563–568, 1973.

Frankel, B. L., Patten, B. M., and Gillin J. C. Restless legs syndrome. Sleep electroencephalographic and neurologic findings. *JAMA* 230: 1302–1303, 1974.

Fraschini, F., Collu, R., and Martini, L. Mechanisms of inhibitory action of pineal principles on gonodotropin secretion, in *Ciba Foundation Symposium on the Pineal Gland*, Wolstenholme, G. E., and Knight, J. (eds.), Churchill Livingstone, London, 1971, pp. 259–273.

Freemon, F. R. *Sleep Research.* Charles C. Thomas, Springfield, Ill., 1972, pp. 111–114.

Freud, S. Project for a scientific psychology (1895) in *The Origins of Psychoanalysis: Letters to Wilhelm Fliess, Drafts and Notes, 1887–1902*, Bonaparte, M., Freud, A., and Kres, E. (eds.), Basic Books, N.Y., 1954, p. 400.

Freund, G. Alcohol withdrawal syndrome in mice. *Arch. Neurol.* 21: 315–320, 1969.

Fullerton, D. T., Wenzel, F. J., Lohrenz, F. N., and Fahs, H. Circadian rhythm of adrenal cortical activity in depression. I. *Arch. Gen. Psychiatry* 19: 674–682, 1968a.

Fullerton, D. T., Wenzel, F. J., Lohrenz, F. N., and Fahs, H. Circadian rhythm of adrenal cortical activity in depression. II. *Arch. Gen. Psychiatry* 19: 682–688, 1968b.

Gallagher, B. B. Regulation of cortisol secretion in Parkinson's syndrome and narcolepsy. *J. Clin. Endocrinol. Metab.* 32: 796–801, 1971.

Gallagher, T. F., Yoshida, K., Roffwarg, H. D., Fukushima, D. K. Weitzman, E. D. and Hellman, L. ACTH and cortisol secretory patterns in man. *J. Clin. Endocrinol. Metab.* 36: 1058–1068, 1973.

Gastaut, H., Duron, B., Tassinari, C., Lyagoubi, S., and Saier, J. Mechanisms of the respiratory pauses accompanying slumber in the Pickwickian syndrome. *Act. Nerv. Super.* 11: 209–215, 1969.

Gelineau, J. De la narcolepsie. *Gas. D. Hop. (Paris)* 53: 626–628, 1880.

Geller, I., Purdy, R., and Merritt, J. H. Alterations in ethanol preference in the rat: The role of brain biogenic amines. *Ann. N.Y. Acad. Sci.* 215: 54–59, 1973.

Gessner, P. K., and Gessner, T. The interaction of barbital and testosterone relative to their hypnotic effects. *Arch. Int. Pharmacodyn.* 201: 52–58, 1973.

Giannelli, A., Penati, G., Pietropolli-Charmet, G. Some considerations on the psychiatric aspects of insomnia, in *The Abnormalities of Sleep in Man*, Gastaut, H., Lugaresi, E., Ceroni, G. B., and Coccogna, G. (eds.), Aulo Gaggi Editore, Bologna, 1968.

Gibbons, R. J., Kalant, H., and LeBlanc, A. E. A technique for accurate measurement of moderate degrees of alcohol intoxication in small animals. *J. Pharmacol. Exp. Ther.* 159: 236–242, 1968.

Giliarorsky, V. A. *Electric Sleep (A Clinical–Physiological Investigation)* (Translation of *Electrosod* (Russia, Moscow, 1958)). Office of Tech. Servs., Washington, D.C. 1960, p. 233.

Gillin, J. C., Jacobs, L. S., Fram, D. H., and Snyder, F. Acute effect of a glucocorticoid on normal human sleep. *Nature 237:* 398–299, 1972a.

Gillin, J., Post, R., Wyatt, R. J., Snyder, F., Goodwin, F., and Bunney, W. E. Infusion of threodihydroxyphenylserine (DOPS) and 5-hydroxytryptophan (5HTP) during human sleep. *Sleep Res. 1:* 45, 1972b.

Gillin, J. C., Post, R. M., Wyatt, R. J., Goodwin, F. K., Snyder, F., and Bunney, W. E. REM inhibitory effect of L-DOPA infusion during human sleep. *Electroencephalogr. Clin. Neurophysiol. 35:* 181–186, 1973.

Gillin, J. C., Jacobs, L. S., Snyder, F., and Henkin, R. I. Effects of decreased adrenal corticosteroids: Changes in sleep in normal subjects and patients with adrenal cortical insufficiency. *Electroencephalogr. Clin. Neurophysiol. 36:* 283–289, 1974a.

Gillin, J. C., Jacobs, L. S., Snyder, F., and Henkin, R. I. Effects of ACTH on the sleep of normal subjects and patients with Addison's disease. *Neuroendocrinology 15:* 21–31, 1974b.

Gillin, J. C., Buchsbaum, M. S., Jacobs, L. S., Fram, D. H., Williams, R. B., Vaughn, T. B., Mellon, E., Snyder, F., and Wyatt, R. J. Partial REM sleep deprivation, schizophrenia, and field articulation. *Arch. Gen. Psychiatry 30:* 653–662, 1974c.

Gillin, J. C., Fram, D. H., Wyatt, R. J., Henkin, R. I., and Snyder, F. L-Histidine: Failure to affect the sleep-waking cycle in man. *Psychopharmacologia 40:* 305–311, 1975a.

Gillin, J. C., van Kammen, D. P., Graves, J., and Murphy, D. Differential effects of D- and L-amphetamine on the sleep of depressed patients. *Life Sci. 17:* 1233–1240, 1975b.

Gillin, J. C., and Wyatt, R. J. Schizophrenia. Perchance a dream? *Int. Rev. Neurobiol. 17:* 297–342, 1975.

Gillin, J. C., Kaplan, J., and Wyatt, R. J. Clinical effects of tryptophan in chronic schizophrenic patients. *Biol. Psychiatry,* 1976, in press.

Gilman, L. *Insomnia and Its Relation to Dreams.* J. B. Lippincott, Philadelphia, 1958, p. 237.

Gitlow, S. E., Bentkover, S. H., Dziedzic, S. W., and Khazan, N. Persistence of abnormal REM sleep response to ethanol as a result of previous ethanol ingestion. *Psychopharmacologia 33:* 135–140, 1973.

Glick, S. M., Roth, J., Yalow, R. S., and Berson, S. A. The regulation of growth hormone secretion. *Recent Prog. Horm. Res. 21:* 241–283, 1965.

Globus, G., Humphries, J., Boyd, R., Gassney, D., and Phoebus, E. The effect of Lorazepam on the sleep of anxious insomniacs recorded in the home. Paper presented at the Annual Meeting of Assoc. for Psychophysiological Study of Sleep, San Diego, California, 1973.

Goldstein, L., Graedon, J., Willard, D., Goldstein, F., and Smith, R. A comparative study of the effects of methaqualone and glutethimide on sleep in male chronic insomniacs. *J. Clin. Pharmacol. 10:* 258–268, 1970.

Goldstein, L., Stoltzfus, N. W., and Smith, R. An analysis of the effects of methaqualone and gluthethimide on sleep in insomniac subjects. *Res. Commun. Chem. Pathol. Pharmacol. 2:* 927–933, 1971.

Goodwin, D. W., and Hill, S. Y. The chronic effects of alcohol and other psychoactive drugs on intellect, learning and memory, in *Alcohol, Drugs and Brain Damage,* Rankin, J. (ed.), Alcoholism and Drug Research Foundation of Ontario, Toronto, 1975, pp. 55–70.

Goodwin, F. K., Dunner, D. L., and Gershon, E. S. Effect of L-DOPA on brain serotonin metabolism in depressed patients. *Life Sci. 10:* 751–759, 1971.

Goodwin, F. K., and Post, R. M. Studies of amine metabolites in affective illness and schizophrenia: A comparative analysis, in *Biology of the Major Psychoses: A Comparative Analysis*, Freedman, D. X. (ed.), Res. Pub. Assoc. Res. Nerv. Ment. Dis., Raven Press, New York, 1975, pp. 299–332.

Graber, A. L., Givens, J. R., Nicholson, W. E., Island, D. P., and Liddle, G. W. Persistence of diurnal rhythmicity in plasma ACTH concentrations in cortisol-deficient patients. *J. Clin. Endocrinol. Metab. 25:* 804–807, 1965.

Green, A. R., and Curzon, G. Decrease of 5-hydroxytryptamine in the brain provoked by hydrocortisone and its prevention of allopurinol. *Nature 220:* 1095–1097, 1968.

Green, W. J., and Stajduher, P. P. The effect of ECT on the sleep-dream cycle in a psychotic depression. *J. Nerv. Ment. Dis. 143:* 123–134, 1966.

Greenberg, R. Dream interruption insomnia. *J. Nerv. Ment. Dis. 144:* 18–21, 1967.

Greenberg, R., and Perlman, C. Delirium tremens and dreaming. *Am. J. Psychiatry 124:* 133–142, 1967.

Greenberg, R., and Perlman, C. A. L-DOPA, parkinsonism, and sleep. *Psychophysiology 7:* 314, 1970.

Greenblatt, D. J., and Greenblatt, M. Which drug for alcohol withdrawal? *J. Clin. Pharmacol. 12:* 429–431, 1972.

Greenwood, M., Friedel, J., Bond, A. J., Curzon, G., and Lader, M. H. The acute effects of intravenous infusion of L-tryptophan in normal subjects. *Clin. Pharmacol. Ther. 16:* 455–464, 1974.

Grelak, R. P., Clark, R., Stump, J. M., and Vernier, V. G. In vivo conversion of [3] H-L-tryptophan into [3] H-serotonin in brain areas of adrenalectomized rats. *Science 169:* 201–204, 1970.

Gresham, S. C., Webb, W. B., and Williams, R. L. Alcohol and caffeine: Effect on inferred visual dreaming. *Science 140:* 1226–1227, 1963.

Gresham, S. C., Agnew, W. F., Jr., and Williams, R. L. The sleep of depressed patients. *Arch. Gen. Psychiatry 13:* 503–507, 1965.

Griesinger, W.; Berliner medicinisch-psychologische Gesellschaft. *Arch. Psychiatr. Nervenkr. 1:* 200–204, 1868.

Griffiths, W. J., Lester, B. K., Coulter, J. D., and Williams, H. L. Tryptophan and sleep in young adults. *Psychophysiology 9:* 345–356, 1972.

Grob, P., and Harvey, J. C. Effects in man of the anticholinesterase compound sarin (isopropyl methyl phosphoro-fluoridate). *J. Clin. Invest. 37:* 350–368, 1958.

Gross, M. M., Goodenough, D., Tobin, M., Halpert, E., Lepore, D., Perlstein, A., Sirota, M., Dibianco, J., Fuller, R., and Kishner I. Sleep disturbances and hallucinations in the acute alcoholic psychoses. *J. Nerv. Ment. Dis. 142:* 493–514, 1966.

Gross, M. M., Goodenough, D. R., Hastey, J., and Lewis, E. Experimental study of sleep in chronic alcoholics before, during and after four days of heavy drinking, with a non-drinking comparison. *Ann. N.Y. Acad. Sci. 215:* 254–275, 1973.

Gruen, P. H., Sachar, E. J., Altman, N., and Sassin, J. Growth hormone responses to hypoglycemia in postmenopausal depressed women. *Arch. Gen. Psychiatry 32:* 31–33, 1975.

Guilleminault, C., Dement, W. C., Wilson, R., and Zarcone, V. Respiration problems and sleep disorders. *Sleep Res. 1:* 151, 1972a.

Guilleminault, C., Eldridge, F., and Dement, W. C. Insomnia, narcolepsy, and sleep apneas. *Bull. Physiopathol. Respir. 8:* 1127–1138, 1972b.

Guilleminault, C., Cathala, J. P., and Castaigne, P. Effects of 5-hydroxytryptophan on sleep of a patient with a brain-stem lesion. *Electroencephalogr. Clin. Neurophysiol. 34:* 177–184, 1973a.

Guilleminault, C., Dement, W., and Monod, N. Nouvelle hypothèse à propos du syndrome "mort subite du nourrisson": Apnées au cours du sommeil. *Nouv. Presse Med.* 2: 1355–1358, 1973b.

Guilleminault, C., Raynal, D., Wilson, R., Dement, W. Continuous polygraphic recording in narcoleptic patients. *Sleep Res.* 2: 152, 1973c.

Guilleminault, C., Eldridge, F. L., and Dement, W. C. Insomnia with sleep apnea: A new syndrome. *Science 181:* 856–858, 1973d.

Guilleminault, C., Smythe, H., and Dement, W. Cataplexy, H-reflex and therapeutic trial. *Sleep Res.* 2: 153, 1973e.

Guilleminault, C., and Dement, W. Pathologies of Excessive Sleep, in *Advances in Sleep Research,* Weitzman, E. (ed.), Spectrum Publications, Flushing, N.Y., 1974, pp. 345–390.

Guilleminault, C., Carskadon, M., Dement, W. C. On the treatment of rapid eye movement narcolepsy. *Arch. Neurol. 30:* 90–93, 1974.

Guilleminault, C., Montplaisir, J., Zarcone, V., and Dement, W. C. Excessive daytime sleepiness (EDS) patients and a sleep disorders clinic. Presented at the Second International Sleep Research Congress, Edinburgh, June 30–July 4, 1975a.

Guilleminault, C., Phillips, R., and Dement, W. C. A syndrome of hypersomnia with automatic behavior. *Electroencephalogr. Clin. Neurophysiol. 38:* 403–413, 1975b.

Gulevich, G., Dement, W., and Johnson, L. Psychiatric and EEG observations on a case of prolonged (264 hours) wakefulness. *Arch. Gen. Psychiatry 15:* 29–35, 1966.

Gulevich, G., Dement, W., and Zarcone, V. All-night sleep recordings of chronic schizophrenics in remission. *Compr. Psychiatry 8:* 141–149, 1967.

Gunderson, C. H., Dunne, P. B., Feyer, T. L. Sleep deprivation seizures. *Neurology (Minneap) 23:* 678–686, 1973.

Gunne, L. M., Lidvall, H. F., and Widen, L. Preliminary clinical trial with L-DOPA in narcolepsy. *Psychopharmacologia 19:* 204–206, 1971.

Gursey, D., and Olson, R. E. Depression of serotonin and norepinephrine levels in brain stem of rabbit by ethanol on noradrenaline, dopamine, or 5-hydroxytryptamine levels in brain. *Acta. Pharmacol. Toxicol. 18:* 278–280, 1961.

Haggendal, F., and Lindqvist, M. Ineffectiveness of ethanol on noradrenaline, dopamine or 5-hydroxytryptamine levels in brain. *Acta Pharmacol. Toxicol. 18:* 278–280, 1961.

Haider, I. Patterns of insomnia in depressive illness: A subjective evaluation. *Br. J. Psychiatry 114:* 1127–1132, 1968.

Hajnšek, F., Dogan, S., Gubarev. N., Durrigl, V., Stojanovic, V., and Jovanovic, U. J. Some characteristics of sleep in depressed patients—a polygraphic study, in *The Nature of Sleep,* Jovanovic, U. J. (ed.), Gustar Fischer Verlag, Stuttgart, 1973.

Halasz, B. The endocrine effects of isolation of the hypothalamus from the rest of the brain, in *Frontiers in Neuroendocrinology,* Ganong, W. F., and Martini, L. (eds.), Oxford University Press, New York, 1969, pp. 307–342.

Hällström, T. Night terror in adults through three generations. *Acta Psychiatr. Scand. 48:* 350–352, 1972.

Halushka, P. V., and Hoffman, P. C. Alcohol addiction and tetrahydropapaveroline. *Science 169:* 1104–1105, 1970.

Harper, C. R., and Kidera, G. J. Aviator performance and the use of hypnotic drugs. *Aerosp. Med. 43:* 197–199, 1972.

Hartmann, E. L. Reserpine: Its effect on the sleep-dream cycle in man. *Psychopharmacologia 9:* 242–247, 1966.

Hartmann, E. Longitudinal studies of sleep and dream patterns in manic-depressive patients. *Arch. Gen. Psychiatry 19:* 312–329, 1968a.

Hartmann, E. The effects of four drugs on sleep in man. *Psychopharmacologia 12:* 346–353, 1968b.

Hartmann, E. The biochemistry and pharmacology of the D-state (dreaming sleep). *Exp. Med. Surg. 27:* 105–120, 1969.

Hartmann, E. L-Tryptophane and 50H-tryptophane: Effects on human sleep. *Psychophysiology 7:* 320–321, 1970.

Hartmann, E. *The Functions of Sleep,* Yale University Press, New Haven, 1973.

Hartmann, E., Verdone, P., and Snyder, F. Longitudinal studies of sleep and dreaming patterns in psychiatric patients. *J. Nerv. Ment. Dis. 142:* 117–126, 1966.

Hartmann, E. L., and Bridwell, T. J. Effects of AMPT, L-DOPA, and L-tryptophane on sleep in the rat. *Psychophysiology 7:* 313, 1970.

Hartmann, E., Chung, R., and Chien, C. P. L-tryptophan and sleep. *Psychopharmacologia 19:* 114–127, 1971.

Hartmann, E., Baekeland, F., and Zwilling, G. R. Psychological differences between long and short sleepers. *Arch. Gen. Psychiatry 26:* 463–468, 1972.

Hartmann, E., and Cravens, J. The effects of long term administration of psychotropic drugs on human sleep: II. The effects of reserpine. *Psychopharmacologia 33:* 169–184, 1973a.

Hartmann, E., and Cravens, J. The effects of long term administration of psychotropic drugs on human sleep, III. The effects of amitriptyline. *Psychopharmacologia 33:* 185–202, 1973b.

Hartmann, E., and Cravens, J. The effects of long term administration of psychotropic drugs on human sleep: IV. The effects of chlorpromazine. *Psychopharmacologia 33:* 203–218, 1973c.

Hartmann, E., and Schildkraut, J. J. Desynchronized sleep and MHPG excretion: An inverse correlation. *Brain Res. 61:* 412–416, 1973.

Hartmann, E., Cravens, J., and List, S. Hypnotic effects of L-tryptophan. *Arch. Gen. Psychiatry 31:* 394–397, 1974a.

Hartmann, E., Orzack, M. H., and Branconnier, R. Deficits produced by sleep deprivation: Reversal by d- and l-amphetamine. *Sleep Res. 3:* 151, 1974b.

Harza, J. Effect of hemicholinium-3 on slow wave and paradoxical sleep of the cat. *Eur. J. Pharmacol. 11:* 395–397, 1970.

Hauri, P., and Hawkins, D. Phasic REM, depression, and the relationship between sleeping and waking. *Arch. Gen. Psychiatry 25:* 56–63, 1971.

Hauri, P., and Hawkins, D. Human sleep after leucotomy: A case study. *Arch. Gen. Psychiatry 26:* 469–473, 1972.

Hauri, P., and Hawkins, D. R. Individual differences in the sleep of depression, in *The Nature of Sleep,* Jovanovic, U. J. (eds.), Gustar Fischer Verlag, Stuttgart, 1973, pp. 193–197.

Hauri, P., Chernik, D., Hawkins, D., and Mendels, J. Sleep of depressed patients in remission. *Arch. Gen. Psychiatry 31:* 386–391, 1974.

Hawkins, D. R., and Mendels, J. Sleep disturbance in depressive syndromes. *Am. J. Psychiatry 123:* 682–690, 1966.

Hawkins, D., and Mendels, J. The psychopathology and psychophysiology of of sleep, in *Biological Psychiatry,* Mendels, J. (ed.), J. Wiley, New York, 1973, pp. 297–330.

Held, R., Schwartz, B. A., and Fischgold, H. Fausse insomnie, étude psychoanalytique et électroencephalographique. *Presse Med. 67:* 141–143, 1959.

Hellman, L., Nakada, F., Curti, J., Weitzman, E. D., Kream, J., Roffwarg, H., Ellman, S., Fukushima, D. K., and Gallagher, T. F. Cortisol is secreted episodically by normal man. *J. Clin. Endocrinol. Metab. 30:* 411–422, 1970a.

Hellman, L., Weitzman, E. D., Roffwarg, H., Fukushima, D. K., Yoshida, K., and Gallagher, T. F. Cortisol is secreted episodically in Cushing's syndrome. *J. Clin. Endocrinol. Metab.* 30: 686–689, 1970b.

Henkin, R. I., Gill, J. R., Warmotts, J. R., Carr, A. A., and Bartter, F. C. Steroid dependent increase in nerve conduction velocity in adrenal insufficiency. *J. Clin. Invest.* 42: 941, 1963.

Henkin, R. I., and Bartter, F. C. Studies on olfactory thresholds in normal man and in patients with adrenal cortical insufficiency: The role of adrenal cortical steroids and of serum sodium concentration. *J. Clin. Invest.* 45: 1631–1639, 1966.

Henkin, R. I., and Daly, R. L. Auditory detection and perception in normal man and in patients with adrenal cortical insufficiency: Effect of adrenal cortical steroids. *J. Clin. Invest.* 47: 1269–1280, 1968.

Hendricksen, S. J., Jacobs, B. L., and Dement, W. E. Dependence of REM sleep PGO waves on cholinergic mechanisms. *Brain Res.* 48: 412–416, 1972.

Hershman, J. M., and Pittman, J. A. Utility of the radioimmunoassay of serum thyrotrophin in man. *Ann. Intern. Med.* 74: 481–490, 1971.

Hess, W. R. Hirnreizversuche über den Mechanismus des Schlafes. *Arch. Psychiatr. Nervenkr.* 86: 287–292, 1929.

Hess, W. R. Das Schlafsyndrom als Folge diencephaler Reizung. *Helv. Physiol. Pharmacol. Acta* 2: 305–344, 1944.

Heston, W. D. W., Erwin, V. G., Anderson, S. M., and Robbins, H. A comparison of the effects of alcohol on mice selectively bred for differences in ethanol sleep-time *Life Sci.* 14: 365–370, 1974.

Hill, S. Y. Intraventricular injection of 5-hydroxytryptamine and alcohol consumption in rats. *Biol. Psychiatry* 8: 151–158, 1974.

Hill, S. Y., and Goldstein, R. Effect of p-chlorophenylalanine and stress of alcohol consumption by rats. *Q.J. Stud. Alcohol.* 35: 34–41, 1974.

Himwich, H. E., and Callison, D. A. The effect of alcohol on evoked potentials of various parts of the central nervous system of the cat, in *The Biology of Alcoholism*, Kissin, B., and Begleiter, H. (eds.), Plenum Press, New York, 1976.

Hinton, J. M. A comparison of the effects of six barbiturates and a placebo on insomnia and motility in psychiatric patients. *Br. J. Pharmacol.* 20: 319–325, 1963a.

Hinton, J. M. Patterns of insomnia in depressive states. *J. Neurol. Neurosurg. Psychiatry* 26: 184–189, 1963b.

Hishikawa, Y., and Keneko, A. Electroencephalographic study on narcolepsy. *Electroencephalogr. Clin. Neurophysiol.* 18: 249–259, 1965.

Ho, A. Sex hormones and sleep of women. *Sleep Res.* 1: 184, 1972.

Hodge, J. V., Oates, J. A., and Sjoerdsma, A. Reduction of the central effects of tryptophan by a decarboxylase inhibitor. *Clin. Pharmacol. Ther.* 5: 149–155, 1964.

Hoffman, J. S., and Domino, E. F. Comparative effects of reserpine on the sleep cycles of man and cat. *J. Pharmacol. Exp. Ther.* 170: 190–198, 1969.

Holmes, J. H., and Gaon, M. D. Observations on acute and multiple exposure to anticholinesterase agents. *Trans. Am. Clin. Climatol. Assoc.* 68: 86–101, 1956.

Honda, Y., Takahashi, K., Takahashi, S., Azumi, K., Irie, M., Tsushima, T., and Shizume, K. Growth hormone secretion during nocturnal sleep in normal subjects. *J. Clin. Endocrinol. Metab.* 29: 20–29, 1969.

Howse, P. M., Rayner, P. H. W., Williams, J. W., and Rudd, B. T. Growth hormone secretion during sleep in short children: A continuous sampling study. *Arch. Dis. Child.* 49: 246, 1974 (abstract).

Hume, K. I., and Mills, J. N. A split sleep investigation of the relative effects of time of day and duration of prior wakefulness on the sleep process. *Sleep Res.* 4: 226, 1975.

Hunter, W. M., Friend, J. A., and Strong, J. A. The diurnal pattern of growth hormone concentration in adults. *J. Endocrinol. Metab.* 34: 139–146, 1966.

Hunter, B. E., Boast, C. A., Walker, D. W., and Zornetyer, S. F. Alcohol withdrawal syndrome in rats: Neural and behavioral correlates. *Pharmacol. Biochem. Behav.* 1: 719–725, 1973.

Illig, R., Stahl, M., Henricks, I., and Hecker, A. Growth hormone release during sleep wave sleep. *Helv. Paediatr. Acta.* 26: 655–663, 1971.

Irie, M., Sakuma, M., Tsushima, T., Shizume, K., and Nakao, K. Effect of nicotinic acid administration on plasma growth hormone concentration. *Proc. Soc. Exp. Biol. Med.* 126: 708–711, 1967.

Iskander, T. W., and Kaebling, R. Catecholamines, a dream sleep model and depression. *Am. J. Psychiatry* 127: 43–50, 1970.

Itil, T. M., Hsu, W., Holden, M. C., and Gannon, P. Digital computer sleep prints in lobotomized and nonlobotomized schizophrenics. *Biol. Psychiatry* 2: 141–152, 1970.

Jacobs, L. S., Green, R., Gillin, J. C. Wyatt, R. J., and Snyder, F. A toxic psychosis and sleep changes in a patient receiving phenelzine. *J. Hawaiian Medical Society* 35: 109–111, 1976.

Jacobson, A., Swearingen, C., Stadel, B., and Scharf, M. Flurazepam (Dalmane R5-6901) as a hypnotic for insomniac psychiatric patients. Paper presented at Annual Meeting of Assoc. for Psychophysiological Study of Sleep. Sante Fe, New Mexico, 1970.

Janowsky, D. S., El-Yousef, M. K., Davis, J. M., and Sekerke, H. J. A cholinergic-adrenergic hypothesis of mania and depression. *Lancet* 2: 632–635, 1972.

Jasper, H. H., and Tessier, J. Acetylcholine liberation from cerebral cortex during para-doxical sleep. *Science* 172: 601–602, 1971.

Jenner, F. A., Gjessing, L. R., Cox, J. R., Davies-Jones, A., Hullin, R. P., and Hanna, S. M. A manic-depressive psychotic with a persistent forty-eight hour cycle. *Br. J. Psychiatry* 113: 895–910, 1967.

Jenner, F. A., Goodwin, J. C., Sheridan, M., Tauber, I. J., and Lobban, M. C. The effect of an altered time regime on biological rhythms in a forty-eight hour periodic psy-chosis. *Br. J. Psychiatry* 14: 215–224, 1968.

Jewett, R. E. Effects of promethazine on sleep stages in the cat. *Exp. Neurol.* 21: 368–382, 1968.

Jick, H., Stone, D., Shapiro, S., and Lewis, G. P. Clinical effects of hypnotics. *JAMA* 209: 2013–2015, 1969.

Johns, M. W., Egan, P., Gay, T. J. A., and Masterson, S. P. Sleep habits and symptoms in male medical and surgical patients. *Br. Med. J.* 2: 509–512, 1970.

Johns, M. W., Masterton, J. P., Paddle-Ledinek, J. E., Winikoff, M., and Makinek, M. Delta-wave sleep and thyroid function in healthy young men. Presented at the Second International Sleep Research Congress, Edinburgh, Scotland, June 30–July 4, 1975.

Johnson, J. H., and Sawyer, C. H. Adrenal steroids and the maintenance of a circadian distribution of paradoxical sleep in rats. *Endocrinology* 89: 507–512, 1971.

Johnson, L. C. Psychological and physiological changes following total sleep deprivation, in *Sleep: Physiology and Pathology*, Kales, A. (ed.), Lippincott, Philadelphia, 1969, pp. 206–220.

Johnson, L. C., Slye, E. S., and Dement, W. Electroencephalographic and autonomic activity during and after prolonged sleep deprivation. *Electroencephalogr. Clin. Neu-rophysiol.* 27: 415–423, 1965.

Johnson, L. C., Burdick, A., and Smith, J. Sleep during alcohol intake and withdrawal in the chronic alcoholic. *Arch. Gen. Psychiatry 22:* 406–418, 1970.

Jones, H. S., and Oswald, I. Two cases of healthy insomnia. *Electroencephalogr. Clin. Neurophysiol. 24:* 378–380, 1968.

Jones, B. E. Catecholamine-containing neurons in the brain stem of the cat and their role in waking. *Imprimerie des Beauxarts,* J. Tixier & Fils, Lyon, 1969.

Jouvet, M. Recherches sur les structures nerveuses et les mécanismes responsables des différentes phases du sommeil physiologique. *Arch. Ital. Biol. 100:* 125–206, 1962.

Jouvet, M. Etude de la dualité des états de sommeil et des mécanismes de la phase paradoxale, in *Aspects Anatomofonctionnels de la Physiologie du Sommeil, a Symposium,* Jouvet, M. (ed.), Centre Natl. Rech. Sci., Paris, 1965a, pp. 393–442.

Jouvet, M. Paradoxical sleep—a study of its nature and mechanisms. *Prog. Brain Res. 18:* 20–62, 1965b.

Jouvet, M. Biogenic amines and the states of sleep. *Science 163:* 32–41, 1969.

Jouvet, M. The role of monoamines and acetylcholine-containing neurons in the regulation of the sleep-waking cycle. *Ergeb. Physiol. 64:* 166–307, 1972.

Jouvet, M., and Michel, F. Correlations électromyographiques du sommeil chez le chat décortique et mésencéphalique chronique. *Comp. Rend. Soc. Biol. (Paris) 153:* 422–425, 1959.

Jouvet, M., and Delorme, F. Locus coeruleus et sommeil paradoxal. *Compt. Rend. Soc. Biol. 159:* 895–899, 1965.

Jouvet, M., and Renault, J. Insomnie persistante après lesions des noyaux du raphe chez le chat. *Compt. Rend. Soc. Biol. 160:* 1461–1465, 1966.

Jovanovic, U. J., Dogan, S., Durrigl, V., Gubarev, N., Hajnsek, F., Rogina, V., and Stojanovic, V. Changes in sleep in manic-depressive patients dependent on the clinical state, in *The Nature of Sleep,* Jovanovic, U. J. (ed.), Gustar Fischar Verlag, Stuttgart, 1973, pp. 208–211.

Judd, H. L., Parker, D. C., Siler, T. M., and Yen, S. S. C. The nocturnal use of plasma testosterone in pubertal boys. *J. Clin. Endocrinol. Metab. 38:* 710–713, 1974.

Jus, A., Jus, K., Villeneuve, A., Gautier, J., Pires, P., Lachance, R., and Villeneuve, R. Influence of reserpine on all night sleep pattern in nonlobotomized and lobotomized chronic schizophrenic patients. *Biol. Psychiatry 10:* 17–25, 1975a.

Jus, K., Kiljan, A., Wilczak, H., Kubacki, A., Rzepecki, J., and Jus, A. Etude polygraphique du sommeil de nuit dans la schizophrénie. *Ann. Med. Psychol. 126:* 713–725, 1968.

Jus, K., Bouchard, M., Jus, A. K., Villeneuve, A., and Lachance, R. Sleep EEG studies in untreated, long term schizophrenic patients. *Arch. Gen. Psychiatry 29:* 386–390, 1973.

Jus, K., Beland, C., Bouchard, M., Jus, A., Fontaine, P., and Branelle, R. Polygraphic sleep pattern during chronic single and multiple neuroleptic dose administration. *Int. Pharmacopsychiatry 10:* 58–63, 1975b.

Jus, K., Jus, A., and Fontaine, P. Polygraphic sleep pattern during penfluridol treatment. *Curr. Ther. Res. 18:* 189–192, 1975c.

Kahn, E., and Fisher, C. The sleep characteristics of the aged male. *J. Nerv. Ment. Dis. 148:* 477–494, 1969.

Kaim, S. C. Prevention of delirium tremens: Use of phenothiazines versus drugs cross-dependent with alcohol, in *The Phenothiazines and Structurally Related Drugs,* Forrest, I. S., Cons. C. J., and Usdin, E. (eds.), Raven Press, New York, 1974, pp. 685–690.

Kaim, S. C., Klett, C. J., and Rothfeld, B. Treatment of the acute alcohol withdrawal state: A comparison of four drugs. *Am. J. Psychiatry 125:* 1640–1646, 1969.

Kaim, S. C., and Klett, C. J. Treatment of delirium tremens: A comparative evaluation of four drugs. *Q. J. Stud. Alcohol 33:* 1065–1072, 1972.

Kales, A., Hoedemaker, F. S., Jacobson, A., and Lichtenstein, E. L. Dream deprivation: An experimental reappraisal. *Nature 204:* 1337–1338, 1964.

Kales, A., Heuser, G., Jacobson, A., Kales, J. D., Hanley, J., Zweizig, J. R., and Paulson, M. J. All night sleep studies in hypothyroid patients, before and after treatment. *J. Clin. Endocrinol. Metab. 27:* 1593–1599, 1967a.

Kales, A., Wilson, T., Kales, J. D., Jacobson, A., Paulson, M. J., Kollar, E., and Walter, R. D. Measurements of all-night sleep in normal elderly persons: Effects of aging. *J. Geriat. Soc. 15:* 405–414, 1967b.

Kales, A., Beall, G. N., Bajor, G. F., Jackson, A., and Kales, J. R. Sleep studies in asthmatic adults; relationship of attack to sleep stage and time of night. *J. Allergy Clin. Immunol. 41:* 164–173, 1968.

Kales, A., Heuser, G., Kales, J. D., Rickles, W. H., Jr., Rubin, R. T., Scharf, M. B., Ungerleider, J. T., and Winters, M. D. Drug dependency. Investigations of stimulants and depressants. *Ann. Intern. Med. 70:* 591–614, 1969a.

Kales, A., Malmstrom, E. J., Scharf, M. B., and Rubin, R. T. Psychophysiological and biochemical changes following use and withdrawal of hypnotics, in *Sleep: Physiology and Pathology*, Kales, A. (eds.), Lippincott, Philadelphia, 1969b, pp. 331–343.

Kales, A., Jacobson, A., Scharf, M., Tan, T. L., Zweizig, J. R., and Alexander, P. Sleep laboratory and clinical studies of the effects of Tofranil, Valium, and placebo on sleep stages and enuresis. Paper presented at Annual Meeting of Assoc. of Psychophysiological Study of Sleep, Sante Fe, N. Mex., 1970a.

Kales, A., Tan, T. L., Killer, E. J., Naitoh, P., Preston, T. A., and Malstrom, E. J. Sleep patterns following 205 hours of sleep deprivation. *Psychosom. Med. 32:* 189–200, 1970b.

Kales, A., and Cary, G. Treating insomnia. *Medical World News Suppl.* 55–56, 1971.

Kales, A., Ansel, R. D., Markham, C. H., Scharf, M. B., and Tan, T. L. Sleep in patients with Parkinson's disease and normal subjects prior to and following levodopa administration. *Clin. Psychopharmacol. Ther. 12:* 397–406, 1971a.

Kales, A., Ritro, E. R., Preston, T. A., Scharf, M. B., and Tan, T. L. Effects of prolonged administration of L-DOPA on the sleep patterns of autistic children. *Psychophysiology 9:* 89–90, 1972.

Kales, A., and Scharf, M. B. Sleep laboratory and clinical studies of the effects of benzodiazepines on sleep: Flurazepam, diazepam, chlordiazepoxide in *The Benzodiazepines*, Garattini, S., Mussini, E., and Randall, L. O. (eds.), Raven Press, New York, 1973, 577–598.

Kales, A., Bixler, E. O., and Kales, J. D. Role of the sleep research and treatment facility: Diagnosis, treatment and education, in *Advances in Sleep Research I*, Weitzman, E. (ed.), Spectrum Publications, Flushing, N.Y., 1974a, pp. 391–417.

Kales, A., Scharf, M., Kales, J. D., Bixler, E. O., and Djoko, M. Sleep laboratory drug evaluation: Thioridazine (Mellaril), a REM enhancing drug. *Sleep Res. 3:* 55, 1974b.

Kales, A., Kales, J. D., Soldatos, C. R., Kotas, K., and Santen, R. Effects of thioridazine (Mellaril) on anterior pituitary secretion: Changes in testosterone and prolactin. Presented at the Second International Sleep Research Congress, Edinburgh, June 30–July 4, 1975.

Kales, J., Kales, A., Bixler, E. O., and Slye, E. S. Effects of placebo and flurazepam on sleep patterns in insomnia subjects. *Clin. Pharmacol. Ther. 12:* 691–697, 1971b.

Kalucy, R. S., Crisp, A. H., Chard, T., and Chen, C. Nocturnal hormonal profiles in obese anorexia nervosa and normal subjects. Presented at Second International Sleep Research Congress, Edinburgh, June 30–July 4, 1975.

Kamberi, I. A., Mical, R. S., and Porter, J. C. Effect of anterior pituitary infusion and intraventricular injection of catecholamines on prolactin release. *Endocrinology 88:* 1012–1020, 1971a.

Kamberi, I. A., Mical, R. S., and Porter, J. C. Effects of melatonin and serotonin on the release of FSH and prolactin. *Endocrinology 88:* 1288–1293, 1971b.

Kanai, T., and Szerb, J. C. Mesencephalic reticular activating system and cortical acetylcholine output. *Nature 205:* 80–82, 1965.

Kapen, S., Boyar, R., Hellman, L., Tucker, K., and Weitzman, E. D. Changes in the sleep stage pattern during the menstrual cycle of normal females. *Sleep Res. 1:* 186, 1972.

Kapen, S., Boyar, R., Perlow, M., Hellman, L., and Weitzman, E. D. Luteinizing hormone: Changes in secretory pattern during sleep in adult women. *Life Sci. 13:* 693–701, 1973.

Kapen, S., Boyar, R. M., Finkelstein, J. W., Hellman, L., and Weitzman, E. D. Effect of sleep-wake cycle reversal on LH secretory pattern in puberty. *J. Clin. Endocrinol. Metab. 39:* 283–289, 1974.

Kapen, S., Boyar, R., Hellman, L., and Weitzman, E. D. Inhibition of LH secretion during the nighttime hours: A subgroup of the amenorrhea–galactorrhea syndrome. Presented at the Second International Sleep Research Congress, Edinburgh, June 30–July 4, 1975.

Kaplan, J., Dawson, S., Vaughan, T., Green, R., and Wyatt, R. J. Effect of prolonged chlorpromazine administration on the sleep of chronic schizophrenics. *Arch. Gen. Psychiatry 31:* 62–66, 1974.

Karacan, I., Williams, N. L., Finley, W. W., and Hursch, C. J. The effects of naps on nocturnal sleep: Influence on the need for stage-1 REM and stage 4 sleep. *Biol. Psychiatry 2:* 391–399, 1970.

Karacan, I., Rosenbloom, A. L., Williams, R. L., Finley, W. W., and Hursch, C. J. Slow wave sleep deprivation in relation to plasma growth hormone concentration. *Behav. Neuropsychiatry 2:* 11–14, 1971.

Karacan, I., Booth, G. H., and Thornby, J. I. The effect of caffeinated and decaffeinated coffee on nocturnal sleep in young adult males. Paper presented at Annual Meeting of Assoc. for the Psychophysiological Study of Sleep, San Diego, California, 1973.

Karacan, I., Warheit, J., Thornby, J., and Schwab, J. Prevalence of sleep disturbance in the general population. Paper presented at the Annual Meeting of Assoc. for the Psychophysiological Study of Sleep, San Diego, California, 1973.

Karacan, I., Rosenbloom, A. L., Londono, J. H., Williams, R. L., and Salis, P. J. Growth hormone levels during morning and afternoon naps. *Behav. Neuropsychiatry 6:* 67–70, 1975.

Karczmar, A. G. Cholinergic influences on behavior, in *Cholinergic Mechanisms,* Waser, P. G., (ed.), Raven Press, New York, 1975, pp. 501–529.

Karfa, J., Karki, N. T., and Tala, E. Inhibition by methysergide of 5-hyydroxytryptophan toxicity to mice. *Acta Pharmacol. Toxicol. 18:* 255–262, 1961.

Karoum, F., Wyatt, R. J., and Costa, E. Estimation of the contribution of peripheral and central noradrenergic neurons to urinary 3-methoxy-4-hydroxyphenylglycol in the rat. *Neuropharmacology 13:* 165–176, 1974.

Karoum, F., Wyatt, R. J., and Majchrowicz, E. Brain concentrations of biogenic amine metabolites in acutely treated and ethanol dependent rats. *Br. J. Pharmacol 56:* 403–411, 1976.

Kastin, A. J., Ehrensing, R. H., Schalch, D. S., and Anderson, M. S. Improvement in mental depression with decreased thyrotropin response after administration of thyrotropin releasing hormone. *Lancet 2:* 740–742, 1972.

Kato, R., Chiesara, E., and Frontino, G. Influence of sex difference on the pharmacological action and metabolism of some drugs. *Biochem. Pharmacol.* 11: 221–227, 1962.

Kawamura, H., and Sawyer, C. H. Elevation in brain temperature during paradoxical sleep. *Science* 150: 912–913, 1965.

Kendel, K., Beck, U., Wita, C., Hohneck, E., and Zimmermann, H. Der Einfluss von L-DOPA auf den Nachtschlaf bei Patienten mit Parkinson-syndrom. *Arch. Psychiatr. Nervenkr.* 216, 82–100, 1972.

Kessler, S., Guilleminault, C., and Dement, W. A family study of narcoleptics. *Acta Neurol. Scand.* 50: 503–512, 1974.

King, D., and Jewett, R. E. The effects of alpha methyl tyrosine on sleep and brain norepinephrine in cats. *J. Pharmacol. Exp. Ther.* 177: 188–194, 1971.

Kingman, R. The insomniac. *New York Med. J. Rec.* 129: 683–687, 1929.

Kinsey, A., Pomeroy, W. B., Martin, C. E., and Gerhard, P. H. *Sexual Behavior in the Human Female*, W. B. Saunders, Philadelphia, 1953.

Kleinberg, D. L., Noel, G. L., and Frantz, A. G. Chlorpromazine stimulation and L-DOPA suppression of plasma prolactin in man. *J. Clin. Endocrinol. Metab.* 33: 873–876, 1971.

Kleitman, N. *Sleep and Wakefulness, as Alternating Phases in the Cycle of Existence*, U. of Chicago Press, Chicago, 1939.

Kleitman, N. *Sleep and Wakefulness*, U. of Chicago Press, Chicago, 1963, p. 274.

Knapp, S., and Mandell, A. J. Parachlorophenylalanine—its three phase sequence of interactions with the two forms of brain tryptophan hydroxylase. *Life Sci.* 11: 761–771, 1972.

Knopf, R. F., Conn, J. W., Fajans, S. S., Floyd, J. C., Guntsche, E. M., and Rull, J. A. Plasma growth hormone response to intravenous administration of amino acids. *J. Clin. Endocrinol. Metab.* 25: 1140–1144, 1965.

Knott, P. J., and Curzon, G. Free tryptophan in plasma and brain tryptophan metabolism. *Nature* 239: 452–453, 1972.

Knowles, J. B., Laverty, S. G., and Kuechler, H. A. The effects of alcohol on REM sleep. *Q. J. Stud. Alcohol* 29: 342–349, 1968.

Koella, W. P. Neurohumoral aspects of sleep control. *Biol. Psychiatry* 1: 161–177, 1969.

Koella, W. P., Feldstein, A., and Czieman, J. S. The effect of parachlorophenylalanine on the sleep of cats. *Electroencephalogr. Clin. Neurophysiol.* 25: 481–490, 1968.

Koranyi, E. K., and Lehmann, H. E. Experimental sleep deprivation in schizophrenic patients. *Arch. Gen. Psychiatry* 2: 534–544, 1960.

Koranyi, L., Beyer, C., and Guzman-Flores, C. Multiple unit activity during habituation, sleepwakefulness cyles and the effect of ACTH and corticosteroid treatment. *Physiol. Behav.* 7: 321–329, 1971.

Koresko, R., Synder, F., and Feinberg, I. 'Dream Time' in hallucinating and nonhallucinating schizophrenic pateitns. *Nature* 199: 1118–1119, 1963.

Kramer, M., Roth, T., and Trindar, J. Noise disturbance and sleep. *Department of Transportation Report No. FAA-NO-70-16*, 1971.

Krieger, D. T., Kreuzer, J., and Rizzo, F. A. Constant light: Effect on circadian pattern and phase reversal of steroid and electrolyte levels in man. *J. Clin. Endocrinol. Metab.* 29: 1634–1638, 1969.

Krieger, I., and Mellinger, R. C. Pituitary function in the deprivation syndrome. *J. Pediatrics* 79: 216–225, 1971.

Krieger, D. T., and Rizzo, F. Circadian periodicity of plasma II-hydroxycorticosteroid levels in subjects with partial and absent light perception. *Neuroendocrinology* 8: 165–179, 1971.

Krieger, D. T., Albin, J., Paget, S., and Glick, S. M. Failure of suppression of nocturnal growth hormone rise by acute corticosteroid administration. *Horm. Metab. Res. 4:* 463–466, 1972.

Krieger, D. T., and Gewirtz, G. P. Recovery of hypothalamic-pituitary-adrenal function, growth hormone responsiveness and sleep EEG pattern in a patient following removal of an adrenal cortical adenoma. *J. Clin. Endocrinol. Metab. 38:* 1075–1082, 1974.

Krieger, D. T., and Glick, S. M. Sleep EEG stages and plasma growth hormone concentration in states of endogenous and exogenous hypercortisolemia or ACTH elevation. *J. Clin. Endocrinol. Metab. 39:* 986–1000, 1974.

Kripke, D. F. Ultradian rhythms in sleep and wakefulness, in *Advances in Sleep Research,* Weitzman, E. S. (ed.), Spectrum Publications, New York, 1975, pp. 305–325.

Kunugi, H. All night sleep EEG in chronic schizophrenia (English Abstract). *Seihin Shinkeigaku Zasshi 72:* 226–227, 1970.

Kupfer, D. J. REM latency: A psychobiologic marker for primary depressive disease. *Biol. Psychiatry II:* 159–174, 1976.

Kupfer, D. J., Wyatt, R. J., and Snyder, F. Comparison between electroencephalographic and systematic nursing observations of sleep in psychiatric patients. *J. Nerv. Ment. Dis. 151:* 361–368, 1970a.

Kupfer, D. J., Wyatt, R. J., Greenspan, K., Scott, J., and Snyder, F. Lithium carbonate and sleep in affective illness. *Arch. Gen. Psychiatry 23:* 35–40, 1970b.

Kupfer, D. J., Wyatt, R. J., Scott, J., and Snyder, F. Sleep disturbance in acute schizophrenic patients. *Am. J. Psychiatry 126:* 1213–1223, 1970c.

Kupfer, D. J., Wyatt, R. J., Snyder, F., and Davis, J. M. Chlorpromazine and sleep in psychiatric patients. *Arch. Gen. Psychiatry 24:* 185–189, 1971.

Kupfer, D. J., and Bowers, M. B. REM sleep and central monoamine oxidase inhibition. *Psychopharmacologia 27:* 183–190, 1972.

Kupfer, D. J., and Foster, F. G. Interval between onset of sleep and rapid eye movement sleep as an indicator of depression. *Lancet 2:* 684–686, 1972.

Kupfer, D. J., and Heninger, E. R. REM activity as a correlate of mood changes throughout the night (EEG sleep patterns in a patient with a 48 hour cyclic mood disturbance). *Arch. Gen. Psychiatry 27:* 368–373, 1972.

Kupfer, D. J., Himmelhook, J., Swartzburg, M., Anderson, C., Byck, R., and Detre, T. P. Hypersomnia in manic depressive disease. *Dis. Nerv. Syst. 33:* 720–724, 1972.

Kupfer, D. J., and Foster, F. G. Sleep and activity in a psychotic depression. *J. Nerv. Ment. Dis. 156:* 341–348, 1973.

Kupfer, D. J., Foster, F. G., and Detre, T. P. Sleep continuity changes in depression, *Dis. Nerv. Syst. 34:* 192–195, 1973.

Kupfer, D. J., Reynolds, C. F., Weiss, B. L., and Foster, F. C. Lithium carbonate and sleep in affective disorders: Further considerations. *Arch. Gen. Psychiatry. 30:* 79–84, 1974.

Kupfer, D. J., and Foster, F. G. The sleep of psychotic patients: Does it all look alike? In *The Biology of the Major Psychosis: A Comparative Analysis,* Freedman, D. X. (ed.), Raven Press, New York, 1975, pp. 143–164.

Kuriyama, K., Rauscher, G. E., and Sze, P. Y. Effect of acute and chronic administration of ethanol on the 5-hydroxytryptamine turnover and tryptophan hydroxylase activity of the mouse brain. *Brain Res. 26:* 450–454, 1971.

Lairy, G., Barte, H., Goldsteinas, L., and Ridjanovic, S. Nocturnal sleep of mental illness. *Somm. Nurt. 2:* 354–381, 1965.

Lasagna, L. A study of hypnotic drugs in patients with chronic diseases. Comparative efficacy of placebo; methyprylon (Noludar); meprobamate (Miltown, Equanil); pentobarbital; phenobarbital; secobarbital. *J. Chronic Dis. 3:* 122–133, 1956.

Lasegue, C. Le délire alcoholique n'est pas un délire, mais un rêve. *Arch. Gen. Med. 88:* 513–536, 1881.

Leaf, A., and Liddle, G. W. Summarization of the effects of hormones on water and electrolyte metabolism, in *Textbook of Endocrinology,* Williams, R. H. (ed.), W. B. Saunders Co., Philadelphia, 1974, pp. 938–947, 1974.

Leckman, J. F., and Gershon, E. S. A genetic model of narcolepsy. *Br. J. Psychiatry 127:* 276–279, 1975.

LeGassiche, J., Ashcroft, G. W., Eccleston, D., Evans, J. I., Oswald, I., and Ritson, E. B. The clinical state, sleep, and amine metabolism of a tranylcypromine ("Parnate") addict. *Br. J. Psychiatry 111:* 357–364, 1965.

Legendre, R., and Pieron, H. Des résultats histo-physiologiques de l'injection intraoccipito-atlantoidedienne des liquides insomniques. *Comptes Rendus Soc. Biol. 68:* 1108–1109, 1910.

Leibowitz, J. O. Studies in the history of alcoholism II. Acute alcoholism in ancient Greek and Roman medicine. *Br. J. Addict. 62:* 83–86, 1967.

Lelek, I., and Danhauser, V. Experience with methaqualone (Moloton) in sleep disorders. *Ther. Hung. 18:* 31–32, 1970.

Lenard, H. G., and Schulte, F. J. Polygraphic sleep study in cranipagus twins (where is the sleep transmitter?). *J. Neurol. Neurosurg. Psychiatry 35:* 756–762, 1972.

Lester, B. K., and Guerrero-Figueroa, R. Effects of some drugs on electroencephalographic fast activity and dream time. *Psychophysiology 2:* 224–236, 1966.

Lester, B. K., Burch, N. R., and Dossett, R. C. Nocturnal EEG-GSR profiles: The influence of presleep states. *Psychophysiology 3:* 238–248, 1967.

Lester, B. K., Chanes, R. E., and Condit, P. T. A clinical syndrome and EEG sleep changes associated with amino acid deprivation. *Am. J. Psychiatry 126:* 185–190, 1969.

Lester, B. K., Coulter, J. D., Cowden, L. C., and Williams, H. L. Chlorpromazine and human sleep. *Psychopharmacologia 20:* 280–287, 1971.

Lester, B. K., Rundell, O. H., Cowden, L. C., and Williams, H. L. Chronic alcoholism, alcohol and sleep. *Adv. Exp. Med. Biol. 35:* 261–279, 1973.

Levin, M. Aggression, guilt and cataplexy. *Am. J. Psychiatry 116:* 133–136, 1959.

Lewis, S. A., and Evans, J. I. Some effects of chlorpromazine on human sleep. *Psychopharmacologia 14:* 342–348, 1969.

Lewis, S. A., and Oswald, I. Overdose of tricyclic antidepressants and deductions concerning their cerebral action. *Br. J. Psychiatry 115:* 1403–1410, 1969.

Liddle, G. W. The adrenal cortex in *Textbook of Endocrinology, 5th edition,* Williams, R. H. (ed.), Saunders, Philadelphia, 1974, pp. 233–283.

Liebreich, O. Das Chloral — ein neues Hypnoticum und Anästheticum.   *Berl. Klin. Wochenschr. 6:* 325–327, 1869.

Lin, T. U., and Tucci, J. R. Provocative tests of growth-hormone release. *Ann. Intern. Med. 80:* 464–469, 1974.

Lipman, R. L., Taylor, A. L., Schenk, A., and Mintz, D. H. Inhibition of sleep-related growth hormone release by elevated free fatty acids. *J. Clin. Endocrinol. Metab. 35:* 592–594, 1972.

Liuzzi, A., Chiodini, P. G., Botalla, L., Cremascoli, G., and Silvestrini, F. Inhibitory effect of L-DOPA on GH release in acromegalic patients. *J. Clin. Endocrinol. Metab. 35:* 941–943, 1972.

Loomis, A. L., Harvey, E. N., and Hobart, G. A. Cerebral states during sleep, as studied by human brain potentials. *J. Exp. Psychol. 21:* 127–144, 1937.

Loosen, P., Achenhell, M., Athen, D., Bechmann, H., Benkert, O., Dittmer, T., Hippius,

H., Matussek, N., Rüther, E., Scheller, M. The therapy of endogenous depression by sleep deprivation. 2. Comparisons of psychopathologic and biochemical parameters. *Arzneim. Forsch.* 24: 1075–1077, 1974.

Lowy, F. H., Cleghorn, J. M., and McClure, D. S. Sleep patterns in depression. *J. Nerv. Ment. Dis.* 153: 10–26, 1971.

Luby, E. D., and Gottlieb, J. S. Sleep deprivation, in *American Handbook of Psychiatry*, Arieti, S. (ed.), Basic Books, New York, 1966, Vol. 3, p. 406.

Luby, E., and Caldwell, D. Sleep deprivation and EEG slow wave activity in chronic schizophrenia. *Arch. Gen. Psychiatry* 17: 361–364, 1967.

Lucke, G., and Glick, S. M. Experimental modification of the sleep-induced peak of growth hormone secretion. *J. Clin. Endocrinol. Metab.* 32: 729–736, 1971a.

Lucke, C., and Glick, S. M. Effect of medroxyprogesterone acetate on the sleep induced peak of growth hormone. *J. Clin. Endocrinol. Metab.* 33: 851–853, 1971b.

Lucke, C., Hoeffken, B., and Morgner, K. D. L-DOPA induced growth hormone secretion. Comparison with insulin tolerance test, arginine infusion and sleep induced GH secretion. *Acta Endocrinologia* 77: 241–249, 1974.

Lugaresi, E., Coccagna, G., Mantovani, M., Cirignotta, F., Ambrosetto, G., and Baturic, P. Hypersomnia with periodic breathing. *J. Neurol. Neurosurg. Psychiatry* 36: 15–26, 1973.

Lukas, J. S. Awakening effects of simulated sonic booms and aircraft noise on men and women. *J. Sound and Vibration* 20: 457–466, 1972.

Lundquist, G. Delirium tremens: A comparative study of pathogenesis, course and prognosis with delirium tremens. *Acta Psychiatr. Scand.* 36: 443–466, 1961.

Lynch, H. J., Wurtman, R. J., Moskowitz, M. A., Archer, M. C., and Ho, M. H. Daily rhythm in human urinary melanin. *Science* 187: 169–171, 1975.

Maas, J. W., and Mednieks, M. Hydrocortisone-mediated increase of norepinephrine uptake by brain slices. *Science* 171: 178–179, 1971.

Mace, J. W., Gotlin, R. W., and Beck, P. Sleep related human growth hormone (GH) release: A test of physiologic growth hormone secretion in children. *J. Clin. Endocrinol. Metab.* 34: 339–341, 1972.

MacIndoe, J. H., and Turkington, R. W. Stimulation of human prolactin secretion by intravenous infusion of L-tryptophan. *J. Clin. Invest.* 52: 1972–1978, 1973.

MacLulich, P. A case of "Circular Insanity" in which the duration of each phase exists for only one day. *J. Ment. Sci.* 45: 554, 1899.

MacWilliam, J. A. Some applications of physiology to medicine III. Blood pressure and heart action in sleep and dreams. *Br. Med. J.* II: 1196–1200, 1923.

Maggini, C., Andreoli, V., and Guazzelli, M. Polygraphic study of sleep in manic and hypomanic patients treated with lithium carbonate. *Rev. Neurol.* 45: 209–1975.

Makipour, H., Iber, F. L., and Hartmann, E. Effects of L-tryptophan on sleep in hospitalized insomniac patients. Paper presented at Annual Meeting of the Assoc. for Psychophysiological Study of Sleep, Lake Minnewaska, New Mexico, 1972.

Malmo, R. B., and Bilanger, D. Related physiological and behavioral changes: What are their determinants?, in *Sleep and Altered States of Consciousness*, Kety, S. S., Evarts, E. V., and Williams, H. C. (eds.), *Research Publication of Assoc. Res. Nerv. Ment. Dis.* 45: 288–313, 1967.

Mandell, A. J., Chaffey, B., Brill, P., Mandell, M. P., Rodnick, J., Rubin, R. T., and Sheff, R. Dreaming sleep in man: Changes in urine volume and osmolality. *Science* 151: 1158–1560, 1966.

Mandell, A. J., and Mandell, M. P. Peripheral hormonal and metabolic correlates of rapid eye movement sleep. *Exp. Med. Surg.* 27: 224–236, 1969.

Mandell, M. P., Mandell, A. J., and Jacobson, A. Biochemical and neurophysiological studies of paradoxical sleep, in *Recent Advances in Biological Psychiatry*, vol. 7, Wortis, J. (ed.), Plenum Press, New York, 1964, pp. 115–122.

Marantz, R., and Rechtshaffen, A. Effect of alpha-methyltyrosine on sleep in the rat. *Percept. Mot. Skills 25:* 805–808, 1967.

Marantz, R., Rechtshaffen, A., Lovell, R. A., and Whitehead, P. K. Effect of alpha-methyltyrosine on the recovery from paradoxical sleep deprivation in the rat. *Commun. Behav. Biol. A2:* 161–164, 1968.

Marczynski, T. J., Yamaguchi, N., Ling, G. M., and Grodzinska, L. Sleep induced by the administration of melatonin (5-methoxy-N-acetyltryptamine) to the hypothalamus in unrestrained cats. *Experientia 20:* 435–437, 1964.

Matsumoto, J., Sogabe, J., and Hori-Santiago, Y. Sleep in parabiosis. *Experientia 15:* 1043–1044, 1972.

Matussek, N., Ackenhill, M., Athen, D., Bechmann, H., Benkert, O., Dittman, T., Hippius, H., Loosen, P., Rüther, E., and Scheller, M. Catecholamine metabolism under sleep deprivation therapy of improved and non-improved depressed patients. Contributions to biochemistry. *Pharmakopsychiatr. Neuropsychopharmakol. 7:* 108–114, 1974.

Maxwell, C., and Seldrup, J. Factors relating to the optimum effect of Imipramine in the treatment of enuresis. *Arzneimittelforschung 21:* 1352–1356, 1971.

McClure, D. J. The diurnal variation of plasma cortisol levels in depression. *J. Psychosom. Res. 10:* 189–195, 1966.

McDonald, D. G. Measures of sleep disturbance in psychiatric patients. *Br. J. Med. Psychol. 48:* 49–53, 1975.

McDonald, R. K., Sollberger, A. R., Mueller, P. S., and Sheard, M. H. The effect of small doses of human ACTH on serum corticosteroid levels in man. *Proc. Soc. Exp. Biol. Med. 131:* 1091–1094, 1969.

McGhie, A. The subjective assessment of sleep patterns in psychiatric illness. *Br. J. Med. Psychol. 39:* 221–230, 1966.

McGhie, A., and Russell, S. M. The subjective assessment of normal sleep patterns. *J. Ment. Sci. 108:* 642–654, 1962.

McGinty, D. J., Harper, R. M., and Fairbanks, M. K. 5-HT-containing neurons: Unit activity in behaving cats, in *Serotonin and Behavior*, Barchas, J., and Usdin, E. (eds.), Academic Press, New York, 1973, pp. 267–279.

Meddis, R., Pearson, A., and Langford, G. An extreme case of healthy insomnia. *Electroencephalogr. Clin. Neurophysiol. 35:* 213–214, 1973.

Medina, M. A., Grachetti, A., and Shore, P. A. On the physiological disposition and possible mechanism of the antihypertensive action of debrisoquine. *Biochem. Pharmacol. 18:* 891–901, 1969.

Meites, J. Control of PRL secretion in animals, in *Human Prolactin: Proceedings of the International Symposium on Human Prolactin*, Brussels, June 12–14, 1973, Pasteels, J. L.; and Robyn, C (eds.), American Elsevier, New York, 1973, pp. 105–118.

Meites, J., and Clemens, J. A. Hypothalamic control of prolactin secretion. *Vitam. and Horm. 30:* 165–221, 1972.

Meites, J., Lu, K. H., Wuttke, W., Welsch, C. W., Nagasawa, H., and Quadri, S. K. Recent studies on function and control of prolactin secretion in rats. *Recent Prog. Horm. Res. 28:* 471–526, 1972.

Mello, N. K., and Mendelson, J. H. Behavioral studies of sleep patterns in alcoholics during intoxication and withdrawal. *J. Pharmacol. Exp. Ther. 175:* 94–112, 1970.

Meltzer, H. Y., Kupfer, D. J., Wyatt, R. J., and Snyder, F. Sleep disturbance and serum CPK activity in acute psychosis. *Arch. Gen. Psychiatry 22:* 398–405, 1970.

Mendels, J., and Hawkins, D. R. Sleep and depression: A controlled EEG study. *Arch. Gen. Psychiatry* 15: 744–754, 1967a.

Mendels, J., and Hawkins, D. R. Sleep and depression: A follow-up study. *Arch. Gen. Psychiatry* 16: 536–542, 1967b.

Mendels, J., and Hawkins, D. R. Sleep and depression: Further considerations. *Arch. Gen. Psychiatry* 19: 445–452, 1968.

Mendels, J., and Hawkins, D. R. Sleep and depression. IV longitudinal studies. *J. Nerv. Ment. Dis.* 153: 251–272, 1971a.

Mendels, J., and Hawkins, D. R. Longitudinal sleep studies in hypomania. *Arch. Gen. Psychiatry* 25: 274–277, 1971b.

Mendels, J., and Chernik, D. A. The effect of L-tryptophan on sleep in man. *Sleep Res.* 1: 66, 1972.

Mendels, J., and Chernik, D. A. The effect of lithium carbonate on the sleep of depressed patients. *Int. Pharmacopsychiatry* 8: 184–192, 1973.

Mendelson, W. B. Review of: Schoenenberger, G. A., Cueni, L. B., Monnier, M., and Hatt, A. M. Humoral transmission of sleep. VII. Isolation and physical–chemical characterization of the "sleep-inducing factor delta." *Sleep Res.* 3: 256, 1974.

Mendelson, W. B., Reichman, J., and Othmer, E. Serotonin inhibition and sleep. *Biol. Psychiatry* 10: 459–464, 1975a.

Mendelson, W. B., Jacobs, L. S., Reichman, J. D., Othmer, E., Cryer, P. E., Trivedi, B., and Daughaday, W. H. Methysergide: Suppression of sleep-related prolactin secretion and enhancement of sleep-related growth hormone secretion. *J. Clin. Invest.* 56: 690–697, 1975b.

Mendelson, W. B., and Hill, S. Y. A dose-response study of the acute effects of ethanol on the sleep of rats. *Sleep Res.* 5, 1976.

Mendelson, W. B., Jacobs, L. S., Sitaram, N., Wyatt, R. J., and Gillin, J. C. Methscopolamine: Suppression of sleep-related growth hormone secretion and dissociation from slow wave sleep. *Sleep Res.* 5, 1976.

Merritt, J. H., and Geller, I. Soporific action of ethanol in mice: Possible role of biogenic amines. *Pharmacol. Biochem. Behav.* 1: 271–276, 1973.

Meyer, J. A., and Kurland, K. Z. Controlled evaluation of flurazepam hydrochloride, a new nonbarbiturate hypnotic. *Milit. Med.* 138: 471–474, 1973.

Michaelis, R., and Hofmann, E. Zur Phänomenologie und Atiopathogenese der Hypersomnie bei endogen-phasischen Depressionen, in *The Nature of Sleep*, Jovanovic, U. J. (ed.), Gustar Fischer Verlag, Stuttgart, 1973, pp. 190–193.

Mirsky, I. A., Piken, P., Rosenbaum, M., and Lederer, H. Adaptation of central nervous system. *Q. J. Stud. Alcohol* 2: 35–45, 1941.

Moir, A. T. B., and Eccleston, D. J. The effects of precursor loading in the cerebral metabolism of 5-hydroxyindoles. *J. Neurochem.* 15: 1093–1108, 1968.

Monnier, M., and Schoenenberger, G. A. Some physical–chemical properties of the rabbit's "sleep hemodialysote." *Experientia* 28: 32–33, 1972.

Monnier, M., Hatt, A. M., Cueni, L. B., and Schoenenberger, G. A. Humoral transmission of sleep VI. *Pflugers Arch.* 331: 257–265, 1974.

Monnier, M., Schoenenberger, G. A., Glatt, A., Dudler, L., Mehlose, W., Gachter, R., and Knappova, L. Distribution of the physiological sleep factor delta in blood and cerebrospinal fluid. Presented at the Second International Sleep Research Congress, Edinburgh, June 30–July 4, 1975.

Monroe, L. J. Psychological and physiological differences between good and poor sleepers. *J. Abnorm. Psychol.* 72: 255–264, 1967.

Monroe, L. J. Transient changes in EEG sleep patterns of married good sleepers: The effects of altering sleeping arrangement. *Psychophysiology* 6: 330–337, 1969.

Morden, B., Conner, R., Mitchell, G., Dement, W., and Levine, S. Effects of rapid eye movement (REM) sleep deprivation on shock-induced fighting. *Physiol. Behav. 3:* 425–432, 1968.

Morgan, H. E. Introduction to endocrine control systems, in *Best and Taylor's Physiological Basis of Medical Practice, Ninth Edition*, Brobeck, J. R. (ed.), Williams and Wilkins, Baltimore, 1973, p. 72.

Morgane, P. J., and Stern, W. C. Relationship of sleep to neuroanatomical circuits, biochemistry and behavior. *Ann. N.Y. Acad. Sci. 193:* 95–111, 1972.

Morgane, P. J., and Stern, W. C. Chemical anatomy of brain circuits in relation to sleep and wakefulness, in *Advances in Sleep Research, Vol. 1,* Weitzman, E. D. (ed.), Spectrum Publications, New York, 1974, pp. 1–131.

Morris, G., and Singer, M. T. Sleep deprivation: Transactional and subjective observations. *Arch. Gen. Psychiatry 5:* 453–465, 1961.

Moruzzi, G. The sleep-waking cycle. *Ergeb. Physiol. 64:* 1–165, 1972.

Moruzzi, G., and Magoun, H. W. Brain stem reticular formation and activation of the EEG. *Electroencephalogr. Clin. Neurophysiol. 1:* 455–473, 1949.

Mouret, J., Bobillier, P., and Jouvet, M. Insomnia following parachlorophenylalanine in the rat. *Eur. J. Pharmacol. 5:* 17–22, 1968.

Mueller, E. E. Nervous control of growth hormone secretion. *Neuroendocrinology 11:* 338–369, 1973.

Mueller, E. E., Pecile, A., Felici, M., and Cocchi, D. Norepinephrine and dopamine injection into lateral brain ventricle of the rat and growth hormone-releasing activity in the hypothalamus and plasma. *Endocrinology 86:* 1376–1382, 1970.

Mueller, P. S., Heninger, G. R., McDonald, R. K. Insulin tolerance test in depression. *Arch. Gen. Psychiatry 21:* 587–594, 1969.

Muratorio, A., and Maggini, C. Caratteristiche struttuveli del sonno dei depressi. *Riv. Neurol. 39:* 101–107, 1967.

Muratorio, A., Maggini, C., and Murri, L. Il sonno notturno delle sindromi depressive, studio poligrafico di 35 casi. *Neopsichiatria 33:* 397, 1967.

Muratorio, A., Maggini, C., and Marcacci, G. Evoluzione del sonno nelle sindromi depressive in corso di trattamento. *Ress. Studi. Psychiatrici. 57:* 351–359, 1968a.

Muratorio, A., Maggini, C., and Murri, L. Effects of P-3693A (Pfizer) on the all night sleep records in depressed patients. *Excerpta Medica International Congress Series* No. 180: 232–233, 1968b.

Muratorio, A., Maggini, C., and Pappagallo, S. Il sonno notturno nelle sindromi maniacali. *Neopsichiatria. 34:* 16–30, 1968c.

Murphree, H. B., and Price, L. M. Electroencephalographic changes in man following smoking. *Ann. N.Y. Acad. Sci. 142:* 245–260, 1967.

Murphree, H. B. Electroencephalographic and other evidence for mixed depressant and stimulant actions of alcoholic beverages. *Ann. N.Y. Acad. Sci. 215:* 325–331, 1973.

Murri, L., Feriozzi, F., Cerone, G., and Piacentino, P. Triptofano e sonno in schizofrenici cronici. *Rev. di Neurobiologia 17:* 184–189, 1971.

Murri, L., Cerone, G., Piacentino, P., and Pirro, R. 5-Idrossitriptofane e sonno in schizofrenici cronici. *Rev. di Neurobiologia 17:* 427–432, 1972.

Murri, L., Cerone, G., Feriozzi, F., Mencini, G. M., and Nurzia, A. Effetto del triptofano sull'Ormone somatotropo durante il sonno in schizofrenici. *Boll. Soc. It. Biol. Sper. 49:* 1490–1495, 1973.

Muzio, J. N., Roffwarg, H. P., and Kaufman, E. Alterations in the nocturnal sleep cycle resulting from LSD. *Electroencephalogr. Clin. Neurophysiol. 21:* 313–324, 1966.

Naftolin, F., Yes, S. S. C., Perlman, D., Tsai, C. C., Parker, D. C., and Vargo, T. Nocturnal patterns of serum gonadotropins during the menstrual cycle. *J. Clin. Endocrinol. Metab.* 37: 6–10, 1973.

Naiman, J., Poitras, R., and Engelsmann, F. Effect of chlorpromazine on REM rebound in normal volunteers. *Can. Psychiatr. Assoc. J.* 17: 463–469, 1972.

Naitoh, P., Kales, A., Dollar, E. J., Smith, J. C., and Jacobson, A. Electroencephalographic activity after prolonged sleep loss. *Electroencephalogr. Clin. Neurophysiol.* 27: 2–11, 1969.

Nakazawa, Y., Tachibana, H., Kotorii, M., Ogata, M. Effects of L-DOPA on natural night sleep and on rebound of REM sleep. *Folia. Psychiatr. Neurol. Jpn.* 27: 223–230, 1973.

Nakazawa, Y., Kotorii, M., Kotorii, T., Tachibana, H., and Nakano, T. Individual differences in compensatory rebound of REM sleep with particular reference to their relationship to personality and behavioral characteristics. *J. Nerv. Ment. Dis.* 161: 18–25, 1975a.

Nakazawa, Y., Kotorii, T., Kotorii, M., Horikawa, S., and Onshima, M. Effects of amitriptyline on human REM sleep as evaluated by using partial differential REM sleep deprivation (PDRD). *Electroencephalogr. Clin. Neurophysiol.* 38: 513–520, 1975b.

Naylor, G. J., and Le Poidevin, D. Sleep patterns in depressive states. *Br. J. Med. Psychol.* 45: 171–176, 1972.

Neff, N. H., and Yang, H. Y. T. Another look at the monoamine oxidase and the monoamine oxidase inhibitor drugs. *Life Sci.* 14: 2061–2074, 1974.

Nevsimalova-Bruhova, S. On the problem of heredity in hypersomnia, narcolepsy, and dissociated sleep disturbances. *Acta Universitatis Carol. Med.* 18: 109–160, 1973.

Nicholson, A. N. Sleep patterns of an airline pilot operating world-wide east-west routes. *Aerosp. Med.* 41: 626–632, 1970.

Nicoloff, J. T. A new method for the measurement of thyroidal iodine release in man. *J. Clin. Invest.* 47: 1912–1921, 1970.

Nicoloff, J. T., Fisher, D. A., and Appleman, M. D. The role of glucocorticoids in the regulation of thyroid function in man. *J. Clin. Invest.* 49: 1922–1929, 1970.

Nokin, J., Vekemans, M., L'Hermite, M., and Robyn, C. Circadian periodicity of serum prolactin concentration in man. *Br. Med. J.* 3: 561–572, 1972.

Nowlin, J. B., Troyer, W. G., Collins, W. S., Silverman, G., Nichols, C. R., McIntosh, H. D., Estes, E. H., Jr., and Bogdonoff, M. D. The association of nocturnal angina pectoris with dreaming. *Ann. Intern. Med.* 63: 1040–1046, 1965.

Oates, J. A., and Sjoerdsma, A. Neurologic effects of tryptophan in patients receiving a monoamine oxidase inhibitor. *Neurology* 10: 1076–1078, 1960.

O'Connor, J. F., Wu, G. Y., Gallagher, T. F., and Hellman, L. The 24-hour plasma thyroxin profile in normal man. *J. Clin. Endocrinol. Metab.* 39: 765–771, 1974.

Ogunremi, O. O., Adamson, L., Brezinova, V., Hunter, W. M., Maclean, A. W., Oswald, I., and Percy-Robb, I. W. Two anti-anxiety drugs: A psychoendocrine study. *Br. Med. J.* 12: 202–205, 1973.

Okuma, T., Hata, N., and Fujii, S. Differential effects of chlorpromazine, imipramine and amobarbital on REM sleep and REM density in man. *Folia Psychiatr. et Neur. Jpn.* 29: 25–37, 1975.

Olden, C. Neurotic disturbances of sleep. *Int. J. Psychoanal.* 23: 52–56, 1942.

Onheiber, P., White, P. T., DeMeyer, M. K., and Ottinger, D. R. Sleep and dream patterns of child schizophrenics. *Arch. Gen. Psychiatry* 12: 568–571, 1965.

Ornitz, E. M., Ritvo, E. R., and Walter, R. D. Dreaming sleep in autistic and schizophrenic children. *Am. J. Psychiatry* 122: 419–424, 1965a.

Ornitz, E., Ritvo, E., and Walter, R. Dreaming sleep in autistic twins. *Arch. Gen. Psychiatry* 12: 77–79, 1965b.

Ornitz, E., Forsythe, A., de la Pena, A. Effect of vestibular and auditory stimulation on the REMs of REM sleep in autistic children. *Arch. Gen. Psychiatry* 29: 786–791, 1973.

Ornstein, P. H., Whitman, R. M., Kramer, H., and Baldridge, B. J. Drugs and dreams. IV. Tranquilizers and their effects upon dreams and dreaming in schizophrenic patients. *Exp. Med. Surg.* 27: 145–156, 1969.

Orth, D. N., Island, D. P., and Liddle, G. W. Experimental alterations of the circadian rhythm in plasma cortisol (17-OHCS) concentration in man. *J. Clin. Endocrinol. Metab.* 27: 549–555, 1967.

Oswald, I. Sleep mechanisms: Recent advances. *Proc. R. Soc. Med.* 55: 910–912, 1962.

Oswald, Ian. Insomnia: The abnormalities of sleep in man. *Proc. of the XVth European Meeting on Electroencephalography*, Bologna, 1967, Gastant, H., Gastaut, H., Lugaria, L., Berti, G., and Coccagna, G. (eds.), 1968, pp. 99–107.

Oswald, I. Sleep and dependence on amphetamine and other drugs, in *Sleep: Physiology and Pathology*, Kales, A. (ed.), J. B. Lippincott, London, 1969a, pp. 317–330.

Oswald, I. Human brain protein, drugs and dreams. *Nature* 223: 893–897, 1969b.

Oswald, I. Sleep, the great restorer. *New Scientist* 46: 170–172, 1970.

Oswald, I., Berger, R. J., Jaramillo, B. A., Keddie, K. M. G., Olley, P. C., and Plunkett, G. B. Melancholia and barbiturates: A controlled EEG, body and eye movement study of sleep. *Br. J. Psychiatry* 109: 66–78, 1963.

Oswald, I., and Thacore, V. R. Amphetamine and phenmetrazine addiction. *Br. Med. J.* 2: 427–431, 1963.

Oswald, I., Berger, R. J., Evans, J. I., and Thacore, V. R. Effects of L-tryptophan upon human sleep. *Electroencephalogr. Clin. Neurophysiol.* 17: 603, 1964.

Oswald, I., and Priest, R. G. Five weeks to escape the sleeping pill habit. *Br. Med. J.* 2: 1093–1095, 1965.

Oswald, I., Ashcroft, G. W., Berger, R. J., Eccleston, D., Evans, J. I., and Thacore, V. R. Some experiments in the chemistry of normal sleep. *Br. J. Psychiatry* 112: 391–399, 1966.

Oswald, I., Adam, K., Allen, S., Burack, R., Spence, M., Thacore, V. Alpha adrenergic blocker, thymoxamine and mesoridazine both increase human REM sleep duration. *Sleep Res.* 3: 62, 1974.

Othmer, E., Goodwin, D., Levine, W., Malarkey, W., Freemon, F., Halikas, J., and Daughaday, W. Sleep related growth hormone secretion in alcoholics. *Clin. Res.* 20: 726, 1972.

Othmer, E., Levine, W. R., Malarkey, W. B., Corvalan, J. C., Hayden-Otto, M. P., Fishman, P. M., and Daughaday, W. H. Body build and sleep-related growth hormone secretion. *Horm. Res.* 5: 156–166, 1974a.

Othmer, E., Mendelson, W. B., Levine, W. R., Malarkey, W. B., and Daughaday, W. H. Sleep-related growth hormone secretion and morning naps. *Steroids Lipids Res.* 5: 380–386, 1974b.

Owen, M., and Bliss, E. L. Sleep loss and cortical excitability. *Am. J. Physiol.* 218: 171–173, 1970.

Palaic, D. J., Desaty, J., Albert, J. M., and Panisset, J. C. Effect of ethanol on metabolism and subcellular distribution of serotonin in the rat brain. *Brain Res.* 25: 381–386, 1971.

Panaccio, L., and Tetreault, L. Comparative study of the hypnotic effects of flurazepam (30 mg), secobarbital (100 mg) and placebo on four different groups of psychotic insomniacs. *Union Med. Can.* 101: 2420–2425, 1972.

Pappenheimer, J. R., Miller, T. B., Goodrich, C. A. Sleep-promoting effects of cerebrospinal fluid from sleep deprived goats. *Proc. Nat. Acad. Sci. USA* 58: 513–517, 1967.

Parker, D. C., Rossman, L. G., and Vanderlaan, E. F. Relation of sleep-entrained human prolactin release to REM-nonREM cycles. *J. Clin. Endocrinol. Metab. 38:* 646–651, 1974.

Parkes, J. D., and Fenton, G. W. Levo (−) amphetamine and dextro (+) amphetamine in the treatment of narcolepsy. *J. Neurol. Neurosurg. Psychiatry 36:* 1076–1081, 1973.

Parmegianni, P. L. A study on the central representation of sleep behavior, in *Progress in Brain Research, Topics in Basic Neurology,* Barsmann, W.; and Schade, J. L. (eds.), Elsevier, Amsterdam, 1964, pp. 180–190.

Pasnau, R. O., Naitoh, P., Stier, S., and Kollar, E. J. The psychological effects of 205 hours of sleep deprivation. *Arch. Gen. Psychiatry 18:* 496–505, 1968.

Passouant, P., Cadilhac, J., and Ribstein, M. Sleep privation with eye movements using antidepressant drugs. *Rev. Neurol. 127:* 173–192, 1972.

Passouant, P., Cadilhac, J., and Billiard, M. Withdrawal of the paradoxical sleep by the chlomipramine, electrophysiological, histochemical, and biochemical study. *Int. J. Neurol. 10:* 186–197, 1975.

Passouant, P., Popoviciu, L., Velok, G., and Baldy-Moulinier, M. Etude polygraphique des narcolepsies au cours du nychémère. *Rev. Neurol. 118:* 431–441, 1968.

Patel, Y. C., Alford, F. P., and Burger, H. G. The 24-hour plasma thryotrophin profile. *Clin. Sci. 43:* 71–77, 1972.

Patel, Y. C., Baker, H. W.G., Burger, H. G., Johns, M. W., and Ledinek, J. E. Suppression of the thyrotrophin circadian rhythm by glucocorticoids. *J. Endocrinol. 62:* 421–422, 1974.

Pattison, J. H., and Allen, R. P. Comparison of the hypnotic effectiveness of secobarbital, pentobarbital, methyprylon and ethchlorvynol. *J. Am. Geriat. Soc. 20:* 398–402, 1972.

Pawel, M. A., Sassin, J. F., and Weitzman, E. D. The temporal relation between HGH release and sleep stage changes at nocturnal sleep onset in man. *Life Sci. 11:* 587–593, 1972.

Payne, R. W., Sorenson, E., Smalley, T., and Brandt, E. Diazepam, meprobamate and placebo in musculoskeletal disorders. *JAMA 188:* 229–232, 1964.

Pegram, V., Robinson, C., Donaldson, P., Beaton, J., and Smythies, J. The effects of chronic use of nicotinamide (three grams/day) on human sleep. Presented at the Second International Sleep Research Congress, Edinburgh, June 30–July 4, 1975.

Pelham, R. W., Vaughn, G. M., Sandock, K. L., and Vaughn, M. H. Twenty-four-hour cycle of a melanin-like substance in the plasma of human males. *J. Clin. Endocrinol. Metab. 37:* 341–344, 1973.

Penati, G., Gianelli, A., Pietropolli-Charmet, G., Bertolini, M. Some considerations about the EEG sleep patterns in schizophrenic psychosis, in *Psicofisciologia del sonno e del sogno,* Bertini, M. (ed.), Editorice Vita e Pensiero, 1970, pp. 213–219.

Perez-Cruit, J., Chase, T. N., and Murphy, D. L. Dietary regulation of brain tryptophan metabolism by plasma ratio of free tryptophan and neutral amino acids in humans. *Nature 248:* 693–695, 1974.

Perlow, M., McGregor, P., Fukushima, D., Hellman, L., and Weitzman, E. Seventy-two-hour polygraphic recording and 24-hour plasma cortisol measurement in the differential diagnosis of sleep disorders. Presented at the 11th annual meeting of the Assn. for the Psychophysiological Study of Sleep, 1971.

Perlow, M., Sassin, J. F., Boyar, R., Hellman, L., MacGregor, P., and Weitzman, E. D. Reduction of twenty-four hour growth growth hormone secretion after clomiphene treatment. *Sleep Res. 1:* 188, 1972.

Pessah, M. A., and Roffwarg, H. P. Spontaneous middle ear muscle activity in man: A rapid eye movement sleep phenomenon. *Science 178:* 773–776, 1972.

Petre-Quadrens, O., and DeGref, A. Effects of 5HTP on sleep in Mongol children. *J. Neurol. Sci. 13:* 115–119, 1971.

Pflug, B. Über den Schlafentzug in der ambulanten endogenen Depression. *Nervenarzt 43:* 614–622, 1972.

Pflug, B. Therapeutic aspects of sleep deprivation, in *Sleep: Physiology, Biochemistry, Psychology, Pharmacology, Clinical Implications,* Koella, W. P., and Levin, P. (ed.). S. Karger, 1973, pp. 185–191.

Pflug, B., and Tölle, R. Therapy of endogenous depression by sleep deprivation: Practical and theoretical consequences. *Nervenarzt 42:* 117–124, 1971a.

Pflug, B., and Tölle, R. Disturbance of the 24-hour rhythm in endogenous depression and the treatment of endogenous depression by sleep deprivation. *Int. Pharmacopsychiatry 6:* 187–196, 1971b.

Phillips, R. L., Mitler, M., and Dement, W. C. Alpha sleep in chronic insomniacs, in *Sleep Research,* Chase, M. H., Stern, W. C., and Walter, P. L. (eds.), Brain Information Service, UCLA, Los Angeles, 1974, p. 143.

Piro, C., Fraioli, F., Sciarra, F., and Conti, C. Circadian rhythm of plasma testosterone, cortisol and gonadotropins in normal male subjects. *J. Steroid Biochem. 4:* 321–329, 1973.

Platman, S. R., and Fieve, R. R. Sleep in depression and mania. *Br. J. Psychiatry 116:* 219–220, 1970.

Poland, R. E., Rubin, R. T., Clank, R. B., and Gouin, P. R. Circadian patterns of urine 17-OHC and VMA excretion during sleep deprivation. *Dis. Nerv. Syst. 33:* 456–458, 1972.

Polzella, D. J. Effects of sleep deprivation on short-term recognition memory. *J. Exp. Psychol. 104:* 194–200, 1975.

Post, R. M., Gillin, J. C., Goodwin, F. K., Wyatt, R. J., and Snyder, F. The effect of orally administered cocaine on sleep of depressed patients. *Sleep Res. 1:* 72, 1972.

Post, R. M., Gillin, J. C., Wyatt, R. J., and Goodwin, F. K. The effect of orally administered cocaine on sleep of depressed patients. *Psychopharmacologia 37:* 59–66, 1974a.

Post, R. M., Kotin, J., and Goodwin, F. K. The effects of cocaine on depressed patients. *Am. J. Psychiatry 131:* 511–517, 1974b.

Post, R. M., Kotin, J., and Goodwin, F. K. Effects of sleep deprivation on mood and central amine metabolism in depressed patients. *Arch. Gen. Psychiatry 33:* 627–632, 1976.

Prange, A. J., Wilson, I. C., Lara, P. P., Alltop, L. B., and Breese, G. R. Effect of thyrotropin releasing hormone in depression. *Lancet 2:* 999–1002, 1972.

Prange, A. J., Breese, G. R., Cott, J. M., Martin, B. R., Cooper, B. R., Wilson, I. C., and Plotnikoff, N. P. Thyrotropin releasing hormone: Antagonism of pentobarbital in rodents. *Life Sci. 14:* 447–455, 1974.

Prinzmetal, M., and Bloomberg, W. The use of benzedrine for the treatment of narcolepsy. *JAMA 105:* 2051–2054, 1935.

Pscheidt, G. R. Monoamine oxidase inhibitors. *Int. Rev. Neurobiol. 7:* 191–229, 1964.

Pscheidt, G. R., Issekuty, B., and Himwich, H. E. Failure of ethanol to lower brain stem concentration of biogenic amines. *Q. J. Stud. Alcohol 22:* 550–553, 1961.

Pujol, J. F., Mouret, J., Jouvet, M., and Glowinsky, J. Increased turnover of cerebral norepinephrine during rebound from paradoxical sleep in the rat. *Science 159:* 112–114, 1968.

Pujol, J. F., Buguet, A., Froment, J. L., Jones, B., and Jouvet, M. The central metabolism of serotonin in the cat during insomnia: A neurophysiological and biochemical study after p-chlorophenyl-alanine or destruction of the raphe system. *Brain Res. 29:* 195–212, 1971.

Quabbe, H. J., Schilling, E., and Helge, H. Pattern of growth hormone secretion during a 24-hour fast in normal adults. *J. Clin. Endocrinol. Metab. 26:* 1173–1177, 1966.

Radulovacki, M. Comparison of effects of paradoxical sleep deprivation and immobilization stress on 5-hydroxyindoleacetic acid in cerebrospinal fluid. *Brain Res. 60:* 255–258, 1973.

Randall, C. L., and Lester, D. Differential effects of ethanol and pentobarbital on sleep time in C57BL and BALB mice. *J. Pharmacol. Exp. Ther. 188:* 27–33, 1974.

Ravenscroft, K., Jr., and Hartmann, E. L. The temporal correlation of nocturnal asthmatic attacks and the D-state. *Psychophysiology 4:* 396–397, 1968.

Rechtschaffen, A. Polygraphic aspects of insomnia: The abnormalities of sleep in man. *Proc. of the XVth European Meeting on Electroencephalography,* Gestaut, H., Lugaresi, L., Berti, G., and Coccagna, G. (eds.), Bologna, 1968.

Rechtschaffen, A., Wolpert, E. A., Dement, W. C., Mitchell, S. A., and Fisher, C. Nocturnal sleep of narcoleptics. *Electroencephalogr, Clin. Neurophysiol. 15:* 599–609, 1963.

Rechtschaffen, A., and Maron, L. The effect of amphetamine on the sleep cycle. *Electroencephalogr. Clin. Neurophysiol. 16:* 438–445, 1964.

Rechtschaffen, A., Schulsinger, F., and Mednick, S. A. Schizophrenia and physiological indices of dreaming. *Arch. Gen. Psychiatry 10:* 89–93, 1964.

Rechtschaffen, A., and Kales, A. A manual of standardized terminology, techniques and scoring system for sleep stages of human subjects. Brain Information Service/Brain Research Institute, Los Angeles, 1968.

Rechtschaffen, A., Lovell, R. A., Freedman, D. W., Whitehead, P. K., and Aldrich, M. Effect of p-chlorophenylalanine on sleep in rats. *Psychophysiology 6:* 223, 1969.

Rechtschaffen, A., and Monroe, L. J. Laboratory studies of insomnia, in *Sleep: Physiology and Pathology,* Kales, A. (ed.), Lippincott Co., Philadelphia and Toronto, 1969, pp. 158–169.

Rechtschaffen, A., Molinari, S., Watson, R., and Wincor, M. Extraocular potentials: A possible indicator of PGO activity in the human. Presented at Association for the Psychophysiological Study of Sleep, Sante Fe, New Mexico, 1970.

Reich, L. H., Kupfer, D. J., Weiss, B. L., McPartland, R. J., Foster, F. G., Detre, T., and Delgado, J. Psychomotor activity as a predictor of sleep efficiency. *Biol. Psychiatry 8:* 253–256, 1974.

Reich, L., Weiss, B. L., Coble, P., McPartland, R., and Kupfer, D. J. Sleep disturbance in schizophrenia: A revisit. *Arch. Gen. Psychiatry 32:* 51–55, 1975.

Reichlin, S. Neuroendocrinology, in *Textbook of Endocrinology, 5th edition,* Williams, R. H. (ed.), Saunders, Philadelphia, 1974, pp. 774–831.

Reinhard, V., Kindel, K., Burmeister, P. L., Boehme, W., and Cramer, H. Melatonin: Influence on afternoon sleep pattern and plasma levels of HGH and cyclic AMP in healthy volunteers. *Proc. 2nd Europ. Cong. Sleep Res.,* Rome, 1974.

Reivich, M., Isaacs, G., Evarts, E., and Kety, S. The effect of slow wave sleep and REM sleep on regional cerebral blood flow in cats. *J. Neurochem. 15:* 301–306, 1968.

Renaud, B., Buda, M., Lewis, B. D., and Pujol, J. F. Effects of 5,6-dehydroxytryptamine on tyrosine-hydroxylase activity in central catecholaminergic neurons of the rat. *Biochem. Pharmacol. 24:* 1739–1742, 1975.

Richter, C. P. Two day cycles of alternating good and bad behavior in psychotic patients. *Arch. Neurol. Psychiatry 39:* 587–598, 1938.

Ritvo, E. R., Ornitz, E. M., LaFranchi, S. C., and Walter, R. D. Effects of imipramine on the sleep dream cycle: An EEG study in boys. *Electroencephalogr. Clin. Neurophysiol. 22:* 465–468, 1967.

Rodden, A., Sinhas, A. K., Dement, W. G., Berchas, J. D., Zarcone, V. P., Macleury, M. R., and DeGrazia, J. A. $^{14}CO_2$ elimination from ^{14}C tyrosine in human sleep and wakefulness. *Brain Res. 59:* 427–431, 1973.

Roffwarg, H. P., Muzio, J. M., and Dement, W. C. Ontogenetic development of the human sleep-dream cycle. *Science 152:* 604–619, 1966.

Roffwarg, H. P., Sachar, E. D., Halpern, F., and Hellman, L. Plasma testosterone and sleep: Relationship to sleep stage variables. *Sleep Res. 3:* 172, 1974.

Ronnekiev, O., Krulich, L., and McCann, S. M. An early morning surge of prolactin in the male rat and its abolition by pinealectomy. *Endocrinology 92:* 1339–1342, 1973.

Rose, R. M., Kreuz, L. E., Holaday, J. W., Sulak, K. J., and Johnson, C. E. Diurnal variation of plasma testosterone and cortisol. *J. Endocrinol. 54:* 177–178, 1972.

Rosenfeld, G. Inhibitory influence of ethanol on serotonin metabolism. *Proc. Soc. Exp. Biol. Med. 103:* 144–149, 1960.

Roth, B., Bruhova, S., and Lehovsky, M. REM sleep and NREM sleep in narcolepsy and hypersomnia. *Electroencephalogr. Clin. Neurophysiol. 26:* 176–182, 1969.

Roth, B., Nevsimalova, S., and Rechtschaffen, A. Hypersomnia with "sleep drunkenness." *Arch. Gen. Psychiatry 26:* 456–462, 1972.

Roth, B., and Nevsimalova, S. Depression in narcolepsy and hypersomnia. Schweitz, *Arch. Neurol. Neurochir. Psychiatr. 116:* 291–300, 1975.

Roth, J., Glick, S. M., Yalow, R. S., and Berson, S. A. Hypoglycemia: Potent stimulus to secretion of growth hormone. *Science 140:* 987–988, 1963.

Roth, N. Problems in narcolepsy. *Bull. Menninger Clin. 10:* 160–170, 1946.

Roth, T., Kramer, M., Leston, W., and Lutz, T. The effects of sleep deprivation on mood. *Sleep Res. 3:* 154, 1974.

Rothenberg, S. Psychoanalytic insight into insomnia. *Psychoanal. Rev. 34:* 141–168, 1947.

Rubin, R. T. Sleep-endocrinology studies in man. *Prog. Brain Res. 42:* 73–80, 1975.

Rubin, R. T., Kales, A., and Clark, B. R. Decreased 17-hydroxycorticosteroid and VMA excretion during sleep following glutethimide administration in man. *Life Sci. 8:* 959–964, 1969.

Rubin, R. T., Kales, A., Adler, R., Fagan, T., and Odell, W. Gonadotropin secretion during sleep in normal adult men. *Science 175:* 196–198, 1972.

Rubin, R. T., Gouin, P. R., Kales, A., and Odell, W. D. Luteinizing hormone, follicle stimulating hormone, and growth hormone secretion in normal adult men during sleep and dreaming. *Psychosom. Med. 35:* 309–321, 1973a.

Rubin, R. T., Gouin, P. R., Arenander, A. T., and Poland, R. E. Human growth hormone release during sleep following prolonged flurazepam administration. *Res. Commun. Chem. Path. Pharmacol. 6:* 331–334, 1973b.

Rubin, R. T., Poland, R. E., Rubin, L. E., and Gouin, P. R. The neuroendocrinology of human sleep. *Life Sci. 14:* 1041–1052, 1974.

Rubin, R. T., Gouin, P. R., Lubin, A., Poland, R. E., and Pirke, K. M. Nocturnal increase of plasma testosterone in men: Relation to gonadotropins and prolactin. *J. Clin. Endocrinol. Metab. 40:* 1027–2033, 1975a.

Rubin, R. T., Poland, R. E., Tower, B. B., and Gouin, P. R. Nocturnal secretion of water and electrolyte-regulating hormones in normal adult men. Presented at the Second International Sleep Research Congress, Edinburgh, June 20–July 4, 1975b.

Rundell, O. H., Lester, B. K., Griffiths, W. J., and Williams H. L. Alcohol and sleep in young adults. *Psychopharmacologia 26:* 201–218, 1972.

Sachar, E. J., Frantz, A. G., Altman, N., and Sassin, J. Growth hormone and prolactin in unipolar and bipolar depressed patients: Responses to hypoglycemia and L-DOPA. *Am. J. Psychiatry 130:* 1362–1367, 1973.

Sagales, T., Erill, S., Domino, E. F. Differential effects of scopolamine and chlorproma-zine on REM and NREM sleep in normal male subjects. *Clin. Pharmacol. Ther. 10:* 522–529, 1969.

Sagales, T., and Domino, E. F. Effects of stress and REM sleep deprivation on the patterns of avoidance learning and brain acetylcholine in the mouse. *Psychopharmacology 29:* 307–315, 1973.

Sagales, T., and Erill, S. Effects of central dopaminergic blockage with pimozide upon the EEG stages of sleep in man. *Psychopharmacologia 41:* 53–56, 1975.

Sampson, H. Deprivation of dreaming sleep by two methods: I. Compensatory REM time. *Arch. Gen. Psychiatry 13:* 79–86, 1965.

Sassin, J. F. Neurological findings following short-term sleep deprivation. *Arch. Neurol.* 22: 54–56, 1970.

Sassin, J. F., Parker, D. C., Mace, J. W., Gotlin, R. W., Johnson, L. C., and Rossman, L. G. Human growth hormone release: Relation to slow-wave sleep and sleep-waking cycles. *Science 165:* 513–515, 1969.

Sassin, J. F., Frantz, A. G., Weitzman, E. D., and Kapen, S. Human prolactin: 24-hour pattern with increased release during sleep. *Science 177:* 1205–1207, 1972a.

Sassin, J., Hellman, L., and Weitzman, E. A circadian pattern of growth hormone secretion in acromegalics. *Sleep Res. 1:* 189, 1972b.

Sassin, J. F., Frantz, A. G., Kapen, S., and Weitzman, E. D. The nocturnal rise of human prolactin is dependent on sleep. *J. Clin. Endocrinol. Metab.* 37: 436–440, 1973.

Sawyer, C. H. Some effects of hormones on sleep. *Exp. Med. Surg.* 27: 177–186, 1969.

Scharf, M., Allen, C., and Kales, A. Hypnotic drugs and their effectiveness: Sleep laboratory studies. Presented at Annual Meeting of Assn. for the Psychophysiological Study of Sleep, Santa Fe, New Mexico, 1970.

Scheiber, S. H. Ein Fall von 7 Jahre lang dauerndem circularem Irresein mit täglich alter-nierendem typus. *Arch. Psychiatry 34:* 225–239, 1901.

Schenck, J. M. Personality components in patients with sleep paralysis. *Psychiatr. Q. 43:* 343–348, 1969.

Schiavi, R. C., Davis, D. M., White, D., Edwards, A., Igel, G., and Fisher, C. Plasma testosterone during nocturnal sleep in normal men. *Steroids 24:* 191–202, 1974.

Schildkraut, J. J. The catecholamine hypothesis of affective disorders: A review of supporting evidence. *Am. J. Psychiatry 122:* 509–522, 1965.

Schildkraut, J. J., and Hartmann, E. Turnover and metabolism of norepinephrine in rat brain after 72 hours on a D-Deprivation Island. *Psychopharmacology 27:* 17–27, 1972.

Schildkraut, J. J., Keeler, B. A., Papousek, M., and Hartmann, E. MHPG excretion in depressive disorders: Relation to clinical subtypes and desynchronized sleep. *Science* 181: 762–764, 1973.

Schmidt, F. O. Macromolecular specificity and biological memory, in *Macromolecular Specificity and Biological Memory,* Schmidt, F. O. (ed.), M.I.T. Press, Cambridge, 1962, pp. 1–6.

Schmidt, H. S., and Knopp, W. Sleep in Parkinson's disease: The effect of L-DOPA. *Psychophysiology 9:* 88–89, 1972.

Schneider, E., Maxion, H., Ziegler, B., and Jacobi, P. Das Schlafverhalten von Parkinson-kranken und seine Beeinflussung durch L-DOPA. *J. Neurol. 207:* 95–108, 1974a.

Schneider, E., Ziegler, B., Maxion, H., and Badawa, M. Long and short-term effects of sulpiride on sleep-EEG of man. *Arzneim Forsch.* 24: 990–993, 1974b.

Schoenenberger, G. A., Gueni, L. B., Monnier, M., and Hatt, A. M. Humoral transmis-sion of sleep. VII. Isolation and physical-chemical characterization of the "sleep-inducing factor delta." *Pflugers Arch. 338:* 1–17, 1972.

Schulte, F. J., and Parmelee, A. H. Thyroid hormone and brain development. An analysis of polygraphic data of hypothyroid babies before and during treatment. *Electroencephalogr. Clin. Neurophysiol. 29:* 212, 1970.

Schulte, F. J., Karsen, J. H., Engelbart, S., Bell, E. F., Castell, R., and Lenard, H. G. Sleep patterns in hyperphenylalaminia: A lesson serotonin learned from phenylketonurea. *Pediatr. Res. 7:* 588–599, 1973.

Schultz, M. A., Schulte, F. J., Akiyama, Y., and Parmelee, A. H. Development of electroencephalographic sleep phenomena in hypothyroid infants. *Electroencephalogr. Clin. Neurophysiol. 25:* 351–358, 1968.

Schwartz, B. A., Guilbaud, G., and Fischgold, H. Etudes electroencephalographiques sur le sommeil de nuit. *Presse Med. 71:* 1474–1476, 1963.

Scollo-Lavizzari, G., Pralle, W., de la Cruz, N. Activation effects of sleep deprivation and sleep in seizure patients. *Eur. Neurol. 13:* 1–5, 1975.

Shaar, C. J., and Clemens, J. A. The role of catecholamines in the release of anterior pituitary prolactin *in vitro. Endocrinology 95:* 1202–1212, 1974.

Shapiro, W. R. Treatment of cataplexy with clomipramine. *Arch. Neurol. 32:* 653–656, 1975.

Shaywitz, B. A., Finkelstein, J., Hellman, L., and Weitzman, E. D. Growth hormone in newborn infants during sleep-wake periods. *Pediatrics 48:* 103–109, 1971.

Sheldon, W. H. *Varieties of Temperament,* Harper, New York, 1942.

Sherman, L., Kin, S., Benjamin, F., and Kolodny, H. D. Effects of chlorpromazine on serum growth-hormone concentration in man. *N. Eng. J. Med. 284:* 72–74, 1971.

Shirakura, K. Effects of isocarboxide on sleep. *Folia Psychiatr. Neurol. Jpn. 27:* 117–142, 1973.

Shute, C. C. D., and Lewis, P. R. The ascending cholinergic reticular system: Neocortical, olfactory and subcortical projections. *Brain 90:* 497–520, 1967.

Simmons, F. B., and Hill, M. W. Hypersomnia caused by upper airway obstruction. *Ann. Otol. 83:* 670–673, 1974.

Sitaram, N., Wyatt, R. J., Dawson, S., and Gillin, J. C. REM sleep induction by physostigmine infusion during sleep in normal volunteers. *Science 191:* 1281–1283, 1976.

Smith, J. W., Johnson, L. C., and Burdick, J. A. Sleep, psychological and clinical changes during alcohol withdrawal in NAD-treated alcoholics. *Q. J. Stud. Alcohol 32:* 982–994, 1971.

Smythe, G. A., and Lazarus, L. Growth hormone regulation by melatonin and serotonin. *Nature 244:* 230–231, 1973.

Smythe, G. A., and Lazarus, L. Suppression of human growth hormone secretion by melatonin and cyproheptadine. *J. Clin. Invest. 54:* 116–121, 1974.

Snyder, F. The new biology of dreaming. *Arch. Gen. Psychiatry 8:* 381–391, 1963.

Snyder, F. Autonomic nervous system manifestations during sleep and dreaming, in *Sleep and Altered States of Consciousness, Res. Publ. Assn. Res. Nerv. Ment. Dis. 45:* 469–487, Williams and Wilkins, Baltimore, 1967.

Snyder, F. Electroencephalographic studies of sleep in depression, in *Computers and Electronic Devices in Psychiatry,* Kline, N. S., and Lasha, E. (eds.), Grune and Stratton, Inc., New York, 1968, pp. 272–301.

Snyder, F. Disturbance of EEG sleep patterns in relation to acute psychosis, in *Schizophrenia: Current Concepts and Research,* Siva Sankar, D. V. (ed.), 1969a, pp. 751–724.

Snyder, F. Dynamic aspects of sleep disturbance in relation to mental illness. *Biol. Psychiatry 1:* 119–130, 1969b.

Snyder, F. NIH Studies of EEG sleep in affective illness, in *Recent Advances in the Psychobiology of the Depressive Illnesses,* Williams, T., Katz, M., and Shields, J. (eds.), DHEW, Washington, 1972a.

Snyder, F. Electroencephalographic studies of sleep in psychiatric disorders, in *The Sleeping Brain*, Chase, M. H. (ed.), Brain Information Service/Brain Research Institute, Los Angeles, 1972b, pp. 376–393.

Snyder, F., Hobson, J. A., Moneson, D. F., and Goldfrank, F. Changes in respiration, heart rate, and systolic blood pressure in human sleep. *J. Appl. Physiol.* 19: 417–422, 1964.

Snyder, S. H. Catecholamines and serotonin, in *Basic Neurochemistry*, Albers, R. W., Siegel, G. J., Katzman, R., and Agranoff, B. W. (eds.), Little, Brown and Co., Boston, 1972, pp. 89–104.

Snyder, S. H. The dopamine hypothesis of schizophrenia: Focus on the dopamine receptor. *Am. J. Psychiatry 133:* 197–202, 1976.

Sourkes, T. L. Psychopharmacology, in *Basic Neurochemistry*, Albers, R. W., Siegel, G. J., Katzman, R., and Agranoff, B. W. (eds.), Little, Brown and Co., Boston, 1972, pp. 581–606.

Sours, J. A. Narcolepsy and other disturbances in the sleep-waking rhythm: A study of 115 cases with review of the literature. *J. Nerv. Ment. Dis.* 137: 525–542, 1963.

Spooner, C. E., and Winters, W. D. Evidence for a direct action of monoamines on the chick central nervous system. *Experientia 21:* 256–258, 1965.

Starobinski, A. Un cas de psychose maniaque-dépressive à un jour d'alternance. *Ann. Med. Psychol. 11:* 344–347, 1921.

Stein, D., Jouvet, M., and Pujol, J-F. Effects of alpha-methyl-para-tyrosine upon cerebral amine metabolism and sleep states in the cat. *Brain Res.* 72: 360–365, 1974.

Stein, L., and Wise, C. D. Possible etiology of schizophrenia: Progressive damage to the noradrenergic reward system by 6-hydroxydopamine. *Science 171:* 1032–1036, 1971.

Steinschneider, A. Prolonged apnea and the sudden infant death syndrome: Clinical and laboratory observations. *Pediatrics 50:* 646–654, 1972.

Stern, E., Parmelee, A. H., Akiyama, Y., Schultz, M. A., and Wenner, W. H. Sleep cycle characteristics in infants. *Pediatrics 43:* 65–70, 1969.

Stern, M., Fram, D., Wyatt, R., Grinspoon, L., and Tursky, B. All-night sleep studies of acute schizophrenics. *Arch. Gen. Psychiatry 20:* 470–477, 1969.

Stern, W. C. The relationship between REM sleep and learning: Animal studies, in *Sleep and Dreaming*, Hartmann, E. (ed.), Little, Brown and Co., Boston, 1970, pp. 249–257.

Stern, W. C., Miller, F. P., Cox, R. H., and Maickel, R. P. Brain norepinephrine and serotonin levels following REM sleep deprivation in the rat. *Psychopharmacologia 22:* 50–55, 1971.

Stern, W. C., and Morgane, P. J. Effects of catecholamine modulating drugs on sleep in the cat. *Psychophysiology 2:* 86, 1972.

Stern, W. C., Jalowiec, J. E., and Morgane, P. J. Growth hormone and sleep in the cat. *Sleep Res. 3:* 173, 1974.

Stern, W. C., Forbes, W. B., Jalowiec, J. E., and Morgane, P. J. Growth hormone administration and sleep in the rat. Presented at the Second International Sleep Research Congress, Edinburgh, June 30–July 4, 1975.

Stewart, J. S., Clarke, C., Shaw, K. M., Ogden, W. S., and Fell, E. A controlled study of night sedation in hospital. *Br. J. Clin. Prac.* 27: 365–371, 1972.

Stiel, J. N., Island, D. P., and Liddle, G. W. Effect of glucocorticoids on plasma growth hormone in man. *Metabolism 19:* 158–164, 1970.

Stonehill, E., and Crisp, A. H. Aspects of the relationship between sleep, weight, and mood. *Psychother. Psychosom.* 22: 148–158, 1973.

Stotsky, B. A., Cole, J. O., Tang, Y. T., and Gahm, I. G. Sodium butabarbital (Butisol Sodium) as an hypnotic agent for aged psychiatric patients with sleep disorders. *J. Am. Geriatr. Soc. 19:* 860–870, 1971.

Stoyva, J., and Metcalf, D. Sleep patterns following chronic exposure to cholinesterase-inhibiting organophosphate compounds. *Psychophysiology 5:* 206, 1968.

Tabushi, K., and Himwich, H. E. Electroencephalographic study of the effects of methysergide on sleep in the rabbit. *Electroencephalogr. Clin. Neurophysiol. 31:* 491–497, 1971.

Takahashi, Y., Kipnis, D. M., and Daughaday, W. H. Growth hormone secretion during sleep. *J. Clin. Invest. 47:* 2079–2090, 1968.

Takahashi, S., and Gjessing, L. R. Studies of periodic catatonia. III. Longitudinal sleep study with urinary excretion of catecholamines. *J. Psychiatr. Res. 9:* 123–139, 1972.

Takahashi, S., Kondo, H., Yoshimura, Ml, Ochi, Y., and Yoshimi, T. Growth hormone responses to administration of L-5-hydroxytryptophan (L-5-HTP) in manic depressive psychoses. *Folia Psychiatr. Neurol. Jpn. 27:* 197–205, 1973.

Takahashi, Y. Growth hormone secretion during sleep: A review, in Biological Rhythms in *Neuroendocrine Activity*, Kawakami, M. (ed.), Igaku-Shoin, Tokyo, 1974, pp. 316–325.

Talwalker, P. K., Ratner, A., and Meites, J. In vitro inhibition of pituitary prolactin synthesis and release of hypothalamic extract. *Am. J. Physiol. 205:* 213–218, 1963.

Tanner, J. M. Human growth hormone. *Nature 237:* 433–439, 1972.

Tanner, J. M., Whitehouse, R. H., Hughes, P. C. R., and Vince, F. P. Effect of human growth hormone treatment for 1 to 7 years on growth of 100 children, with growth hormone deficiency, low birthweight, inherited smallness, Turner's syndrome and other complaints. *Arch. Dis Child. 46:* 745–782, 1971.

Taub, J. M., Globus, G. G., Phoebus, E., and Drury, R. Extended sleep and performance. *Nature 233:* 142–143, 1971.

Taub, J. M., and Berger, R. J. Sleep stage patterns associated with acute shifts in the sleep-wakefulness cycle. *Electroencephalogr. Clin. Neurophysiol. 35:* 613–619, 1973.

Teutsch, G., Mahler, D. L. Brown, C. R., Forrest, W. H., Jr., James, K. E., and Brown, B. W. Hypnotic efficacy of diphenhydramine, methapyriline, and pentobarbital. *Clin. Pharmacol. Ther. 17:* 195–201, 1975.

Tiller, P. M. Bed rest, sleep, and symptoms: Study of older persons. *Ann. Int. Med. 61:* 98–105, 1964.

Tissot, R. The effects of certain drugs on the sleep cycles in man, in *Progress in Brain Research*, Akert, K., Bally, C., and Schade, J. P. (eds.), Elsevier Publishing Co., New York, 1965, pp. 175–177.

Tomlinson, D. R., and Mayor, D. The effects of quanethidine, bretylium and debrisoquine on the accumulation of noradrenaline in constricted postganglionic sympathetic nerves *in vitro. Eur. J. Pharmacol. 21:* 161–170, 1973.

Torda, C. Effect of serotonin depletion on sleep in rats. *Brain Res. 6:* 375–377, 1967.

Torda, C. Contribution to serotonin theory of dreaming (LSD infusion). *N.Y. State J. Med. 68:* 1135–1138, 1968.

Toyoda, J. The effects of chlorpromazine and imipramine on the human nocturnal sleep electroencephalogram. *Folia Psychiatr. Neurol. Jpn. 18:* 198–221, 1964.

Toyoda, J., Saraki, K., and Kurihara, M. A polygraphic study on the effect of atropine on human nocturnal sleep. *Folia Psychiatr. Neurol. Jpn. 20:* 275–289, 1966.

Traub, A. C. Sleep stage deficits in chronic schizophrenia. *Psychol. Rep. 31:* 815–820, 1972.

Tsuchiya, K., Tora, M., and Kobayaski, T. Sleep deprivation: Changes of monoamines and acetylcholine in rat brain. *Life Sci. 8:* 867–873, 1969.

Tune, G. S. The influence of age and temperament on the adult human sleep–wakefulness pattern. *Br. J. Psychol. 60:* 431–441, 1969a.

Tune, G. S. Sleep and wakefulness in 509 normal human adults. *Br. J. Psychol.* 42: 75–80, 1969b.

Turkington, R. W. Prolactin secretion in patients treated with various drugs. *Arch. Intern. Med.* 130: 349–354, 1972.

Tyler, D. B. Psychological changes during experimental sleep deprivation. *Dis. Nerv. Syst.* 16: 293–299, 1955.

Underwood, L. E., Azumi, K., Voina, S. J., and Van Wyk, J. J. Growth hormone levels during sleep in normal and growth-hormone deficient children. *Pediatrics* 48: 946–954, 1971.

Ungerstedt, U. Stereotaxic mapping of the monoamine pathways in the rat brain. *Acta Physiol. Scand., Supp.* 367: 1–48, 1971.

Ursin, R. Differential effect of para-chlorophenylalanine on the two slow wave stages in the cat. *Acta Physiol. Scand.* 86: 278–285, 1972.

Van den Burg, W., and van den Hoofdakker, R. H. Total sleep deprivation on endogenous depression. *Arch. Gen. Psychiatry* 32: 1121–1125, 1975.

Vanhaelst, L., Van Cauter, E., Degaute, J. P., and Golstein, J. Circadian variations of serum thyrotropin levels in man. *J. Clin. Endocrinol. Metab.* 35: 479–482, 1972.

Vanhaelst, L., Golstein, J., Van Cauter, E., L'Hermite, M., and Robyn, C. Etude simultanée des variations circadiennes des taux sanguins de la thyréotripine (THS) et de la prolactine hypophysaires chez l'homme. *C.R. Acad. Sci. Paris* 276: 1875–1877, 1973.

Van Loon, G. R. Brain catecholamines and ACTH secretion, in *Frontiers in Neuroendocrinology*, Ganong, W. F., and Martini, L. (eds.), Oxford University Press, New York, 1973, pp. 209–247.

Vaughan, T., Wyatt, R. J., and Green, R. Changes in REM sleep of chronically anxious depressed patients givan alpha-methyl-paratyrosine (AMPT). *Psychophysiology* 9: 96, 1972.

Verdone, P. Sleep satiation: Extended sleep in normal subjects. *Electroencephalogr. Clin. Neurophysiol.* 24: 417–423, 1968.

Vesell, E. S. Pharmacogenetics. *N. Engl. J. Med.* 287: 904–909, 1972.

Vigneri, R., and D'Agata, R. Growth hormone release during the first year of life in relation to sleep-wake periods. *J. Clin. Endocrinol. Metab.* 33: 561–563, 1971.

Vigneri, R., Pezzino, V., Squatrito, S., Calandra, A., and Maricchiolo, M. Sleep-associated growth hormone (GH) release in schizophrenia. *Neuroendocrinology* 14: 356–361, 1974.

Vincent, J. D., Favarel-Garrigues, B., Bourgeois, M., and Dufy, B. Night sleep of the schizophrenic at the start of evolution (translated). *Ann. Med. Psychol.* (Paris) 2: 227–235, 1968.

Vogel, G. W. REM deprivation III. Dreaming and psychoses. *Arch. Gen. Psychiatry* 18: 312–329, 1968.

Vogel, G. W. A review of REM sleep deprivation. *Arch. Gen. Psychiatry* 32: 749–761, 1975.

Vogel, G. W., and Traub, A. C. REM deprivation. I. The effect on schizophrenic patients. *Arch. Gen. Psychiatry* 18: 287–300, 1968.

Vogel, G. W., Traub, A. C., and Ben-Horin, P. REM deprivation II: The effects on depressed patients. *Arch. Gen. Psychiatry* 18: 301–311, 1968.

Vogel, G. W., Hickman, S., Thurmond, J., and Barrowclough, A. The effect of Dalmane (flurazepam) on the sleep cycle of good and poor sleepers. Paper presented at Annual Meeting of the Assoc. for the Psychophysiological Study of Sleep. Bruges, Belgium, 1971.

Vogel, G. W., Rudman, D., Thurmond, A., Barrowclough, B., Giesler, D., and Hickman, J. Human growth hormone and slow-wave sleep. *Psychophysiology* 9: 102, 1972.

Vogel, G. W., Schultz, E. N., and Swenson, G. S. Quoted in *Federal Register* 40 (236), 1975a,

p. 57306.

Vogel, G. W., Thurmond, S., Gibbons, P., Sloan, K., and Walker, M. REM sleep reduction effects on depression syndromes. *Arch. Gen. Psychiatry 32:* 765–777, 1975b.

Von Economo, C. Schlaftheorie. *Ergeb. Physiol. 28:* 312–339, 1929.

Von Hoffmeister, W., and Koller, S. Clinical trial of a combination of methaqualone and diphenhydramine HCL and methaqualone alone in a double blind test. *Arzeneim. Forsch. 20:* 261–264, 1970.

Voss, A., and Kind, H. Ambulante Behandlung endogener Depression durch schlafentzug. *Praxis 63:* 564–565, 1974.

Wagman, A. M. I., and Allen, R. P. Effects of alcohol ingestion and abstinence on slow wave sleep of alcoholics. *Adv. Exp. Med. Biol. 59:* 453–466, 1974.

Walls, P., Bigelow, L., Rauscher, F., Gillin, J. C., and Wyatt, R. J. The clinical effects of L-5-hydroxytryptophan plus haloperidol administration to chronic schizophrenics. Unpublished, 1976.

Ware, J. Treatment of delirium tremens. *Med. Commun. Mass. Med. Soc. 6:* 175–182, 1841.

Watson, R., Hartmann, E., and Schildkraut, J. J. Amphetamine withdrawal: Affective state, sleep patterns, and MHPG excretion. *Am. J. Psychiatry 129:* 263–269, 1972.

Webb, W. B., and Agnew, H. W. Sleep stage characteristics of long and short sleepers. *Science 168:* 146–147, 1970.

Webb, W. B., and Friel, J. Sleep stage and personality characteristics of "natural" long and short sleepers. *Science 171:* 587–588, 1971.

Webb, W. B., and Agnew, H. W. Effects on performance of high and low energy-expenditure during sleep deprivation. *Percept. Mot. Skills 37:* 511–514, 1973.

Webb, W. B., and Agnew, H. W. Sleep efficiency for sleep-wake cycles of varied length. *Psychophysiology 12:* 637–641, 1975.

Webb, W. B., and Agnew, H. W. Stage 4 sleep: Influence of time course variables. *Science 174:* 1354–1356, 1971.

Webster, B. R., Guansing, A. R., and Paice, J. C. Absence of diurnal variation of serum TSH. *J. Clin. Endocrinol. Metab. 34:* 899–901, 1972.

Weeke, J. Circadian variation of the serum thyrotropin level in normal subjects. *Scand. J. Clin. Lab. Invest. 31:* 337–342, 1973.

Weiss, B. L., McPartland, R. J., and Kupfer, D. J. Once more: The inaccuracy on non EEG estimations of sleep. *Am. J. Psychiatry 130:* 1282–1285, 1973.

Weiss, B. L., Kupfer, D. J., Foster, F. G., and Delgado, J. Psychomotor activity, sleep, and biogenic amine metabolites in depression. *Biol. Psychiatry 9:* 45–54, 1974.

Weiss, H. G., Kasinoff, B. H., and Bailey, M. A. An exploration of reported sleep disturbance. *J. Nerv. Ment. Dis. 134:* 528–534, 1962.

Weiss, M. F. The treatment of insomnia through the use of electrosleep: An EEG study. *Sleep Res. 2:* 174, 1973.

Weitzman, E. D., Goldmacher, D., Kripke, D., MacGregor, P., Kream, J., and Hellman, L. Reversal of sleep-waking cycle: Effect on sleep stage pattern and certain neuroendocrine rhythms. *Trans. Am. Neurol. Assoc. 93:* 153–157, 1968a.

Weitzman, E. D., Rapport, M. M., McGregor, P., and Jacobs, J. Sleep patterns of the monkey and brain serotonin concentration: Effect of p-chlorophenylalanine. *Science 160:* 1361–1363, 1968b.

Weitzman, E. D., McGregor, P., Moore, C., and Jacobs, J. The effects of alpha-methyl-paratyrosine on sleep patterns of the monkey. *Life Sci. 8:* 751–757, 1969.

Weitzman, E. D., Kripke, D. F., Goldmacher, D., McGregor, P., and Nogeire, C. Acute reversal of the sleep-waking cycle in man. *Arch. Neurol. 22:* 483–489, 1970.

Weitzman, E. D., Fukushima, D., Nogeire, C., Roffwarg, H., Gallagher, T. F., and Hellman, L. Twenty-four hour pattern of the episodic secretion of cortisol in normal subjects. *J. Clin. Endocrinol. 33:* 14–22, 1971.

Weitzman, E. D., Perlow, M., Sassin, F. J., Fukushima, D., Burack, B., and Hellman, L. Persistance of the twenty-four hour pattern of episodic cortisol secretion and growth hormone release in blind subjects. *Trans. Am. Neurol. Assoc. 97:* 197–199, 1972.

Weitzman, E. D., Nogeire, C., Perlow, M., Fukushima, D., Sassin, J., McGregor, P., Gallagher, T. F., and Hellman, L. Effects of a prolonged 3-hour sleep-wake cycle on sleep stages, plasma cortisol, growth hormone and body temperature in man. *J. Clin. Endocrinol. Metab. 38:* 1018–1030, 1974.

Weitzman, E. D., deGraaf, A. S., Sassin, J. F., Hansen, T., Gotlibsen, O. B., Perlow, M., and Hellman, L. Seasonal patterns of sleep stages and secretion of cortisol and growth hormone during 24 hour periods in northern Norway. *Acta Endocrinol. 78:* 65–76, 1975.

Weldon, V. W., Gupta, S. K., Haymond, M. W., Paliara, A. S., Jacobs, L. S., and Daughaday, W. H. The use of L-DOPA in the diagnosis of hyposomatotropism in children. *J. Clin. Endocrinol. Metab. 36:* 42–46, 1973.

Westphal, C. Eigenthümliche mit Einschlafen verbundene Anfälle. *Arch.Psychiatry 7:* 631–635, 1877.

Wetterberg, L., Arendt, J., Paunier, L., Sizonenko, P. C., van Donselaar, W., and Heyden, T. Human serum melatonin changes during the menstrual cycle. *J. Clin. Endocrinol. Metab. 42:* 185–188, 1976.

Wexburg, L. E. Insomnia as related to anxiety and ambition. *J. Clin. Psychopath. 10:* 373–375, 1949.

Wiesel, F. Un cas de psychose manique-dépressive (forme circulaire) a phases alternantes quotidiennes. *Acta Psychiat. Neurol. 2:* 146–166, 1927.

Williams, H. L., Lubin, A., and Goodnow, J. J. Impaired performance with acute sleep loss. *Psychol. Monogr. 73:* 1–26, 1959.

Williams, H. L., Lester, B. K., and Coulter, J. D. Monoamines and the EEG stages of sleep. *Acta Nerv. Super. 11:* 188–192, 1969.

Williams, H. L., and Salamy, A. Alcohol and sleep, in *The Biology of Alcoholism*, Kissin, B., and Begleiter, H. (eds.), Plenum Press, New York-London, 1972, pp. 435–483.

Wilson, R., Raynal, D., Guilleminault, C., Zarcone, V., and Dement, W. REM sleep latencies in daytime sleep recordings of narcoleptics. *Sleep Res. 2:* 166, 1973.

Wise, C. D., and Stein, L. Dopamine-beta-hydroxylase deficits in the brains of schizophrenic patients. *Science 181:* 344–347, 1973.

Wolff, G., and Money, J. Relationship between sleep and growth in patients with reversible somatotropin deficiency (psychosocial dwarfism). *Psychol. Med. 3:* 18–27, 1973.

Wolin, S. J., and Mello, N. K. The effects of alcohol on dreams and hallucinations in alcohol addicts. *Ann. N.Y. Acad. Sci. 215:* 266–302, 1973.

Woolley, D. W., and Shaw, E. A biochemical and pharmacological suggestion about certain mental disorders. *Ann. N.Y. Acad. Sci. 40:* 228–231, 1954.

Wurtman, R. J., and Romero, J. A. Effects of Levo-DOPA on nondopaminergic brain neurons. *Neurology 22:* 72–81, 1972.

Wurtman, R. J., and Cardinali, D. P. The pineal organs, in *Textbook of Endocrinology*, Williams, R. H. (ed.), W. B. Saunders, Philadelphia, 1974, pp. 832–840.

Wyatt, R. J. The serotonin-catecholamine dream bicycle: A clinical study. *Biol. Psych. 5:* 33–63, 1972.

The effects of L-tryptophan (a natural sedative) on human sleep. *Lancet 2:* 842–846, 1970a.

Wyatt, R. J., Chase, T. N., Scott, J., Snyder, F., and Engelman, K. Effect of L-Dopa on the sleep of man. *Nature 228:* 999–1001, 1970b.

Wyatt, R. J., Stern, M., Fram, D. H., Tursky, B., and Greenspoon, L. Abnormalities in skin potential fluctuations during the sleep of acute schizophrenic patients. *Psychosom. Med. 32:* 301–308, 1970c.

Wyatt, R. J., Chase, T. N., Kupfer, D. J., Scott, J., Snyder, F., Sjoerdsma, A., and Engelman, K. Brain catecholamine and human sleep. *Nature 233:* 63–65, 1971a.

Wyatt, R. J., Fram, D. H., Buchbinder, R., and Snyder, F. Treatment of intractable narcolepsy with a monoamine oxidase inhibitor. *N. Engl. J. Med. 285:* 987–991, 1971b.

Wyatt, R. J., Fram, D., Kupfer, D. J., and Snyder, F. Total prolonged drug-induced REM sleep suppression in anxious-depressed patients. *Arch. Gen. Psychiatry 24:* 145–155, 1971c.

Wyatt, R. J., Zarcone, V., Engelman, K., Dement, W. C., Snyder, F., and Sjoerdsma, A. Effects of 5-hydroxytryptophan on the sleep of normal human subjects. *Electroencephalogr. Clin. Neurophysiol. 30:* 505–509, 1971d.

Wyatt, R. J., Gillin, J. C., and Vaughan, T. Adrenal corticol and neuro-transmitter activity during human sleep. *Proc. Fifth Int. Cong. of Pharmacology,* San Francisco 4: 134–144, 1972a.

Wyatt, R. J., Vaughan, T., Galanter, M., Kaplan, J., and Green, R. Behavioral changes of chronic schizophrenic patients given L-5-hydroxytryptophan. *Science 177:* 1124–1126, 1972b.

Wyatt, R. J., Kaplan, J., and Vaughan, T. Tolerance and dependence to serotonin. *Arch. Gen. Psychiatry 29:* 597–599, 1973.

Wyatt, R. J., Neff, N. H., Vaughan, T., Franz, J., and Ommaya, A. Ventricular fluid 5-hydroxyindoleacetic acid concentrations during human sleep. *Adv. Biochem. Psychopharmacol. 11:* 193–197, 1974.

Wyatt, R. J., and Gillin, J. C. Development of tolerance to and dependence on endogenous neurotransmitters, in *Neurobiological Mechanisms of Adaption and Behavior,* Mandell, A. J. (ed.), Raven Press, New York, 1975, pp. 47–59.

Wyatt, R. J., Cantor, F., Gillin J. C., Gordon, E., Karoum, F., McCulloch, D., Neff, N., Ommaya, A., Rauscher, F. P., Seaborg, J. B., and Slaby, A. Ventricular fluid metabolites of phenolic and catecholamines, in *Trace Amines in the Brain,* Usdin, E., and Sander, M. (eds.), Marcel Dekker, Inc., New York, 1976.

Wyler, A. R., Wilkus, R. J., and Troupin, A. S. Methysergide in the treatment of narcolepsy, *Arch. Neurol. 32:* 265–268, 1975.

Yamamoto, K. I., and Domino, E. F. Cholinergic agonist-antagonist interaction on neocortical and limbic EEG activation. *Int. J. Neuropharmacol. 6:* 357–375, 1967.

Yen, S. S. C., Tsai, C. S., Naftolin, F., Vandenberg, G., and Ajabor, L. Pulsatile patterns of gonadotropin release in subjects with and without ovarian function. *J. Clin. Endocrinol. Metab. 34:* 671–675, 1972.

Yoss, E. R., and Daly, D. D. Criteria for the diagnosis of the narcoleptic syndrome. *Proc. Staff Meetings of the Mayo Clinic 32:* 320–328, 1957.

Yoss, R. E., and Daly, D. D. Narcolepsy. *Med. Clin. North Am. 44:* 953–968, 1960a.

Yoss, R. E., and Daly, D. D. Narcolepsy. *Arch. Int. Med. 106:* 168–171, 1960b.

Yules, R. B., Ogden, J. A., Gault, F. P., and Freedman, D. X. The effect of ethyl alcohol on electroencephalographic sleep cycles in cats. *Psychonom. Sci. 5:* 97–98, 1966a.

Yules, R. B., Freedman, D. X., and Chandler, K. A. The effect of ethyl alcohol on man's electroencephalographic sleep cycle, *Electroencephalogr. Clin. Neurophysiol. 20:* 109–111, 1966b.

Yules, R. B., Lippman, M. E., and Freedman, D. X. Alcohol administration prior to sleep: The effect on EEG sleep stages. *Arch. Gen. Psychiatry 16:* 94–97, 1967.

Zarcone, V. Narcolepsy. *N. Engl. J. Med. 288:* 1156–1166, 1973.

Zarcone, V., Gulevich, G., Pivok, T., and Dement, W. Partial REM phase deprivation and schizophrenia. *Arch. Gen. Psychiatry 18:* 194–202, 1968.

Zarcone, V., Hollister, L., and Dement, W. C. The effect of L-dihydroxyphenylalanine (L-Dopa) on the sleep of two depressed patients. *Psychophysiology 7:* 314–315, 1970.

Zarcone, V. P., Hoddes, E., and Smythe, H. Oral 5-hydroxytryptophan effects on sleep, in *Serotonin and Behavior*, Barchas, J., and Usdin, E. (eds.), Academic Press, New York, 1973a, pp. 499–509.

Zarcone, V., Kales, A., Scharf, M., Tan, T. L., Simmons, J. Q., and Dement, W. C. Repeated oral ingestion of 5-hydroxytryptophan: The effect on behavior and sleep processes in two schizophrenic children. *Arch. Gen. Psychiatry 28:* 843–846, 1973b.

Zarcone, V., Azumi, K., Dement, W. C., Gulevich, G., Kraemer, H., and Pivik, T. REM phase deprivation and schizophrenia II. *Arch. Gen. Psychiatry 32:* 1431–1436, 1975.

Zarcone, V. P., and Hoddes, E. Effects of 5-hydroxytryptophan on fragmentation of REM sleep in alcoholics. *Am. J. Psychiatry 132:* 74–76, 1975.

Zimanova, J., and Vojtechovsky, M. Sleep deprivation as a potentiation of antidepressive pharmacotherapy. *Acta Nerv. Super. (Praha) 16:* 188–189, 1974.

Zung, W. W. K., Wilson, W. P., and Dodson, W. E. Effect of depressive disorders on sleep EEG responses. *Arch. Gen. Psychiatry 10:* 439–445, 1964.

Zung, W. W. K. Effect of antidepressant drugs on sleeping and dreaming. II. On the adult male. *Proceedings of the IV World Congress of Psychiatry.* Reprinted from *Excerpta Medica International Congress Series No. 150:* 1824–1826, 1966.

Zung, W. W. K. The treatment of insomnia with antidepressant drugs. *Psychophysiology 5:* 234–235, 1968.

Zung, W. W. K. Antidepressant drugs and sleep. *Exp. Med. Surg. 27:* 124–137, 1969a.

Zung, W. W. K. Effect of antidepressant drugs on sleeping and dreaming III. On the depressed patient. *Biol. Psychiatry 1:* 283–287, 1969b.

Index